APPLYING CONCEPTUAL MODELS
OF NURSING

Jacqueline Fawcett, PhD, ScD (Hon), RN, FAAN, ANEF, is a professor in the University of Massachusetts at Boston Department of Nursing. She has been an educator for more than 40 years, and previously has held faculty positions at the University of Connecticut and the University of Pennsylvania. She is a prolific writer, and has served as lead or coauthor for 15 books, more than 200 journal articles, and 97 chapters and monographs. Three of Dr. Fawcett's books have won *American Journal of Nursing* Book of the Year Awards—*The Relationship of Theory and Research* (1992, with Florence S. Downs), *Contemporary Nursing Knowledge* (2005), and *Evaluating Research for Evidence-Based Nursing Practice* (2009, with Joan Garity). She has been elected to Sigma Theta Tau, Pi Lambda Theta, and the American Academy of Nursing. She continues to serve on the editorial review panels of several journals. She received her baccalaureate degree in nursing from Boston University (1964), and her master of arts degree in parent–child nursing with a minor in nursing education (1970) and a PhD in nursing (1976), both from New York University. Dr. Fawcett received a doctor of science degree Honoris Causa from Université Laval, in Quebec, Canada (2013). She was named a Living Legend by the Massachusetts Association of Registered Nurses (2012), and received the Betty Neuman Award for Nursing Leadership from Walsh University Byers School of Nursing in North Canton, Ohio (2015).

APPLYING CONCEPTUAL MODELS OF NURSING

Quality Improvement, Research, and Practice

Jacqueline Fawcett, PhD, ScD (Hon), RN, FAAN, ANEF

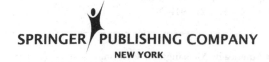

SPRINGER PUBLISHING COMPANY
NEW YORK

Springer Publishing Company, LLC
11 West 42nd Street
New York, NY 10036
www.springerpub.com

Acquisitions Editor: Joseph Morita
Composition: Newgen KnowledgeWorks

ISBN: 978-0-8261-8005-6
e-book ISBN: 978-0-8261-8006-3
PowerPoint Slides: 978-0-8261-8007-0

Instructor's Materials: Qualified instructors may request supplements by e-mailing textbook@springerpub.com

16 17 18 / 5 4 3 2 1

The author and the publisher of this Work have made every effort to use sources believed to be reliable to provide information that is accurate and compatible with the standards generally accepted at the time of publication. Because medical science is continually advancing, our knowledge base continues to expand. Therefore, as new information becomes available, changes in procedures become necessary. We recommend that the reader always consult current research and specific institutional policies before performing any clinical procedure. The author and publisher shall not be liable for any special, consequential, or exemplary damages resulting, in whole or in part, from the readers' use of, or reliance on, the information contained in this book. The publisher has no responsibility for the persistence or accuracy of URLs for external or third-party Internet websites referred to in this publication and does not guarantee that any content on such websites is, or will remain, accurate or appropriate.

Library of Congress Cataloging-in-Publication Data
Names: Fawcett, Jacqueline, author.
Title: Applying conceptual models of nursing: quality improvement, research, and practice / Jacqueline Fawcett.
Description: New York, NY: Springer Publishing Company, LLC, [2017] | Includes bibliographical references.
Identifiers: LCCN 2016025689 | ISBN 9780826180056 | ISBN 9780826180063 (e-book ISBN) |
    ISBN 9780826180070 (PowerPoint Slides)
Subjects: | MESH: Models, Nursing | Nursing Process | Quality Assurance, Health Care
Classification: LCC RT51 | NLM WY 20.5 | DDC 610.73—dc23
LC record available at https://lccn.loc.gov/2016025689

Printed in the United States of America by McNaughton & Gunn.

CONTENTS

PREFACE

Inasmuch as some nurses are advocating use of conceptual models from non-nursing disciplines rather than nursing conceptual models, nursing students and nurses at all levels of education and expertise are now rejecting nursing conceptual models even more than in the past. I believe that the major reason for rejection of nursing conceptual models is the lack of understanding of how these abstract and general perspectives of the discipline of nursing can be used to guide nursing practice, nursing quality improvement (QI) projects, and nursing research. Therefore, the purpose of this book is to present a practical guide for the application of nursing conceptual models to nursing practice, nursing QI projects, and several types of research, including literature reviews; instrument development; and descriptive, correlational, experimental, and mixed-methods designs for each of the nine conceptual models included in the book.

This book evolved from more than 40 years of teaching nursing students about the value of applying nursing discipline-specific knowledge to all nursing activities. It is the product of what I have learned from my students and faculty colleagues about the pragmatics of constructing conceptual–theoretical–empirical (CTE) structures to better understand and appreciate how the starting point for all practice, QI projects, and research always is a nursing conceptual model.

The first chapter of this book is an introduction to conceptual models of nursing and their use as guides for practical nursing activities. This chapter includes the definition and functions of a conceptual model of nursing, a discussion of the need for use of conceptual models to guide practical nursing activities, guidelines for selection of a conceptual model, and discussion of how to construct and apply the CTE structures that are used to guide practical nursing activities.

Each of the next nine chapters focuses on one nursing conceptual model. The nine conceptual models of nursing included in this book are: Johnson's Behavioral Systems Model, King's Conceptual System, Levine's Conservation Model, Neuman's Systems Model, Orem's Self-Care Framework, Rogers's Science of Unitary Human Beings, Roy's Adaptation Model, the Synergy

Model, and the Transitions Framework. A concise yet comprehensive summary of the content of each conceptual model is given, including concepts, definitions of the concepts (non-relational propositions), and associations between the concepts (relational propositions). **The practice methodology, QI methodology, and research methodology for each conceptual model are explicated, and downloadable templates for use of the methodologies are available, in the ancillary online material that accompanies this book. Qualified instructors can obtain this material by e-mailing Springer Publishing Company at textbook@springerpub.com.** The methodologies are applied in the form of CTE structures to a practice situation, a QI project, a literature review, an instrument development study, a descriptive qualitative study, a correlational study, an experimental study, and a mixed-methods study for each of the nine conceptual models. Applications of each conceptual model have been drawn from available published literature; if relevant literature was not available, a hypothetical application was constructed.

This book is designed as a required or recommended text for undergraduate and graduate students, nurse educators, nurse researchers, and practicing nurses, including novice nurses and advanced practice nurses. Specifically, the book is intended for associate degree, baccalaureate degree, master's degree, practice doctoral degree (e.g., doctor of nursing practice [DNP]), and research doctoral degree (e.g., PhD) nursing students, as well as for nurse educators, nurse researchers, and any other nurses who are interested in applying distinctive nursing knowledge to their particular practical nursing activities. The book may be used for any required or elective academic course and for continuing education workshops and courses for which the focus is the application of nursing discipline-specific knowledge to practice, QI, and/or research activities.

In undergraduate programs, the book is best used as part of the first clinical course or a course that is a pre- or corequisite of the first clinical course. The portion of each chapter of the book focusing on nursing practice is most appropriate for undergraduate students, although the portions focusing on nursing QI projects and nursing research could be used as required or recommended content for baccalaureate degree program undergraduate nursing research courses, as a companion to an undergraduate nursing research textbook. For graduate programs, this book would be best used in the first course addressing nursing knowledge in master's and DNP programs, or as a required or recommended book in master's, DNP, and PhD program research courses as a companion to a graduate-level nursing research textbook.

No other book includes the wide scope of examples of practical applications that are included in this book and no other book includes downloadable or printed templates for CTE structures for practice, QI projects, literature reviews, instrument development studies, descriptive qualitative studies, correlational studies, experimental studies, and mixed-methods studies.

Non-nursing conceptual models are not included in this book. As a champion of distinctive nursing knowledge, I do not believe that nursing practice, nursing QI projects, and nursing research should be guided by non-nursing knowledge.

I understand that many other nurses do not agree with me. Therefore, I encourage anyone who believes that non-nursing knowledge can and, perhaps, should guide nurses' practical activities to apply the content of Chapter 1 of this book to provide examples of application of those non-nursing conceptual models.

In addition, this book focuses on nursing conceptual models and the construction of CTE structures. Therefore, the book deliberately does not include chapters addressing nursing or non-nursing theories. When the starting point is theory, the conceptual model (C) component of the CTE structure may not be known and, therefore, a complete CTE structure cannot be constructed. Theories of change and theories of QI are, however, included in the book as methodological theories that guide the conduct of the methods portion of the QI projects included in Chapters 2 through 10 of this book.

I acknowledge the continuing stimulation to my thinking from colleagues and students. Their questions about more examples of explicit CTE structures were the catalyst for this book. I acknowledge and am grateful to the University of Massachusetts Boston for granting me a sabbatical leave, which provided the concentrated time to write much of this book. I also acknowledge the supportive comments of the peer reviewers for this book and for the continuing support of the editors and staff of Springer Publishing Company, especially Joseph Morita and Rachel Landes.

As always, I acknowledge the continuing love and support from my husband, John S. Fawcett. I wrote this book at our home in Maine, at a time during which we celebrated our 50th wedding anniversary.

Jacqueline Fawcett

CHAPTER 1

USING CONCEPTUAL MODELS TO GUIDE PRACTICAL NURSING ACTIVITIES

The content of this chapter provides an introduction to the use of conceptual models of nursing as guides for practical nursing activities. These activities encompass nursing practice; nursing quality improvement (QI) projects; and nursing research, including literature reviews, instrument development, and descriptive, correlational, experimental, and mixed-methods studies.

WHAT IS A CONCEPTUAL MODEL?

A conceptual model is an abstract and general representation for phenomena—things or circumstances (Parse, 2014)—that are of interest to the members of a discipline. Conceptual models of nursing address these things within the context of the concepts of the metaparadigm of nursing, namely, human beings, the environment, health, and nursing (Fawcett & DeSanto-Madeya, 2013). Thus, a conceptual model of nursing is defined as a set of relatively abstract and general concepts and propositions about those concepts that address the concepts of the nursing metaparadigm.

Concepts

A concept is a word or phrase that is "shorthand" for a thing. Each conceptual model of nursing typically includes at least one concept that is shorthand for nursing interventions and other concepts that are shorthand for what is to be assessed and what the outcomes of interventions are.

Propositions

Propositions are statements about concepts. A statement that is a definition of a concept is called a non-relational proposition. A statement that links two or more concepts is called a relational proposition. Some relational propositions are statements of the relation between two or more concepts; others are statements of the effect of one concept—usually an intervention—on one or more other concepts that are considered outcomes.

Conceptual Models of Nursing

The conceptual models included in this book are Johnson's (1990) Behavioral System Model, King's (1999) Conceptual System, Levine's (1996) Conservation Model, Neuman's (Neuman & Fawcett, 2011) Systems Model, Orem's (2001) Self-Care Framework, Rogers's (1994) Science of Unitary Human Beings, Roy's (2009) Adaptation Model, the Synergy Model (Curley, 2007), and the Transitions Framework (Meleis, 2010). The concepts and propositions of these conceptual models are identified in Chapters 2 through 10 of this book.

WHAT IS THE FUNCTION OF A CONCEPTUAL MODEL?

The starting point for all practical nursing activities is a conceptual model. Each conceptual model of nursing is a distinctive frame of reference—what Popper (1965) called "a horizon of expectations" (p. 47)—for thinking about things that matter to nurses. In particular, each conceptual model provides a different way of thinking about the nursing metaparadigm concepts—human beings, environment, health, and nursing—and a different way to guide practical activities, such as nursing practice, nursing QI projects, and nursing research. To date, there is no indication that any one conceptual model is any better than another, although some conceptual models may be more appropriate for application to certain people, situations, and events than others.

The broad function of conceptual models is articulated in general guidelines for practical nursing activities, including practice, QI projects, and research. These general guidelines are listed in Boxes 1.1 to 1.3. The function provided by the distinctive frame of reference of each conceptual model included in this book is evident in its particular guidelines for practical nursing activities, which are given in Chapters 2 through 10.

WHY ARE CONCEPTUAL MODELS OF NURSING NEEDED TO GUIDE PRACTICAL NURSING ACTIVITIES?

All practical nursing activities have value and make contributions to advancement of the knowledge needed to care for those who seek nursing services, and all practical nursing activities are guided by some conceptual model. However, the conceptual models that guide many nurses' practical activities remain more implicit than explicit in nurses' thoughts and publications.

BOX 1.1 General Guidelines for Nursing Practice

- The first guideline stipulates the purposes to be fulfilled by nursing practice.
- The second guideline stipulates the general nature of the practice problems to be considered.
- The third guideline stipulates the settings in which nursing practice occurs.
- The fourth guideline stipulates the characteristics of legitimate participants in nursing practice.
- The fifth guideline stipulates the nursing process to be employed and the technologies to be used, including [areas] for assessment, labels for results of assessment, a strategy for planning, a typology of interventions, and criteria for evaluation of outcomes.
- The sixth guideline describes the nature of contributions that nursing practice makes to the well-being of nursing participants.

Adapted from Fawcett and DeSanto-Madeya (2013), with permission.

BOX 1.2 General Guidelines for Quality Improvement Projects

- The first guideline stipulates the purpose to be fulfilled by the quality improvement project.
- The second guideline stipulates something of interest for the quality improvement project and the anticipated outcome(s).
- The third guideline stipulates the source of the data for the quality improvement projects (such as individuals, a group, or an organization) and the setting in which the project is to be conducted.
- The fourth guideline stipulates the methods to be used to collect data, including the methodological theory of change or quality improvement that will guide the project design and times of data collection, the instruments to be used to collect the data, and the technique(s) used to analyze the data.
- The fifth guideline describes the nature of contributions that the quality improvement project will make to the advancement of nursing knowledge.

Private Images and Implicit and Explicit Frames of Reference for Nursing

Decades ago, Reilly (1975) stated, "We all have a private image (concept) of nursing practice. In turn, this private image influences our interpretation of data, our decisions, and our actions" (p. 567). Similarly, Johnson (1987) and Kalideen (1993) pointed out that many nurses use implicit frames of reference for their activities. Johnson (1987) commented:

It is important to note that some kind of implicit framework is used by every practicing nurse, for we cannot observe, see, or describe, nor can we prescribe anything for which we do not already have some kind of mental image or concept. (p. 195)

BOX 1.3 General Guidelines for Nursing Research

- The first guideline stipulates the purposes to be fulfilled by the research.
- The second guideline stipulates the phenomena that are to be studied.
- The third guideline stipulates the nature of the problems to be studied.
- The fourth guideline stipulates the source of the data (individuals, groups, animals, documents) and the settings in which data are to be gathered.
- The fifth guideline stipulates the research designs, instruments, and procedures that are to be employed.
- The sixth guideline stipulates the methods to be employed in reducing and analyzing the data.
- The seventh guideline describes the nature of contributions that the research will make to the advancement of nursing knowledge.

Adapted from Fawcett and DeSanto-Madeya (2013), with permission.

Kalideen (1993) added,

> Whatever you may think, we all use models to guide our actions, be it the way we conduct our personal lives or the way we nurse. These are based on the beliefs and values of family, friends, peers, and those we respect or those who have influenced us greatly. (p. 4)

Reilly's (1975), Johnson's (1987), and Kalideen's (1993) words of so long ago remain current, despite the requirement of the American Nurses Credentialing Center Magnet Recognition Program® for articulation of a professional practice model that makes explicit nurses' private images and implicit frames of reference for their practical activities.

There is an obvious limitation for using a private image or an implicit frame of reference for practical nursing activities—what is not shared with others cannot be known to the others and, therefore, the context in which the activities are performed is not known. Lack of knowledge of context leads to lack of continuity of nursing practice, lack of understanding of the reasons for and outcomes of QI projects, and lack of understanding of the progression of knowledge about something through research. Perhaps even more important, using a private image or implicit frame of reference for practical nursing activities prevents nurses from articulating a "nursing voice" that will be heard by others (Pridmore, Murphy, & Williams, 2010, p. 25).

Added Value of Conceptual Models of Nursing

Use of an explicit conceptual model of nursing overcomes the limitation of a private image or implicit frame of reference and adds substantial value to all practical nursing activities (Fawcett, 2008). The content of an explicit conceptual model is the best way to articulate nursing's voice within a particular context so that the activities nurses do and why they do these activities can be known by others, and that the contributions made by these nurses will clearly advance the distinctive nursing knowledge needed for the highest possible quality of care of individuals, families and other groups, and communities who certainly deserve enhancement of the quality of their existence.

HOW IS A CONCEPTUAL MODEL SELECTED?

The process of selecting an explicit conceptual model of nursing encompasses four steps:

1. Analyze and evaluate the content of several conceptual models of nursing
2. Determine whether the content of one or more conceptual models is congruent with your personal perspective of nursing
3. Review the literature about the use of the conceptual model as a guide for practical nursing activities with various patient populations and for various situations and events
4. Select the conceptual model that most closely matches your personal perspective of nursing and the patient population experiencing the health-related condition, situation, or event of special interest to you (Fawcett & DeSanto-Madeya, 2013)

Analyses and evaluations of several nursing conceptual models are available in various nursing textbooks, such as *Contemporary Nursing Knowledge: Analysis and Evaluation of Nursing Models and Theories* (Fawcett & DeSanto-Madeya, 2013); *Nursing Theories and Nursing Practice* (Parker & Smith, 2015); *Nursing Theory: Utilization and Application* (Alligood, 2014); and *Theories Guiding Nursing Practice and Research: Making Nursing Knowledge Explicit* (Fitzpatrick & McCarthy, 2014). All of these books include bibliographies of the use of conceptual models as guides for some practical nursing activities targeted to people of diverse cultures who are experiencing various health-related conditions, situations, and events.

HOW DOES A CONCEPTUAL MODEL GUIDE PRACTICAL NURSING ACTIVITIES?

Using a conceptual model to guide practical nursing activities requires construction and application of a conceptual–theoretical–empirical (CTE) structure. In this book, examples of CTE structures for practical nursing activities for nine conceptual models are given in Chapters 2 through 10—Johnson's Behavioral System Model, King's Conceptual System, Levine's Conservation Model, Neuman's Systems Model, Orem's Self-Care Framework, Rogers's Science of Unitary Human Beings, Roy's Adaptation Model, The Synergy Model, and The Transitions Model.

Components of CTE Structures

The C component of a CTE structure is the conceptual model, which serves as the overall frame of reference for the activities and guides development of the T and E components. The T component is the theory that is the direct guide for certain practical nursing activities. Theories are linked with conceptual models, and, like conceptual models, are made up of concepts and propositions. However, the concepts and propositions of a theory are more concrete and specific than those of a conceptual model.

The E component is the empirical methods, including all elements of the methodology that is used to implement the activities. These elements, which are directly accessible to the senses, include the focus of a practice activity—such as assessment or intervention and evaluation of outcomes—or the design of a QI project or a study; the patient population or study sample; the setting for the activities; assessment tools, interview guides, or questionnaires used to gather clinical information or collect QI or research data and document outcomes; the protocol for a practice intervention or an experimental research treatment; and techniques used to analyze the information or data obtained. Examples of CTE structures for nursing practice, QI projects, and research for the conceptual models included in this book are given in Chapters 2 through 10.

Templates for Inductive and Deductive CTE Structures

A theory must be linked to the conceptual model because the concepts and propositions of the conceptual model are too abstract for direct guidance of practical activities. In contrast, the concepts and propositions of a theory and the elements of the E component are directly linked. Templates for two basic CTE structures for practical nursing activities are shown in Figures 1.1A and 1.1B. Figure 1.1A illustrates an inductive approach to practical nursing activities, which is used to generate a new theory. An inductive approach means that the theory—typically in the form of one concept, any dimensions, and the definition(s) (non-relational proposition[s])—is induced from the data collected; that is, the theory concept, any dimensions, and the definition(s) are discovered or emerge as the data are analyzed. Figure 1.1B illustrates a deductive approach, which is used to test an existing theory. A deductive approach means that the theory concepts, any dimensions, definitions, and any associations between the concepts (relational propositions) are deduced from concepts and propositions of a conceptual model, and then the theory is tested by means of analysis of the data that are collected.

Terminology for CTE Structures

The narrative description of the CTE structure is an explanation of the C, T, and E components, including the name of the conceptual model, the name of

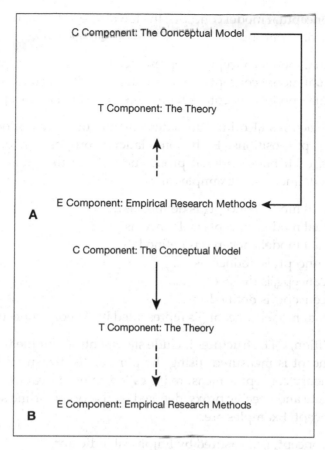

FIGURE 1.1 (A) Template for conceptual–theoretical–empirical (CTE) structures for practical nursing activities: Induction—generation of a new theory. (B) Template for basic CTE structures for practical nursing activities: Deduction—testing of an existing theory.

the theory, and all linkages among the C, T, and E components illustrated in the CTE structure diagram, along with the conceptual model and theory concepts and any dimensions, their definitions (non-relational propositions), and any statements of associations between conceptual model concepts, between theory concepts, and between empirical indicators (relational propositions). The narrative description also includes all elements of the E component of the CTE.

CTE structures also include the name of each relevant conceptual model concept and the name of each theory concept that is linked with a relevant conceptual model concept. The phrase "is represented by" is used to indicate the linkage between a conceptual model concept and a theory concept. Examples are given in the following. The letters A and B and a and b are symbols used to indicate different concepts; N and n are symbols used to indicate any other number of different concepts. The uppercase letters A, B, and N are used to indicate conceptual model concepts; the lowercase letters a, b, and n are used to indicate theory concepts.

- Conceptual model concept$_A$ is represented by Theory concept$_a$.
- Conceptual model concept$_B$ is represented by Theory concept$_b$.
- Conceptual model concept$_N$ is represented by Theory concept$_n$.

CTE structures also include statements of conceptual model propositions and theory propositions. Each non-relational proposition of the conceptual model and each non-relational proposition of the theory is stated using the phrase, "is defined as."[1] Examples are:

- Conceptual model concept$_A$ is defined as....
- Conceptual model concept$_B$ is defined as....
- Conceptual model concept$_N$ is defined as....
- Theory concept$_a$ is defined as....
- Theory concept$_b$ is defined as....
- Theory concept$_n$ is defined as....
- Conceptual model concept$_N$ is represented by Theory concept$_n$.

In addition, CTE structures include statements about the way in which each theory concept is measured, using the phrase, "is measured by." The way in which a theory concept is measured is called an empirical indicator, which is a very concrete and specific proxy, denoted by use of the prime symbol ('), for the theory concept. Examples are:

- Theory concept$_a$ is measured by Empirical indicator$_{a'}$.
- Theory concept$_b$ is measured by Empirical indicator$_{b'}$.
- Theory concept$_n$ is measured by Empirical indicator$_{n'}$.

When empirical indicators are for theory concepts that are interventions, QI project programs, or experimental treatments, the phrase "is operationalized by..." typically is used instead of "is measured by.... " The empirical indicators for concepts that are interventions, QI project programs, or experimental treatments may be referred to as protocols. Examples are:

- Theory concept$_a$ is operationalized by Protocol$_{a'}$.
- Theory concept$_b$ is operationalized by Protocol$_{b'}$.
- Theory concept$_n$ is operationalized by Protocol$_{n'}$.

Each relational proposition of a conceptual model and each relational proposition of a theory is a statement of the association between two or more concepts. The association is stated using the phrase, "is related to" for concepts that are related or correlated. The association is stated using the phrase, "has an effect on" for concepts that are interventions or experimental treatments and their outcomes. Examples are:

- Conceptual model concept$_A$ is related to Conceptual model concept$_B$.
- Conceptual model concept$_A$ has an effect on Conceptual model concept$_B$.

- Theory concept$_a$ is related to Theory concept$_b$.
- Theory concept$_a$ has an effect on Theory concept$_b$.

The connection between a relational proposition of a conceptual model concept and a corresponding relational proposition of a theory typically is explained by use of the word, "therefore." Examples are:

- Conceptual model concept$_A$ is related to Conceptual model concept$_B$.

  Therefore, Theory concept$_a$ is related to Theory concept$_b$.

- Conceptual model concept$_A$ has an effect on Conceptual model concept$_B$.

  Therefore, Theory concept$_a$ has an effect on Theory concept$_b$.

Furthermore, CTE structures include statements of the relational propositions between empirical indicators. Examples are:

- Scores on Empirical indicator$_{a'}$ are related to scores on Empirical indicator$_{b'}$.
- Participants who receive Protocol$_{a'}$ will have higher (or lower) scores on Empirical indicator$_{a'}$ than participants who receive Protocol$_{b'}$.

Diagramming Conventions for CTE Structures

Diagrams of CTE structures typically include the name of the conceptual model, the names of the conceptual model concepts and any dimensions, the names of the theory concepts and any dimensions, and the names of the empirical indicators or protocols; other elements of the methodology also may be included in the diagram. The name of the theory usually is given in the label for the diagram.

Dimensions of conceptual model concepts and theory concepts are illustrated by solid lines connecting the concept with its dimensions:

Empirical indicators that measure theory concepts that have a various number of dimensions are made up of subscales, which are illustrated by dashed lines connecting the empirical indicator with its subscales.

The links between the C component concept and the E component—for inductive structures—or the C component concepts and the T component concepts—for deductive structures—are illustrated by vertical solid lines with arrowheads:

For inductive structures, the links between the E component empirical indicators and the T component concepts are illustrated by vertical dashes with upward arrowheads:

For deductive structures, the links between the T component concepts and the E component empirical indicators are illustrated by vertical dashes with downward arrowheads:

Diagrams of relational propositions also may be included in the CTE diagram. Relational propositions for the C and T components are illustrated by horizontal solid lines with arrowheads:

Relational propositions for the E component are illustrated by horizontal dashes with arrowheads:

CTE Structures for Nursing Practice

The C component of a CTE structure for nursing practice includes the name of the conceptual model selected by a practicing nurse or groups of practicing nurses, as well as the names and the definitions (non-relational propositions) of relevant conceptual model concepts and any dimensions. The C component also includes statements of association between the concepts of the conceptual model (relational propositions) if the focus of nursing practice is to determine the effect of an intervention on outcomes.

The T component includes the name of a theory of assessment or a theory of the effect of an intervention on one or more outcomes. The T component also includes names of relevant concepts and any dimensions and their definitions (non-relational propositions). In addition, if the CTE is for a practice intervention and its outcomes, a statement about the effects of an intervention on one or more outcomes (relational proposition[s]) is included. The E component of the CTE structure for nursing practice is the empirical indicators for the theory concepts and any dimensions, including assessment tools, intervention protocols, and the way to evaluate the outcomes of the intervention, which typically is done by again using the assessment tool that was initially used to identify the need for the intervention.

Templates for the linkages of conceptual model concepts with theory concepts and theory concepts with empirical indicators for nursing practice are shown in Figures 1.2A and 1.2B. As can be seen in the figures, the CTE structures are deductive, proceeding from the C component to the T component and then to the E component. Examples of nursing practice CTE structures for nine conceptual models are given in Chapters 2 through 10 of this book.

CTE Structures for Nursing QI Projects[2]

QI is "Use [of] data to monitor the outcomes of care processes and use [of] improvement methods to design and test changes to continuously improve the quality and safety of health care systems" (Cronenwett et al., 2007, p. 127; Cronenwett et al., 2009, p. 344). The purpose of nursing QI projects is to determine what nurses can do to improve nursing care of people and are, therefore, crucial to the advancement of the quality of nursing practice and ultimately to improving the quality of life of people who seek nursing services.

The C component of CTE structures for QI projects includes the name of a conceptual model that guides selection of the QI topic and the names of the conceptual model concepts and any dimensions that guide selection of the specific QI project intervention and its outcomes. The relevant conceptual model concepts and propositions for QI projects are those that address interventions and the outcomes of interventions. Definitions of the conceptual model concepts and any dimensions are non-relational propositions. Statements of the effects of the conceptual model concepts and any dimensions on conceptual model concepts that are the outcomes are relational propositions.

The T component includes the name of a theory of the effects of a QI intervention on outcomes, as well as the concepts and any dimensions and the propositions of the theory. These concepts and propositions are deduced from the relevant conceptual model concepts and propositions. Definitions of the theory concepts are non-relational propositions. Statements of the effects of the QI intervention on theory concepts that are the outcomes are relational propositions.

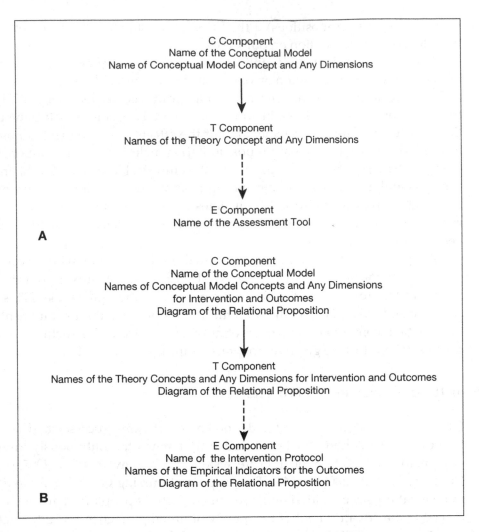

FIGURE 1.2 (A) Template for conceptual–theoretical–empirical (CTE) structures for nursing practice: Assessment—name of a theory of assessment. (B) Template for CTE structures for nursing practice: Effects of an intervention on outcomes—name of a theory of the effects of an intervention on outcomes.

The E component encompasses all methodological elements of a QI project, including the name of the QI intervention protocol and the names of the empirical indicators for the theory concepts that are outcomes. The relational proposition for the effects of the QI intervention protocol and the empirical indicators also is included.

The way in which the QI project is conducted is based on a theory of QI or a theory of change. These theories are methodological theories; as such, they are part of the E component of CTE structures for QI projects, rather than the T component. The theories of QI developed by Florence Nightingale, Ernest Codman, Avedis Donabedian, W. Edwards Deming, Joseph M. Juran, and Philip B. Crosby include five shared characteristics (Anderson, 2015). Two of

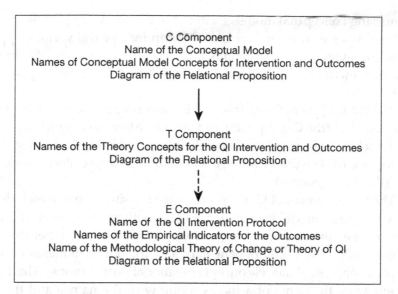

FIGURE 1.3 Template for conceptual–theoretical–empirical (CTE) structures for nursing QI projects—name of a theory of the effects of a QI intervention on outcomes.

QI, quality improvement.

the characteristics—emphasis on process improvement and formal process improvement methods and tools—address the methodological aspects of QI projects. The other three characteristics—quality is driven by organization leaders, customer-mindedness permeates the organization, and involvement of all employees—refer to the context or culture of the organization, which should be considered when designing a QI project.

Theories of change developed by Lewin, Rogers, and Lippitt (Mitchell, 2013) and the Plan-Do-Study-Act (PDSA) method address stages of change experienced by human beings (Taylor et al., 2014). Other relevant theories, which focus on readiness for and processes of changes in behavior, include the health belief model, the theories of reasoned action and planned behavior, the integrated behavioral model, the transtheoretical stages of change theory, social cognitive theory, social ecological models, and the representational approach to patient education (Glanz, Burke, & Rimer, 2015).

A template for CTE structures for QI projects is illustrated in Figure 1.3. As can be seen in this figure, the CTE structure is deductive, proceeding from the C component to the T component and then to the E component. Examples of QI project CTEs for nine conceptual models are given in Chapters 2 through 10 of this book.

CTE Structures for Nursing Research[3]

Nursing research encompasses literature reviews, instrument development, and descriptive, correlational, experimental, and mixed-methods research designs.

All nursing conceptual models included in this book support the conduct of all of these types of nursing research. Descriptions of the various approaches to literature reviews and the various research designs used by the authors of the examples included in Chapters 2 through 10 are given in Appendix A of this book.

The starting point for all research is the conceptual model that is selected by the researcher (the C component of the CTE structure) to guide theory development, including generation of new theories and testing of existing theories (the T component). The theories are generated or tested by collection and analysis of data (the E component).

The C component of CTE structures for nursing research includes the name of a conceptual model and the names and definitions (non-relational propositions) of the concepts and any dimensions that the researcher deems relevant for the study. The C component may also include statements of associations between conceptual model concepts (relational propositions). The T component encompasses the name of a theory along with the names and the definitions (non-relational propositions) of the theory concepts and any dimensions, as well as any statements of associations between concepts (relational propositions).

The E component refers to the methods used to conduct the study. The research methods encompass five elements: (a) the research design, which may be descriptive, correlational, experimental, or mixed method; (b) the sample of research participants, which is the source of data, typically human beings, but may be documents, organizations, or animals; (c) the instruments and any experimental conditions that serve as very concrete and specific real-world substitutes, or proxies, for theory concepts; (d) the procedures used to collect data and protect research participants from harm; and (e) the techniques used to analyze the data.

CTE Structures for Systematic Literature Reviews[4]

Systematic literature reviews, which may be considered a type of nursing research, are done to identify the existing knowledge about something. The C component of a CTE structure for a systematic literature review is the conceptual model that guides the selection of the topic for the literature review. This component is what Popper (1968) called a net "to catch what we call 'the world': to rationalize, to explain, and to master it" (p. 59). Together, the concepts and propositions of a nursing conceptual model are the net used to catch the available literature about the topic. The literature may include theoretical works and reports of research that are directly derived from the conceptual model, or theoretical works and research reports that are not explicitly connected to a particular conceptual model but reflect one or more concepts of that conceptual model.

The C component includes the name of a conceptual model along with the names and any dimensions of the concepts and their definitions (non-relational propositions) and any statements of associations between conceptual model concepts (relational propositions). The T component is a formalization of the results of the literature review as a theory. The T component includes the name of the theory, along with the names and any dimensions of the concepts and their definitions (non-relational propositions) extracted from the literature that was reviewed, as well as statements of any associations between the theory concepts (relational propositions) that were found in the literature.

The E component includes the type of systematic literature review conducted, such as a concept analysis, a scoping review, a realist review, or an integrative review. The goal of a concept analysis is to clarify the meaning of a concept. The goal of a scoping review of literature is to examine all available literature about a broad topic and identify gaps in knowledge about the topic. The goal of a realist review is to synthesize literature that will facilitate understanding of why an assessment tool does or does not provide accurate clinical information about certain people in a certain setting or why an intervention does or does not lead to the expected outcomes for certain people in a certain setting. The goal of an integrative review is to compare and contrast the contents of the literature included in the review.

The E component also includes the sample (a portion) or population (all) of literature reviewed. The literature selected for review, which typically encompasses reports of theoretical work and/or research reports published as journal articles, book chapters, or entire books, may be all of the available publications or only a portion of all available publications about the topic.

In addition, the E component includes the technique used to synthesize the results of the obtained literature. A basic technique for integrating the available publications is a detailed narrative description of the results of the literature review, which may also include a simple tally of consistent and conflicting results. Any one of several approaches to concept analysis may be used (Rodgers & Knafl, 2000). Other techniques, which are more complex, include meta-summary, meta-synthesis, and meta-analysis. Meta-summary and meta-synthesis are appropriate if the literature review results are qualitative, that is, results that are words. In contrast, meta-analysis is appropriate if the results are quantitative, that is, results that are numbers. Critical interpretive synthesis is a technique that facilitates synthesizing results that include both words and numbers.

The results of a systematic literature review provide direction for the next step required to fill gaps in or extend knowledge about a topic. The next step may be development of one or more instruments to measure theory concepts. For example, if the literature review results reveal that a concept of the theory about the topic has not yet been measured, then an instrument such as an interview guide or a questionnaire needs to be developed. Alternatively, the next step may be the design and conduct of a certain type of study. If, for example, the results of a literature review reveal that several experimental studies of the effects of an intervention on outcomes have been conducted but that an explanation for the effects of the intervention on the outcomes is not yet understood, then a correlational study should be conducted to determine the explanation.

Examples of coding sheets that can be used to record the results of a literature review are shown in Tables 1.1A and 1.1B. A template for CTE structures for literature reviews is shown in Figure 1.4. As can be seen in Figure 1.4, the CTE structure is inductive, proceeding from the C component to selection of the elements of the E component and then to the T component, which emerges from the results of the literature review. Examples for nine conceptual models are given in Chapters 2 through 10 of this book.

TABLE 1.1A An Example of a Coding Sheet for Literature Reviews

NAME OF CONCEPTUAL MODEL			
LITERATURE REVIEWED	CONCEPTUAL MODEL CONCEPT$_A$	CONCEPTUAL MODEL CONCEPT$_B$	CONCEPTUAL MODEL CONCEPT$_N$
Citation$_1$			
Theory concept studied			
Sample size and characteristics			
Instruments			
Results			
Comments			
Citation$_2$			
Theory concept studied			
Sample size and characteristics			
Instruments			
Results			
Comments			
Citation$_n$			
Theory concept studied			
Sample size and characteristics			
Instruments			
Results			
Comments			

TABLE 1.1B An Example of a Coding Sheet for Literature Reviews

LITERATURE REVIEWED	THEORY CONCEPT STUDIED	SAMPLE SIZE AND CHARACTERISTICS	INSTRUMENTS	RESULTS	COMMENTS
		NAME OF CONCEPTUAL MODEL			
Citation$_1$					
	Conceptual model Concept$_A$				
	Conceptual model Concept$_B$				
	Conceptual model Concept$_N$				
Citation$_2$					
	Conceptual model Concept$_A$				
	Conceptual model Concept$_B$				
	Conceptual model Concept$_N$				
Citation$_n$					
	Conceptual model Concept$_A$				
	Conceptual model Concept$_B$				
	Conceptual model Concept$_N$				

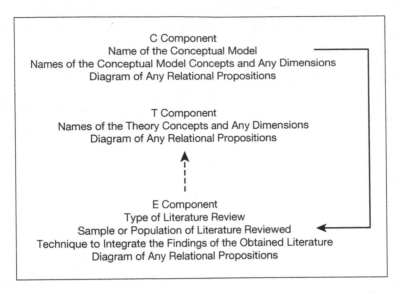

C Component
Name of the Conceptual Model
Names of the Conceptual Model Concepts and Any Dimensions
Diagram of Any Relational Propositions

T Component
Names of the Theory Concepts and Any Dimensions
Diagram of Any Relational Propositions

E Component
Type of Literature Review
Sample or Population of Literature Reviewed
Technique to Integrate the Findings of the Obtained Literature
Diagram of Any Relational Propositions

FIGURE 1.4 Template for conceptual–theoretical–empirical (CTE) structures for systematic literature reviews—name of the theory.

CTE Structures for Instrument Development[5]

Instrument development research is a type of quantitative descriptive research that is conducted to test a theory of how to measure a concept (Fawcett & Garity, 2009). Instruments are needed for collection of accurate clinical information and research data. Therefore, instrument development is a very important aspect of nursing research.

A conceptual model should be used to guide the development of every instrument used for collection of clinical information or research data, as well as for development of intervention protocols or experimental treatment protocols. Instruments used to collect clinical information typically are called practice tools or assessment tools, whereas instruments used to collect research data are referred to as interview guides, which may be referred to as interview schedules, or questionnaires. Intervention protocols and experimental treatment protocols are instruments in the form of scripts that specify exactly what the nurse is to do when implementing the intervention or experimental treatment.

Use of a conceptual model to guide development of an instrument requires selection of a concept of the conceptual model from which a theory concept is derived. The theory concept should, of course, clearly reflect the definition of the conceptual model concept. The theory concept may be one-dimensional or multidimensional. Items for the instrument, which is the empirical indicator for the theory concept, are generated to capture the definition of the theory concept, and ultimately, to clearly reflect the definition of the conceptual model concept. Items may be generated from a review of literature about the concept and/or from data provided by people who represent the population for whom the instrument is intended.

The C component of a CTE structure for instrument development includes the name of the conceptual model, as well as the name of the one relevant conceptual model concept, any dimensions, and the definition(s) (non-relational proposition[s]). The C component is necessary to provide a context for the instrument that will allow the practicing nurse or nurse researcher to view all practical activities of interest within the same frame of reference.

The T component includes the name of the theory along with the names and definitions (non-relational propositions) of the one relevant theory concept and any dimensions of the concept, which are directly derived from the conceptual model concept and its dimensions, if any. Each concept of a theory is measured by one instrument. If the theory concept is one-dimensional—that is, complete without any parts—all of the instrument items cluster together with no subscales. If, however, the theory concept is multidimensional—that is, has more than one part—the instrument items are clustered in separate subscales that measure the separate dimensions of the theory concept.

The E component includes the name of the instrument and any subscales. The entire instrument is the way in which a theory concept is measured. Subscales are the way in which any dimensions of a theory concept are measured. The E component also includes the sample of people who are recruited for testing the adequacy of the instrument, the procedures used for instrument testing, and the techniques used to analyze the data. Analysis of data for instrument development is done to estimate the trustworthiness of instruments that yield word (qualitative) data and the psychometric properties of instruments that yield number (quantitative) data. Estimating the trustworthiness of instruments requires consideration of the dependability and credibility of word data. Estimating the psychometric properties of instruments requires consideration of the reliability and validity of the data. Dependability and reliability refer to the extent to which all of the instrument items provide a consistent measure of a theory concept. Credibility and validity refer to the extent to which all of the instrument items actually measure the theory concept that the instrument is intended to measure. An important and frequently overlooked consideration when estimating credibility or validity is the extent to which the theory concept and the instrument items actually reflect the definition of the conceptual model concept that was the starting point for the instrument development.

A template for CTE structures for instrument development is shown in Figure 1.5. As can be seen in Figure 1.5, the CTE structure is deductive, proceeding from the C component to the T component and then to the E component. Examples of instrument development CTE structures for nine conceptual models are given in Chapters 2 through 10 of this book.

CTE Structures for Descriptive, Correlational, Experimental, and Mixed-Methods Research

There are two general types of CTE structures for descriptive, correlational, experimental, and mixed-methods research. One type of CTE structure depicts

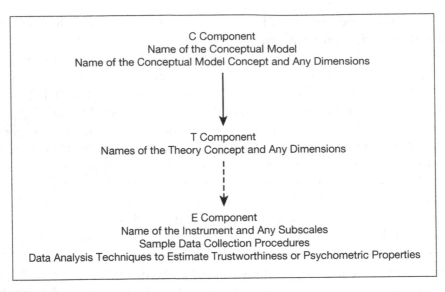

FIGURE 1.5 Template for conceptual–theoretical–empirical (CTE) structures for instrument development nursing research—name of the theory.

theory-generating research. Descriptive research designs are used to generate new theories that usually are made up of one concept and any dimensions and the definition(s) (non-relational proposition[s]). The concept may be one-dimensional or multidimensional. Qualitative (word) data typically are collected using interview guides containing open-ended questions. The word data are analyzed using a general or a particular approach to content analysis. Descriptions of the various approaches to content analysis used by the authors of the examples included in Chapters 2 through 10 are given in Appendix B of this book.

The other type of CTE structure depicts theory-testing research. Correlational and experimental research designs are used to test existing theories. Correlational research is conducted to test theories that are about relations between two or more concepts. Experimental research is conducted to test theories about the effects of an experimental treatment on one or more outcomes. Number (quantitative) data are collected using questionnaires containing fixed-choice items that usually are rated on numerical scales. Descriptions of the various statistical techniques used by the authors of the examples included in Chapters 2 through 10 are given in Appendix B of this book.

Mixed-methods studies are a combination of theory-generating research and theory-testing research that include collection of both word data and number data (Creswell, 2015). The symbols for qualitative (word) data are QUAL and qual. The symbols for quantitative (number) data are QUAN and quan. Uppercase letters denote an emphasis on one type of data, and lowercase letters denote that the other type of data is supplementary.

When mixed-methods research designs emphasize word data (QUAL + quan), the number data are used to supplement the word data. When

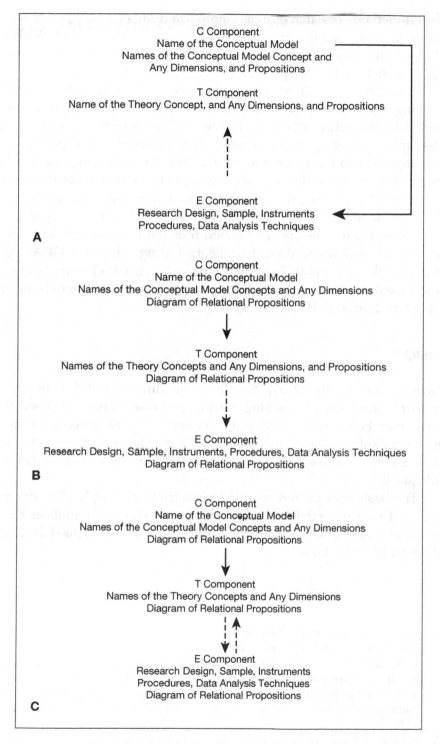

FIGURE 1.6 (A) Template for conceptual–theoretical–empirical (CTE) structures for theory-generating descriptive qualitative nursing research—name of the theory. (B) Template for CTE structures for theory-testing quantitative correlational and experimental nursing research—name of the theory. (C) Template for CTE structures for equal emphasis (QUAN + QUAL) mixed-methods nursing research—name of the theory.

mixed-methods research designs emphasize number data (QUAN + qual), the word data are used to clarify the number data. Some mixed-methods research designs give equal emphasis to both word data and number data (QUAN + QUAL), such that each type of data amplifies the other type.

Templates for CTE structures for theory-generating and theory-testing nursing research are shown in Figures 1.6A and 1.6B. A template for mixed-methods research is shown in Figure 1.6C. As can be seen in Figure 1.6A, descriptive theory-generating research is inductive, proceeding from the C component to the E component, and then to the T component, which is a new theory that was discovered or emerged from analysis of the data. As can be seen in Figure 1.6B, theory-testing research is deductive, proceeding from the C component to the T component and then to the E component. As can be seen in Figure 1.6C, mixed-method research is a combination of inductive theory generation and deductive theory testing (QUAN + QUAL, QUAN + qual, or QUAL + quan). Examples of descriptive, correlational, experimental, and mixed-method CTE structures for nine conceptual models are given in Chapters 2 through 10 of this book.

CONCLUSION

Fawcett and Garity (2009) described the direct parallel between nursing research processes and nursing practice processes. They explained that each encounter between a nurse and a patient may be considered single-case research (Rolfe, 2006), which allows the nurse to test a theory of assessment or a theory of the effects of an intervention on outcomes to determine its adequacy.

The basic information needed to construct and apply CTE structures for practical nursing activities is provided in this chapter. Templates for various practical nursing activities given in this chapter are applied in Chapters 2 through 10 of this book.

NOTES

1. For the examples used in Chapters 2 through 10 of this book, the definitions (non-relational propositions) of relevant conceptual model concepts and their dimensions are those listed at the beginning of the chapter unless explicit definitions for those concepts are given by the authors of the examples. The definitions of relevant theory concepts and their dimensions are taken from the examples; when no definitions are given by the authors of the examples, other sources are used, such as *Taber's Cyclopedic Medical Dictionary* (Venes, 2013).
2. Portions of this section of the chapter are from Fawcett (2014).
3. Portions of this section of the chapter are from Fawcett and Garity (2009).
4. Portions of this section of the chapter are from Fawcett (2012, 2013b).
5. Portions of this section of the chapter are from Fawcett and Garity (2009) and Fawcett (2013a).

REFERENCES

Alligood, M. R. (2014). *Nursing theory: Utilization and application* (5th ed.). St. Louis, MO: Mosby Elsevier.

Anderson, P. (2015). Theoretical approaches to quality improvement. In J. B. Butts & K. L. Rich (Eds.), *Philosophies and theories for advanced nursing practice* (2nd ed., pp. 355–373). Burlington, MA: Jones & Bartlett.

Creswell, J. W. (2015). *A concise introduction to mixed methods research.* Los Angeles, CA: Sage.

Cronenwett, L., Sherwood, G., Barnsteiner, J., Disch, J., Johnson, J., Mitchell, P.,...Warren, J. (2007). Quality and safety education for nurses. *Nursing Outlook, 55,* 122–131.

Cronenwett, L., Sherwood, G., Pohl, J., Barnsteiner, J., Moore, S., Sullivan, D. T., & Warren, J. (2009). Quality and safety education for advanced practice nursing. *Nursing Outlook, 57,* 338–348.

Curley, M. A. Q. (2007). *Synergy: The unique relationship between nurses and patients. The AACN synergy model for patient care.* Indianapolis, IN: Sigma Theta Tau International.

Fawcett, J. (2008). The added value of nursing conceptual model-based research. *Journal of Advanced Nursing, 61,* 583.

Fawcett, J. (2012). Thoughts about concept analysis: Multiple approaches, one result. *Nursing Science Quarterly, 25,* 285–287.

Fawcett, J. (2013a). Thoughts about conceptual models and measurement validity. *Nursing Science Quarterly, 26,* 189–191.

Fawcett, J. (2013b). Thoughts about conceptual models, theories, and literature reviews. *Nursing Science Quarterly, 26,* 285–288.

Fawcett, J. (2014). Thoughts about conceptual models, theories, and quality improvement projects. *Nursing Science Quarterly, 27,* 336–339.

Fawcett, J., & DeSanto-Madeya, S. (2013). *Contemporary nursing knowledge: Analysis and evaluation of nursing models and theories* (3rd ed.). Philadelphia, PA: F. A. Davis.

Fawcett, J., & Garity, J. (2009). *Evaluating research for evidence-based nursing practice.* Philadelphia, PA: F. A. Davis.

Fitzpatrick, J. J., & McCarthy, G. (Eds.). (2014). *Theories guiding nursing practice and research: Making nursing knowledge explicit.* New York, NY: Springer Publishing.

Glanz, K., Burke, L. E., & Rimer, B. K. (2015). Health behavior theories. In J. B. Butts & K. L. Rich (Eds.), *Philosophies and theories for advanced nursing practice* (2nd ed., pp. 235–256). Burlington, MA: Jones & Bartlett.

Johnson, D. E. (1987). Guest editorial: Evaluating conceptual models for use in critical care nursing practice. *Dimensions of Critical Care Nursing, 6,* 195–197.

Johnson, D. E. (1990). The behavioral system model for nursing. In M. E. Parker (Ed.), *Nursing theories in practice* (pp. 23–32). New York, NY: National League for Nursing.

Kalideen, D. (1993). Is there a place for nursing models in theatre nursing? *British Journal of Theatre Nursing, 3*(5), 4–6.

King, I. M. (1999). A theory of goal attainment: Philosophical and ethical implications. *Nursing Science Quarterly, 12,* 292–296.

Levine, M. E. (1996). The conservation principles: A retrospective. *Nursing Science Quarterly, 9,* 38–41.

Meleis, A. I. (Ed.). (2010). *Transitions theory: Middle-range and situation-specific theories in nursing research and practice.* New York, NY: Springer Publishing.

Mitchell, G. (2013). Selecting the best theory to implement planned change. *Nursing Management, 20*(1), 32–37.

Neuman, B., & Fawcett, J. (Eds.). (2011). *The Neuman systems model* (5th ed.). Upper Saddle River, NJ: Pearson.

Orem, D. E. (2001). *Nursing: Concepts of practice* (6th ed.). St. Louis, MO: Mosby.

Parse, R. R. (2014). Research language: A call for consistency. *Nursing Science Quarterly, 27,* 273.

Popper, K. R. (1965). *Conjectures and refutations: The growth of scientific knowledge*. New York, NY: Harper and Row.

Popper, K. R. (1968). *The logic of scientific discovery*. New York, NY: Harper Torchbooks.

Pridmore, J. A., Murphy, F., & Williams, A. (2010). Nursing models and contemporary nursing 2: Can they raise standards of care? *Nursing Times, 106*(24), 22–25.

Reilly, D. E. (1975). Why a conceptual framework? *Nursing Outlook, 23*, 566–569.

Rodgers, B. L., & Knafl, K. A. (2000). *Concept development in nursing: Foundations, techniques, and applications* (2nd ed.). Philadelphia, PA: Saunders.

Rogers, M. E. (1994). The science of unitary human beings: Current perspectives. *Nursing Science Quarterly, 7*, 33–35.

Rolfe, G. (2006). Nursing praxis and the science of the unique. *Nursing Science Quarterly, 19*, 39–43.

Roy, C. (2009). *The Roy adaptation model* (3rd ed.). Upper Saddle River, NJ: Pearson.

Smith, M. C., & Parker, M. E. (2015). *Nursing theories and practice* (4th ed.). Philadelphia, PA: F. A. Davis.

Taylor, M. J., McNicholas, C., Nicolay, C., Darzi, A., Bell, D., & Reed, J. E. (2014). Systematic review of the application of the plan-do-study-act method to improve quality in healthcare. *BMJ Quality & Safety, 23*, 290–298.

Venes, D. (Ed.). (2013). *Taber's cyclopedic medical dictionary* (22nd ed.). Philadelphia, PA: F. A. Davis.

CHAPTER 2

JOHNSON'S BEHAVIORAL SYSTEM MODEL[1]

Dorothy E. Johnson's Behavioral System Model focuses on human beings as behavioral systems, which are made up of all the patterned, repetitive, and purposeful ways of behavior that characterize life (Johnson, 1980, 1990). The goal of Johnson's Behavioral System Model nursing is to restore, maintain, or attain behavioral system balance and dynamic stability at the highest possible level for the person.

JOHNSON'S BEHAVIORAL SYSTEM MODEL: CONCEPTS AND NON-RELATIONAL PROPOSITIONS

This section of the chapter includes the concepts of Johnson's Behavioral System Model and the definitions (non-relational propositions) of the concepts and dimensions of the multidimensional concepts.

Behavioral System is defined as the whole person. The seven dimensions of the concept are attachment subsystem, dependency subsystem, ingestive subsystem, eliminative subsystem, sexual subsystem, aggressive–protective subsystem, and achievement subsystem. The definitions of the concept dimensions indicate their functions.

Attachment subsystem is defined as behaviors required to attain the security needed for survival as well as social inclusion, intimacy, and the formation and maintenance of social bonds.

Dependency subsystem is defined as succoring behavior that calls for a response of nurturance as well as approval, attention, or recognition, and physical assistance.

Achievement subsystem is defined as mastery or control behaviors for some aspect of self or environment with regard to intellectual, physical, creative, mechanical, social, and caretaking (of children, partner, home) skills, and as measured against some standard of excellence.

Ingestive subsystem is defined as appetite satisfaction behaviors, with regard to when, how, what, how much, and under what conditions the person eats, which is governed by social and psychological considerations as well as biological requirements for food and fluids.

Eliminative subsystem is defined as elimination behaviors, with regard to when, how, and under what conditions the person eliminates wastes within the context of socially accepted behaviors.

Aggressive–protective subsystem is defined as protection and preservation of self and society behaviors.

Sexual subsystem is defined as procreation and gratification behaviors, with regard to behaviors dependent on the person's biological sex and gender role identity, including but not limited to courting and mating.

Structural Components is defined as elements of each of the subsystems of the behavioral system. The four dimensions of the concept are drive or goal, set, choice, and action.

Drive or goal is defined as motivation for behavior.

Set is defined as the person's predisposition to act in certain ways, rather than in other ways, to fulfill the function of each subsystem.

Choice is defined as the person's total behavioral repertoire for fulfilling subsystem functions and achieving particular goals, including the person's recognition of alternatives for behavior.

Action is defined as the person's actual behavior.

Functional Requirements is defined as requirements that must be met for all of the subsystems of the behavioral system to fulfill functions. The three dimensions of the concept are protection, nurturance, and stimulation.

Protection is defined as a requirement that protects the person from noxious influences.

Nurturance is defined as a requirement that provides appropriate environmental resources.

Stimulation is defined as a requirement that enhances the person's growth and prevents stagnation.

System Environment is defined as the person's internal and external surroundings. The two dimensions of the concept are internal environment and external environment.

Internal environment is defined as fluids within the body, including their temperature, quantity, and composition.

External environment is defined as objects, events, situations, and forces that impinge on the person and to which the person adjusts and adapts.

Behavioral System Balance and Stability is defined as behavior that has a purpose and is orderly and predictable.

Behavioral System Imbalance and Instability is defined as a malfunction of the behavioral system.

External Regulatory Force is defined as nursing activities that preserve behavioral system balance and stability or overcome behavioral system imbalance and instability. The three dimensions of the concept are impose external regulatory or control mechanisms, change structural components, and fulfill functional requirements.

Impose external regulatory or control mechanisms is defined as nursing activities that are directed toward inhibition, stimulation, or reinforcement of certain behaviors.

Change structural components is defined as nursing activities that involve changes in any one or more of the behavioral system structural components by means of reduction of drive strength, redirection of goals, alteration of set, and addition of choices.

Fulfill functional requirements is defined as nursing activities that provide one or more of the behavioral system functional requirements by means of protection, nurturance, or stimulation.

JOHNSON'S BEHAVIORAL SYSTEM MODEL: RELATIONAL PROPOSITIONS

The statements of associations (relational propositions) among concepts of Johnson's Behavioral System Model are listed here.

- The subsystems of the Behavioral System are interrelated, such that a disturbance in any one subsystem is related to a disturbance in one or more of the other subsystems.
- The extent and type of disturbance in any one or more of the Behavioral System subsystems are related to the use of a specific structural element.
- The extent and type of disturbance in any one or more of the Behavioral System subsystems are related to the type of Functional Requirement needed.
- The extent of disturbance in any one or more of the Behavioral System subsystems is related to the extent of Behavioral System Imbalance and Instability.
- The condition of the internal and external system environments is related to the extent of Behavioral System Balance and Stability.
- External Regulatory Force has an effect on the extent of Behavioral System Balance and Stability.

JOHNSON'S BEHAVIORAL SYSTEM MODEL: APPLICATION TO NURSING PRACTICE

The guidelines for Johnson's Behavioral System Model nursing practice are listed in Box 2.1. A diagram of the practice methodology for Johnson's Behavioral System Model, which is called the Nursing Diagnostic and Treatment Process, is illustrated in Figure 2.1.

A practice tool that includes all parts of the practice methodology is given in Box 2.2.

BOX 2.1   Guidelines for Johnson's Behavioral System Model Nursing Practice

The purpose of nursing practice is to facilitate restoration, maintenance, or attainment of behavioral system balance and stability.

Practice problems of particular interest include all conditions in which behavior is a threat to health or in which illness is found.

Nursing practice occurs in diverse settings, ranging from people's homes to practitioners' private offices to ambulatory clinics to the critical care units of tertiary medical centers.

Legitimate participants in nursing practice are those persons who are experiencing actual or potential threats to behavioral system balance and stability.

The nursing process is Johnson's Nursing Diagnostic and Treatment Process.

Behavioral System Model–based nursing practice contributes to the well-being of people by promoting behavioral system balance and stability.

Adapted from Fawcett and DeSanto-Madeya (2013), with permission.

A Conceptual–Theoretical–Empirical Structure for Assessment

A journal article by Ma and Gaudet (1997) provides an example of Johnson's Behavioral System Model nursing practice focused on assessment. The purpose of their article was to describe how they used Johnson's Behavioral System Model to assess quality of life experienced by people who had end-stage renal disease.

The theory used to guide practice is assessment of patients receiving dialysis or kidney transplantation. The conceptual model concept is Behavioral System and its dimensions—attachment subsystem, dependency subsystem, achievement subsystem, ingestive subsystem, eliminative subsystem, aggressive-protective subsystem, and sexual subsystem. The theory concept is Quality of Life and its seven dimensions—fear of loss, employment status, sense of control, dietary regimen, lack of voiding and constipation, health-related stressors, and sexual function.

Each subsystem of the Behavioral System is represented by a dimension of Quality of Life. For example, the attachment subsystem is represented by fear of loss, and the dependency subsystem is represented by employment status. Each dimension of Quality of Life was assessed by an analysis of a clinical situation about a person with end-stage renal disease receiving dialysis or kidney transplantation.

The conceptual–theoretical–empirical (CTE) structure that was constructed from the content of Ma and Gaudet's (1997) article is illustrated in Figure 2.2. The non-relational propositions for each component of the CTE structure are listed in Box 2.3.

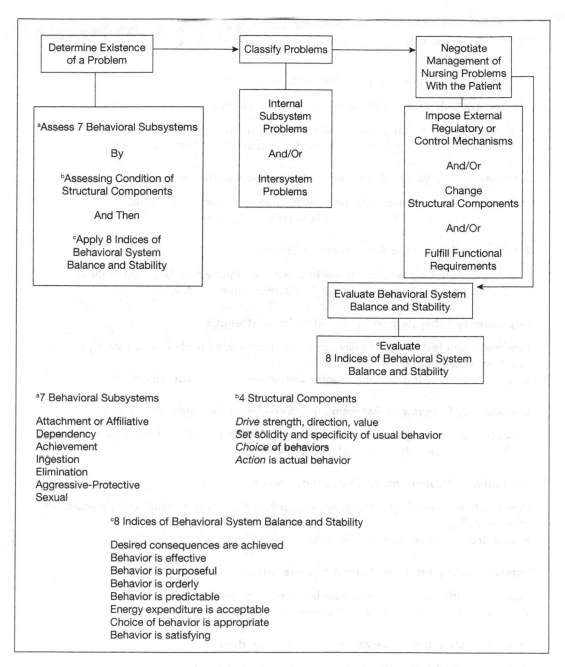

FIGURE 2.1 Johnson's Behavioral System practice methodology.
Adapted from Fawcett and DeSanto-Madeya (2013, p. 63), with permission.

BOX 2.2   The Johnson's Behavioral System Practice Methodology Tool

DETERMINATION OF THE EXISTENCE OF A PROBLEM

Attachment Subsystem: Assessment of Drive Strength

How important is the time you spend with family members and friends?
Very important   Important   Somewhat important   Not important

Attachment Subsystem: Assessment of Set—Usual Behavior

How much time do you usually spend with family members and friends?
A lot of time   Some time   Very little time   No time

Attachment Subsystem: Assessment of Choice

How much more time would you like to spend with family members and friends?
A lot more time   Some more time   No more time   A lot less

Dependency Subsystem: Assessment of Drive Strength

How important is it to have family members and friends on whom you can rely to help you meet your needs?
Very important   Important   Somewhat important   Not important

Dependency Subsystem: Assessment of Set—Usual Behavior

How often do you rely on family members and friends to help you meet your needs?
All the time   Usually   Sometimes   Never

Dependency Subsystem: Assessment of Choice

How much more would you like to rely on family members and friends to help you meet your needs?
A lot more   Some more   No more   A lot less

Ingestive Subsystem: Assessment of Drive Strength

How important is it to consume your favorite foods and drinks?
Very important   Important   Somewhat important   Not important

Ingestive Subsystem: Assessment of Set—Usual Behavior

How often do you consume your favorite foods and drinks?
All the time   Usually   Rarely   Never

Ingestive Subsystem: Assessment of Choice

How much more would you like to consume your favorite foods and drinks?
A lot more   Some more   No more   A lot less

(continued)

BOX 2.2 The Johnson's Behavioral System Practice Methodology Tool (continued)

Eliminative Subsystem: Assessment of Drive Strength

How important is it to have control over your bladder and bowel elimination (urination and defecation)?
Very important   Important   Somewhat important   Not important

Eliminative Subsystem: Assessment of Set—Usual Behavior

How often do you experience difficulties with urination and defecation?
A lot   Sometimes   Rarely   Never

Eliminative Subsystem: Assessment of Choice

How much more often would you like to control your urination and defecation?
A lot more   Some more   No more   A lot less

Sexual Subsystem: Assessment of Drive Strength

How important is it to feel good about yourself as a (female or male)?
Very important   Important   Somewhat important   Not important

Sexual Subsystem: Assessment of Set—Usual Behavior

How often do you feel good about yourself as a (female or male)?
All the time   Usually   Sometimes   Never

Sexual Subsystem: Assessment of Choice

How much more often would you like to feel good about yourself as a (female or male)?
A lot more   Some more   No more   A lot less

Aggressive–Protective Subsystem: Assessment of Drive Strength

How important is it to you to feel safe?
Very important   Important   Somewhat important   Not important

Aggressive–Protective Subsystem: Assessment of Set—Usual Behavior

How often do you feel safe?
All the time   Usually   Sometimes   Never

Aggressive–Protective Subsystem: Assessment of Choice

How much more often would you like to feel safe?
A lot more   Some more   No more   A lot less

(continued)

BOX 2.2   The Johnson's Behavioral System Practice Methodology Tool   (continued)

Achievement Subsystem: Assessment of Drive Strength

How important is it to you to achieve your goals?
Very important   Important   Somewhat important   Not important

Achievement Subsystem: Assessment of Set—Usual Behavior

How often do you achieve your goals?
All the time   Usually   Sometimes   Never

Achievement Subsystem: Assessment of Choice

How much more often would you like to achieve your goals?
A lot more   Some more   No more   A lot less

CLASSIFY PROBLEMS

The nurse and the patient discuss the patient's behaviors in each behavioral subsystem and compare the behaviors with the indices of behavioral balance and stability. They agree that a diagnosis of [insert relevant diagnosis] is appropriate.
   The indices of behavioral system balance and stability are:

   Desired consequences are achieved
   Behavior is effective, purposeful, orderly, predictable, and satisfying
   Energy expenditure is acceptable
   Choice of behavior is appropriate

NEGOTIATE MANAGEMENT OF NURSING PROBLEMS WITH THE PATIENT

The patient and the nurse discuss which approaches to management of the identified nursing problems will be appropriate for and acceptable to the patient and develop appropriate timelines and strategies to reach the desired level of behavioral system balance and stability.
   Management approaches are:

   Impose external regulatory or control mechanisms
   Change structural components
   Fulfill requirements

EVALUATE BEHAVIORAL SYSTEM BALANCE AND STABILITY

After the problems are managed, the nurse meets with the patient to compare then–current behaviors in the relevant subsystems with the indices of behavioral system balance and stability to determine whether the desired level of behavioral system balance and stability has been attained.

Adapted from Fawcett and DeSanto-Madeya (2013), with permission.

BOX 2.3   An Example of a Conceptual–Theoretical–Empirical Structure for Johnson's Behavioral System Model Nursing Practice: Assessment

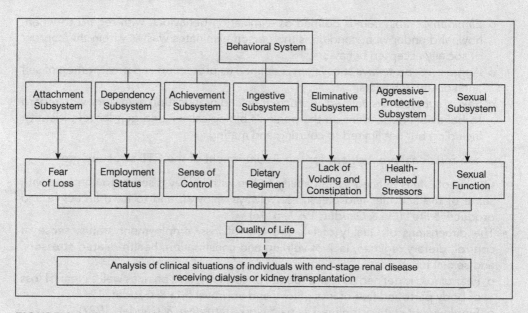

FIGURE 2.2 Conceptual–theoretical–empirical (CTE) structure for Johnson's Behavioral System Model nursing practice: Assessment—theory of assessment of patients receiving dialysis or kidney transplantation.

The *non-relational propositions* for the C component of the conceptual–theoretical–empirical (CTE) structure are:

- *Behavioral System* is defined as the whole person.
- The dimensions of the concept, Behavioral System, are attachment subsystem, dependence subsystem, achievement subsystem, ingestive subsystem, eliminative subsystem, aggressive–protective subsystem, and sexual subsystem.
  - o *Attachment subsystem* is defined as behaviors required to attain the security needed for survival as well as social inclusion, intimacy, and the formation and maintenance of social bonds.
  - o *Dependency subsystem* is defined as succoring behavior that calls for a response of nurturance as well as approval, attention or recognition, and physical assistance.
  - o *Achievement subsystem* is defined as mastery or control behaviors for some aspect of self or environment, with regard to intellectual, physical, creative, mechanical, social, and care-taking (of children, spouse, home) skills, and as measured against some standard of excellence.
  - o *Ingestive subsystem* is defined as appetite satisfaction behaviors, with regard to when, how, what, how much, and under what conditions the person eats, which is governed by social and psychological considerations as well as biological requirements for food and fluids.

(continued)

BOX 2.3 An Example of a Conceptual–Theoretical–Empirical Structure for Johnson's Behavioral System Model Nursing Practice: Assessment *(continued)*

o *Eliminative subsystem* is defined as elimination behaviors, with regard to when, how, and under what conditions the person eliminates wastes within the context of socially accepted behaviors.

o *Aggressive–protective subsystem* is defined as protection and preservation of self and society behaviors.

o *Sexual subsystem* is defined as procreation and gratification behaviors, with regard to behaviors dependent on the person's biological sex and gender role identity, including but not limited to courting and mating.

The *non-relational propositions* for the *T* component of the CTE structure are:

• *Quality of Life* is defined as "an ability to live with kidney disease, to continue with some of the activities and pleasures…always enjoyed, and to have an active and productive life" (Ma & Gaudet, 1997, p. 16).

• The dimensions of Quality of Life are fear of loss, employment status, sense of control, dietary regimen, lack of voiding and constipation, health-related stressors, and sexual function.

o *Fear of loss* is defined as fear of death, uncertainty, and pain, as well as fear of loss of body parts and fear of loss of love and approval (Ma & Gaudet, 1997).

o *Employment status* is defined as paid work status (Ma & Gaudet, 1997).

o *Sense of control* is defined as ability to control life circumstances (Ma & Gaudet, 1997).

o *Dietary regimen* is defined as "patterns of eating, likes and dislikes, and taking availability of all types of food for granted" (Ma & Gaudet, 1997, p. 14).

o *Lack of voiding and constipation* is defined as the inability to produce urine and infrequent bowel movements (Ma & Gaudet, 1997).

o *Health-related stressors* is defined as problems associated with hemodialysis, peritoneal dialysis, and kidney transplantation (Ma & Gaudet, 1997).

o *Sexual function* is defined as "[extent of] libido and frequency of intercourse, impotence, and infertility" (Ma & Gaudet, 1997, p. 15).

The *non-relational proposition* for the *E* component of the CTE structure is:

• All of the dimensions of the theory concept, Quality of Life, were assessed by analysis of clinical situations of people with a medical diagnosis of end-stage renal disease who were receiving dialysis or kidney transplantation (Ma & Gaudet, 1997).

Source: Ma and Gaudet (1997).

A CTE Structure for Intervention

An example of Johnson's Behavioral System Model nursing practice focused on intervention was extracted from a practice exemplar of nursing care of a man who had a medical diagnosis of small cell lung cancer (White, 2010). Assessment of the Behavioral System dimension of ingestive subsystem revealed that the man had experienced a loss of appetite due to chemotherapy.

The theory used to guide practice is the effect of appetite enhancement on appetite. The two conceptual model concepts are the External Regulatory Force concept dimension of fulfill functional requirements–stimulation, and the Behavioral System concept dimension of ingestive subsystem. The two theory concepts are Appetite Enhancement and Appetite.

The fulfill functional requirements–stimulation dimension of External Regulatory Force is represented by Appetite Enhancement. The Behavioral System dimension of ingestive subsystem is represented by Appetite. Appetite Enhancement is operationalized by a protocol for consumption of liquid nutritional supplements. Appetite is measured by the amount of intake of liquid nutritional supplements and other fluids and food.

The CTE structure constructed from the content of White's (2010) practice exemplar is illustrated in Figure 2.3. The non-relational and relational propositions for each component of the CTE structure are listed in Box 2.4.

BOX 2.4   An Example of a Conceptual–Theoretical–Empirical Structure for Johnson's Behavioral System Model Nursing Practice: Intervention

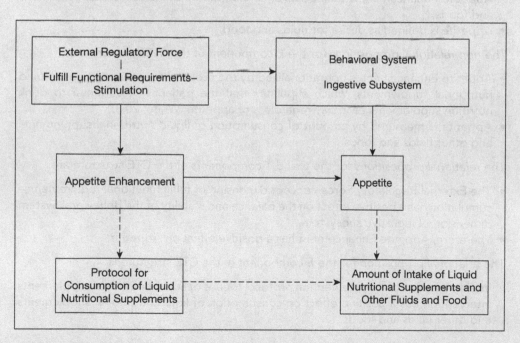

FIGURE 2.3 Conceptual–theoretical–empirical (CTE) structure for Johnson's Behavioral System Model nursing practice: Intervention—theory of the effect of appetite enhancement on appetite.

(continued)

BOX 2.4   An Example of a Conceptual–Theoretical–Empirical Structure for Johnson's Behavioral System Model Nursing Practice: Intervention   *(continued)*

The *non-relational propositions* for the *C component* of the conceptual–theoretical–empirical (CTE) structure are:

- *External Regulatory Force* is defined as nursing activities that preserve behavioral system balance and stability or overcome behavioral system imbalance and instability.
- The relevant dimension of External Regulatory Force is fulfill functional requirements–stimulation.
  - o *Fulfill functional requirements–stimulation* is defined as nursing activities that provide stimulation.
- *Behavioral System* is defined as the whole person.
- The relevant dimension of the Behavioral System is ingestive subsystem.
  - o *Ingestive subsystem* is defined as appetite satisfaction behaviors, with regard to when, how, what, how much, and under what conditions the person eats, which is governed by social and psychological considerations as well as biological requirements for food and fluids.

The *non-relational propositions* for the *T component* of the CTE structure are:

- *Appetite Enhancement* is defined as an intervention that increases desire for fluids and foods.
- *Appetite* is defined as desire for fluids and food.

The *non-relational propositions* for the *E component* of the CTE structure are:

- Appetite Enhancement is operationalized by the protocol for consumption of liquid nutritional supplements, which stipulates that the patient will continue to drink nutrition supplements each day regardless of appetite (White, 2010).
- Appetite is measured by amount of consumption of liquid nutritional supplements and other fluids and foods.

The *relational propositions* for the *C* and *T components* of the CTE structure are:

- The External Regulatory Force concept dimension of fulfill functional requirements–stimulation has a positive effect on the balance and stability of the Behavioral System dimension of ingestive subsystem.
- Therefore, Appetite Enhancement has a positive effect on Appetite.

The *relational proposition* for the *E component* of the CTE structure is:

- Implementation of the intervention protocol for use of liquid nutritional supplements intervention has a positive effect on consumption of liquid nutritional supplements and other fluids and foods.

Source: White (2010).

JOHNSON'S BEHAVIORAL SYSTEM MODEL: APPLICATION TO QUALITY IMPROVEMENT

The guidelines for Johnson's Behavioral System Model quality improvement (QI) projects are listed in Box 2.5.

A CTE Structure for a QI Project

No explicit QI projects guided by Johnson's Behavioral System Model were located in the literature. An example of a CTE structure for a hypothetical Johnson's Behavioral System Model QI project is based on the report of a managed care evaluation project by Dee, van Servellen, and Brecht (1998). The purpose of the hypothetical QI project is to encourage psychiatric mental health nurses to conduct comprehensive behavioral system assessments to determine the degree of behavioral system balance and stability of people with a medical diagnosis of a psychiatric illness.

The theory is nurses' conduct of comprehensive behavioral system assessments. The two conceptual model concepts are the External Regulatory Force

---

BOX 2.5   Guidelines for Johnson's Behavioral System Model Quality Improvement Projects

The purpose of quality improvement (QI) projects is to test the effectiveness of a dimension of the External Regulatory Control concept of the Johnson Behavioral System Model on nurses' use of a particular step of the Johnson's Behavioral System practice methodology—Determine existence of a problem, Classify problems, Negotiate management of nursing problems with the patient, Evaluate behavioral system balance and stability.

The phenomenon of interest for QI projects is the extent of nurses' use of a particular step of the Johnson's Behavioral System Model practice methodology.

Data for QI projects are to be collected from nurses working in various settings, such as patients' homes, practitioners' private offices, ambulatory clinics, and hospitals.

Any methodological theory of change or QI may be used to guide the design of the QI project and the times for data collection. Checklists, rating scales, and responses to open-ended questions may be used to determine the extent to which nurses actually implement a particular step of the Johnson's Behavioral System Model practice methodology. Descriptive statistics may be used to analyze data obtained from checklists or rating scales, and content analysis may be used to identify categories or themes found in responses to open-ended questions.

The results of Johnson's Behavioral System–based QI projects enhance understanding of the extent to which nurses implement certain steps of the Johnson's Behavioral System Model practice methodology.

concept dimension of change structural components–choice, and the Behavioral System concept dimension of achievement subsystem. The two theory concepts are QI Comprehensive Behavioral System Assessment Program and Comprehensive Behavioral System Assessment.

The change structural component–choice dimension of External Regulatory Force is represented by the QI Comprehensive Behavioral System Assessment Program, which is operationalized by a hypothetical QI Comprehensive Behavioral Assessment Program protocol that is guided by Rogers's (2003) methodological theory of planned change (see Appendix A). The Behavioral System dimension of achievement subsystem is represented by Comprehensive Behavioral System Assessment, which is measured by the extent to which psychiatric-mental health nurses use the Behavioral System Assessment Tool (BSAT; Dee et al., 1988). Descriptive statistics (numbers, percents) are used to determine the extent of nurses' use of the BSAT (see Appendix B).

The CTE structure constructed for the hypothetical QI project is illustrated in Figure 2.4. The non-relational and relational propositions for each component of the CTE structure are listed in Box 2.6.

JOHNSON'S BEHAVIORAL SYSTEM MODEL: APPLICATION TO NURSING RESEARCH

The guidelines for Johnson's Behavioral System Model nursing research are listed in Box 2.7.

A CTE Structure for a Systematic Literature Review

No published explicit Johnson's Behavioral System Model–guided systematic literature reviews could be located. A review of the research literature was, therefore, conducted to provide an example. The Behavioral System concept dimension of the attachment subsystem was selected as the starting point for an integrative review of literature.

The literature review was limited to a search of the Complete Cumulative Index to Nursing and Allied Health Literature (CINAHL Complete) electronic database, which includes publications from 1937 to the present. The search for this literature review included publications from 1937 to August 2014. The search terms "Johnson's Behavioral System Model" AND "attachment" yielded one publication (Oyedele, Wright, & Maja, 2013). Inasmuch as that publication was a report of a study of teenage pregnancy, the decision was made to focus the literature review on research about the attachment behaviors of teenagers. The search terms "attachment behavior" AND "teenager" yielded nine additional publications. Four of the nine publications were eliminated; one because it was a book review, one because it was a brief practice case study, one because it was a theoretical framework for educational practice, and one because it was an analysis of a national policy. Therefore, the literature reviewed encompassed

BOX 2.6   An Example of a Conceptual–Theoretical–Empirical Structure for Johnson's Behavioral System Model Quality Improvement Project

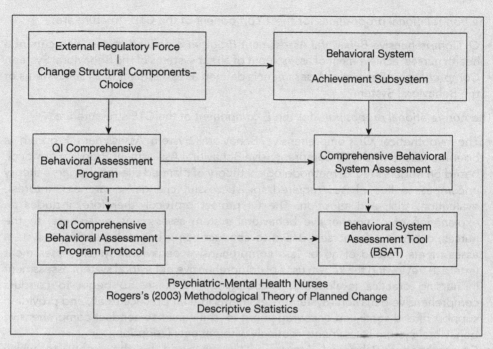

FIGURE 2.4 Conceptual–theoretical–empirical (CTE) structure for a hypothetical Johnson's Behavioral System Model QI project—theory of nurses' conduct of comprehensive behavioral system assessments.

The *non-relational propositions* for the C *component* of the conceptual–theoretical–empirical (CTE) structure are:

- *External Regulatory Force* is defined as nursing activities that preserve behavioral system balance and stability or overcome behavioral system imbalance and instability.
- The relevant dimension of External Regulatory Force is change structural components–choice.
  - o *Change structural components–choice* is defined as nursing activities that involve change by means of addition of choices.
- *Behavioral System* is defined as the whole person.
- The relevant dimension of the Behavioral System is achievement subsystem.
  - o *Achievement subsystem* is defined as mastery or control behaviors for some aspect of self or environment, with regard to intellectual, physical, creative, mechanical, social, and care-taking skills, and as measured against some standard of excellence.

(continued)

BOX 2.6   An Example of a Conceptual–Theoretical–Empirical Structure for Johnson's Behavioral System Model Quality Improvement Project   (continued)

The *non-relational propositions* for the *T component* of the CTE structure are:

- *QI Comprehensive Behavioral Assessment Program* is defined as psychiatric-mental health nurses' achievement of assessment of all subsystems of the Behavioral System.
- *Comprehensive Behavioral Assessment* is defined as assessment of all subsystems of the Behavioral System.

The *non-relational propositions* for the *E component* of the CTE structure are:

- The hypothetical QI Comprehensive Behavioral System Assessment Program is operationalized by the QI Comprehensive Behavioral Assessment Program protocol, based on Rogers's (2003) methodological theory of planned change. Rogers's theory encompasses five phases required for successful change—awareness, interest, evaluation, trial, and adoption. The QI project protocol, therefore, includes an explanation of comprehensive behavioral system assessment (awareness) to the nurses, catalyzing the nurses' desire to conduct comprehensive behavioral system assessments instead of no or less comprehensive behavioral system assessment (interest), reviewing the known uses of comprehensive behavioral system assessment in nursing practice (evaluation), encouraging the nurses to begin to conduct comprehensive behavioral system assessments in their practice (trial), and providing support of and continued encouragement for the nurses to conduct comprehensive behavioral system assessments routinely with patients (adoption).
- Comprehensive Behavioral Assessment is measured by the extent to which psychiatric-mental health nurses use the Behavioral System Assessment Tool (BSAT; Dee et al., 1988). The BSAT is a comprehensive tool that allows assessment of degree of balance and stability of behaviors associated with each subsystem of the behavioral system—attachment, dependency, achievement, ingestive, eliminative, aggressive–protective, and sexual, as well as the restorative subsystem, which was added by Grubbs in 1974. Each BSAT subscale is rated on a scale of 1 = effective to 5 = critically ineffective. Overall severity of illness is rated on a scale of "1= health, 2 = potential for health deviation, 3 = illness, 4 = serious illness, [and] 5 = critical illness" (Dee et al., 1988, p. 60).

The *relational propositions* for the *C and T components* of the CTE structure are:

- The External Regulatory Force concept dimension of change structural components—choice has a positive effect on the balance and stability of the Behavioral System dimension of achievement subsystem.
- Therefore, a QI Comprehensive Behavioral System Assessment Program has a positive effect on Comprehensive Behavioral Assessment.

The *relational proposition* for the *E component* of the CTE structure is:

- Psychiatric-mental health nurses who participate in the Comprehensive Behavioral System Assessment Program protocol will use the BSAT.

Source: Constructed for this chapter based on a journal article by Dee, van Servellen, and Brecht (1998).

BOX 2.7 Guidelines for Johnson's Behavioral System Model Research

One purpose of Behavioral System Model–based research is to explore problems in the structure or function of the behavioral system and its subsystems. The task is to identify, describe, and explain these problems. Another purpose of Behavioral System Model–based research is to understand prevention and treatment of problems in the structure or function of the behavioral system and its subsystems. The task is to develop the scientific bases for intervention, as well as specific methodologies for intervention.

The phenomena of interest are the behavioral system as a whole, as well as the structural components and the functional requirements of the behavioral subsystems.

The precise problems to be studied are those that represent actual or potential imbalance and instability in the behavioral system and subsystems.

Study participants may be persons of all ages in various settings.

Data may be collected via interview; observation, including participant observation, film, and photography; and projective technique using research instruments and practice tools derived from or consistent with the Behavioral System Model. Research may be conducted using descriptive, correlational, experimental, and/or mixed-methods designs. Descriptive designs include literature reviews, instrument development, and descriptive qualitative designs.

Qualitative and quantitative data analysis techniques may be used.

Behavioral System Model–based research findings enhance understanding of factors that affect behavioral system functioning.

Adapted from Fawcett and DeSanto-Madeya (2013), with permission.

six reports of research (Figueiredo, Bifulco, Pecheco, Costa, & Magarinho, 2006; Maxwell, Proctor, & Hammond, 2011; Oyedele et al., 2013; Schreck & Fisher, 2004; Smith, 1997; Yi, Pan, Chang, & Chan, 2006). The results of the literature review were entered into a coding sheet (see Table 2.1) and are written here as a brief narrative.

The literature reviewed was published by researchers from various disciplines—nursing, psychology, social work, family sociology, and criminology—reflecting widespread interest in teenagers' attachment behaviors. The international interest in teenagers' attachment behaviors is evident in samples drawn from populations in England (Maxwell et al., 2011), Portugal (Figueiredo et al., 2006), South Africa (Oyedele et al., 2013), Taiwan (Yi et al., 2006), and the United States (Schreck & Fisher, 2004; Smith, 1991). Study sample sizes ranged from six to 3,500 teenagers. The smaller sample sizes were appropriate for the descriptive, primarily qualitative study designs used; the larger sample sizes were drawn from respondents to quantitative surveys. Instruments included interview schedules with open-ended questions developed by the researchers and national surveys. Details about each research report are given in Table 2.1.

The theory of teenager attachment was generated from the results of the literature review. The conceptual model concept is the attachment subsystem

TABLE 2.1 Coding Sheet for Review of Literature About Teenagers' Attachment Behaviors

			JOHNSON'S BEHAVIORAL SYSTEM MODEL			
			BEHAVIORAL SYSTEM—ATTACHMENT SUBSYSTEM			
LITERATURE REVIEWED	THEORY CONCEPTS STUDIED	SAMPLE SIZE AND CHARACTERISTICS	INSTRUMENTS	RESULTS	COMMENTS	
Oyedele, Wright, & Maja, 2013	Knowledge and perception of teenage pregnancy Study guided by Johnson's Behavioral System Model	30 sexually active female teenagers, aged 14 to 19 years, residing in a township in South Africa	A semi-structured interview schedule containing questions about demographic characteristics and the attachment subsystem, as well as questions about the dependency, sexual, and achievement subsystems	Eight themes were extracted from the data: 1. Family background 2. Family and partner's attitude toward pregnancy 3. Sexual development and relationship history 4. High-risk behavior 5. Prevention of pregnancy 6. Pregnancy history 7. Termination of pregnancy 8. Dependence and achievement	Could be considered QUAL + QUAN mixed-methods design Included number and percent of participations who gave each response for each theme Offered practice guidelines for the attachment, dependency, sexual, and achievement subsystems	
Maxwell, Proctor, & Hammond, 2011	Teenagers' experience of themselves as mothers, their relationship with their child, and their understanding of their child's experiences	6 female teenagers who had left care provided by a local authority organization in England, aged 18–20 years at time of study participation and aged 17–19 years at the time of childbirth	Semi-structured interviews with open-ended questions about childbirth, milestones, and separation, as well as participants' 2-week diary entries about their thoughts and feelings about the child	Four dialectical themes were extracted from the data: 1. Ideal and reality 2. Motherhood as building positive views of self and other, but also highlighting vulnerability	Could be considered QUAL + QUAN mixed-methods design The "mothers' experiences of themselves and their children [were] dynamic and often conflicting, changing over time and	

	Study guided by functional and neurobiological perspectives		and the thoughts and feelings they imagined the child had	3. Identification with the child but also feeling taken over by the child 4. External world as needed but also unwanted and destabilizing	with the context" (p. 31) Included number of participants whose responses reflected each aspect of each theme Theme 1—5+3 Theme 2—6+6 Theme 3—6+6 Theme 4—5+6
Figueiredo, Bifulco, Pecheco, Costa, & Magarinho, 2006	Attachment style Depression Study guided by attachment theory	66 Portuguese pregnant teenagers and 64 Portuguese pregnant adults	Attachment Style Interview measures support and attachment style Support includes assessment of the quality of relationships with partner and one or two family members or friends Attachment style is rated as type of insecure attachment: Enmeshed, Fearful, Angry-Dismissive, Withdrawn, or Clearly Secure Edinburgh Postnatal Depression Scale	Pregnant teenagers had substantially higher levels of insecure attachment style than pregnant adults for Enmeshed, Angry-Dismissive, and Fearful types Only one twelfth of teenagers were Clearly Secure vs. almost one third of the adults The Enmeshed type of insecure attachment and poor partner support were related to depression for both pregnant teens and adults	Authors recommended that insecure attachment style should be a component of prevention and intervention strategies designed for pregnant teenagers

(continued)

TABLE 2.1 Coding Sheet for Review of Literature About Teenagers' Attachment Behaviors *(continued)*

| | JOHNSON'S BEHAVIORAL SYSTEM MODEL | | | | |
| | BEHAVIORAL SYSTEM—ATTACHMENT SUBSYSTEM | | | | |
LITERATURE REVIEWED	THEORY CONCEPTS STUDIED	SAMPLE SIZE AND CHARACTERISTICS	INSTRUMENTS	RESULTS	COMMENTS
Yi, Pan, Chang, & Chan, 2006	Intergenerational relations (emotional attachment)—teenagers, their parents, and their grandparents Study guided by an intergenerational relations perspective	2,500 female and male Taiwanese teenagers	Taiwan Youth Project survey	Grandparent–parent relationships and grandparent–grandchild relationships influence teenager–parent relationships. Early care by paternal grandparents is positively related to teenager–father relationships, whereas early care by maternal grandparents is negatively related to teenager–father relationships	Secondary analysis of data from a national survey Researchers recommended that the influence of early family processes on later family relations warrants further study Taiwanese families are more likely to include coresidence of paternal grandparents with their sons, daughters-in-law, and grandchildren than coresidence of maternal grandparents with their daughters, sons-in-law, and grandchildren; the latter is more common in Western societies

Smith, 1997	Early sexual activity High-risk sexual activity Life context Study guided by life span and ecological frameworks	237 female teenagers (205 African American and 32 Hispanic) 566 male teenagers (443 African American and 123 Hispanic) All residing in an eastern city in the United States	Structured interviews Items for: Sexual behavior—Sexuality, Fertility Neighborhood Sociodemographic status Family variables—Parent attachment Child maltreatment Supervision School context—School aspirations Reading achievement Individual factors—Depression Early substance use	There was a positive association between lack of presence of two biological parents in the home and early intercourse Hispanic ethnicity was associated with early sexual activity Lower parent attachment, lack of parental supervision, and substance abuse were associated with early intercourse for both female and male teenagers Low school achievement aspirations and depression were associated with early sexual activity for girls	Large sample longitudinal study that began in 1987 Secondary analysis of data "The findings strongly suggest that sexual activity at young age is more problematic than sexual activity initiated in later adolescence. Teenagers who initiated intercourse early were more likely to engage in unprotected sex and to have multiple partners and risk markers for exposure to STDs. Teenage boys were more likely to have sexual intercourse early, thus prolonging their exposure to disease. Teenage girls who initiated sex earlier were substantially more likely to become pregnant in addition to risking STDs; in fact, more than half of those who had sex early became teenage parents" (p. 341).

STDs, sexually transmitted diseases.

dimension of Behavioral System, and the theory concept is Attachment Behaviors and its seven dimensions—attachment with child, attachment with family, attachment with mother, attachment with father, attachment with grandparents, attachment with partner, and attachment with peers.

The attachment dimension of Behavioral System guided the selection of literature to review and the analysis of the qualitative data extracted from the literature review. Analysis of these data indicated that the attachment subsystem dimension of Behavioral System is represented by Attachment Behaviors and its dimensions.

Examination of the six research reports reviewed yielded one explicit definition of attachment behavior (Oyedele et al., 2013). Dimensions of Attachment Behaviors were extracted from the various research reports. Maxwell et al. (2011) focused on English female teenagers' perceptions of their attachment to their child; Oyedele et al. (2013) found that sexually active South African female teenagers were attached to their families and their partners, as did Figueiredo et al. (2005) for pregnant Portuguese teenagers. Yi et al. (2006) reported various degrees of Taiwanese female and male teenagers' attachment with their mothers, fathers, and grandparents. Schreck and Fisher (2004) found that male and female teenagers residing in the United States reported attachments to their families and peers. Smith (1997) found a range of degree of attachment with parents for a sample of female and male African American and Hispanic teenagers living in the United States.

The CTE structure for the literature review is illustrated in Figure 2.5. The non-relational propositions for each component of the CTE structure are listed in Box 2.8.

A CTE Structure for Instrument Development

Wilmoth and Tingle's (2001) report of the development and testing of the Wilmoth Sexual Behaviors Questionnaire—Female (WSBQ-F) provides a source for construction of a Johnson's Behavioral System Model CTE structure for instrument development. The theory is female sexual behaviors. The conceptual model concept is Behavioral System, and the relevant dimension is sexual subsystem, and the theory concept is Female Sexual Behavior and its seven dimensions—communication, techniques, sexual response, body scar, self-touch, relationship quality, and masturbation.

The sexual system dimension of Behavioral System is represented by Female Sexual Behavior and its seven dimensions, which are measured by the WSBQ-F. Wilmoth and Tingle (2001) reported adequate estimates of reliability and validity for the WSBQ-F. Internal consistency reliability was estimated with Cronbach's alpha, and stability reliability was estimated with test–retest reliability. Content validity, using the Content Validity Index, was estimated with a panel of two experts in sexuality, two experts in oncology, and two experts in nursing theory. Exploratory factor analysis and the known group's technique were used to estimate construct validity (see Appendix B).

BOX 2.8   An Example of a Conceptual–Theoretical–Empirical Structure for Johnson's Behavioral System Model Systematic Literature Reviews

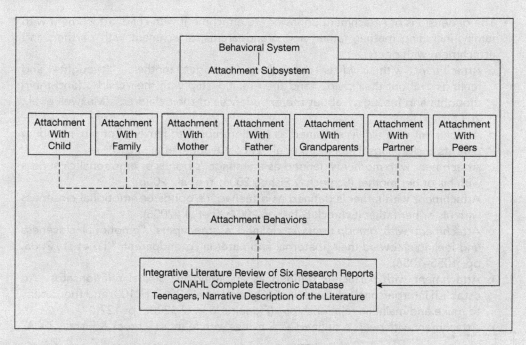

FIGURE 2.5 Conceptual–theoretical–empirical (CTE) structure for Johnson's Behavioral System Model literature review—theory of teenager attachment.
CINAHL, Complete Comprehensive Index to Nursing and Allied Health Literature.

The *non-relational propositions* for the *C component* of the conceptual–theoretical–empirical (CTE) structure are:

• *Behavioral System* is defined as the whole person.
• The relevant dimension of Behavioral System is attachment subsystem.
  o *Attachment subsystem* is defined as behaviors required to attain the security needed for survival as well as social inclusion, intimacy, and the formation and maintenance of social bonds.

The *non-relational propositions* for the *T component* of the CTE structure are:

• *Attachment Behavior* is defined as

  The ability of a teenager to master or control herself [or himself] and [the] environment in order to achieve the desired expectation of life, including setting short and long term goals, building up personal strength and being knowledgeable about her [or his] weaknesses (Oyedele et al., 2013, p. 105).

(continued)

BOX 2.8 An Example of a Conceptual–Theoretical–Empirical Structure for Johnson's Behavioral System Model Systematic Literature Reviews (continued)

- The dimensions of Attachment Behavior are attachment with child; attachment with family, including mother, father, and grandparents; attachment with partner; and attachment with peers.
  - o *Attachment with child* is defined as teenager mothers' "thoughts and feelings...about their child...and their relationship with their child...[and their] thoughts and feelings...about the experiences of their children" (Maxwell et al., 2011, p. 31).
  - o *Attachment with family* is defined as relationships with family of origin, including parents and siblings (Figueiredo et al., 2006; Oyedele et al., 2013).
  - o *Attachment with mother* is defined as a teenager's bonds or emotional closeness with his or her mother (Schreck & Fisher, 2004; Yi et al., 2006).
  - o *Attachment with father* is defined as a teenager's bonds or emotional closeness with his or her father (Schreck & Fisher, 2004; Yi et al., 2006).
  - o *Attachment with grandparents* is defined as teenagers' "emotional closeness and feeling[s] toward their [maternal and paternal] grandparents" (Yi et al., 2006, pp. 1055–1056).
  - o *Attachment with partner* is defined as engaging in "sexual relationships...to establish interpersonal relationships" (Oyedele et al., 2012, p. 103) and the "ability to make and maintain relationships" (Figueiredo et al., 2006, p. 127).
  - o *Attachment with peers* is defined as activities with friends (Schreck & Fisher, 2004).

The *non-relational proposition* for the *E component* of the CTE structure is:

- The concept of Attachment Behavior and its dimensions were extracted from an integrative literature review of six research reports about types of teenagers' attachment.

Source: Constructed for this chapter based on a journal article by Oyedele, Wright, and Maja (2013).

The CTE structure constructed for Wilmoth and Tingle's (2001) instrument development study is illustrated in Figure 2.6. The non-relational propositions for each component of the CTE structure are listed in Box 2.9.

A CTE Structure for Descriptive Qualitative Research

A journal article by Wang and Palmer (2010) is an example of a report of Johnson's Behavioral System Model descriptive qualitative research. The purpose of their study was to analyze "the concept of women's toileting behavior related to urinary elimination" (p. 1875).

The theory of women's toileting behavior related to urinary elimination was generated from their concept analysis, which is a type of descriptive qualitative research (see Appendix A). Wang and Palmer (2010) used Walker and Avant's (2005) approach to concept analysis (see Appendix B).

BOX 2.9   An Example of a Conceptual–Theoretical–Empirical Structure for Johnson's Behavioral System Model Instrument Development

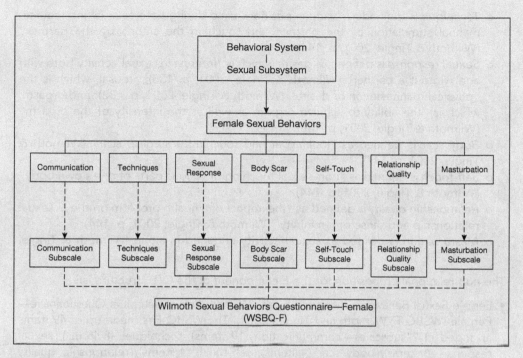

FIGURE 2.6 Conceptual–theoretical–empirical (CTE) structure for Johnson's Behavioral System Model instrument development research—theory of female sexual behaviors.

The *non-relational propositions* for the *C component* of the conceptual–theoretical–empirical (CTE) structure are:

- *Behavioral System* is defined as the whole person.
- The relevant dimension of Behavioral System is sexual subsystem.
  - o *Sexual subsystem* is defined as procreation and gratification, with regard to behaviors dependent on the person's biological sex and gender role identity, including but not limited to courting and mating.

The *non-relational propositions* for the *T component* of the CTE structure are:

- *Female Sexual Behavior* "is defined as the range of behaviours in which [a female] can engage, alone or with another person, to reduce sexual tensions and achieve satisfaction" (Wilmoth & Tingle, 2001, p. 138).
- The dimensions of Female Sexual Behavior are communication, techniques, sexual response, body scar, self-touch, relationship quality, and masturbation.
  - o *Communication* is defined as various verbal and nonverbal behaviors focusing on sexual gratification (Wilmoth & Tingle, 2001).

(continued)

BOX 2.9   An Example of a Conceptual–Theoretical–Empirical Structure for Johnson's Behavioral System Model Instrument Development   *(continued)*

- o *Technique* is defined as "various positions used during heterosexual intercourse, manual stimulation by the partner, and touching the clitoris by the partner" (Wilmoth & Tingle, 2001, p. 144).
- o *Sexual response* is defined as desire, which is "interest in sexual activity both with and without a partner" (Wilmoth & Tingle, 2001, p. 138); arousal, which is the "physical manifestation of desire" (Wilmoth & Tingle, 2001, p. 138); and orgasm, which is "the ability to achieve orgasm as well as the intensity of the orgasm" (Wilmoth & Tingle, 2001, p. 138).
- o *Body scar* is defined as "looking at and touching a surgical scar" (Wilmoth & Tingle, 2001, p. 147).
- o *Self-touch* is defined as "non-sexual touching of various parts of one's own body" (Wilmoth & Tingle, 2001, p. 144).
- o *Relationship quality* is defined as "the impact of a health problem on the . . . sexual relationship and sense of femininity" (Wilmoth & Tingle, 2001, p. 144).
- o *Masturbation* is defined as sexual activity engaged in alone (Wilmoth & Tingle, 2001).

The *non-relational proposition* for the *E component* of the CTE structure is:

- • Female Sexual Behavior is measured by the Wilmoth Sexual Behaviors Questionnaire—Female (WSBQ-F; Wilmoth and Tingle, 2001). The WSBQ-F is made up of 49 items arranged in 7 subscales—communication (19 items), techniques (8 items), sexual response (8 items), body scar (4 items), self-touch (4 items), relationship quality (3 items), and masturbation (3 items). Items are rated on a 7-point Likert scale of 0 to 6, with 0 = not applicable, 1 = never, and 6 = always. Wilmoth and Tingle (2001) explained that "The *not applicable* choice was included to distinguish between items that were not part of a [person's] set of sexual behaviours and items that were part of [her] set of sexual behaviors but were not being currently used, which would receive a *never* response" (p. 139).

Source: Wilmoth and Tingle (2001).

The conceptual model concept is Behavioral System and the relevant dimension is eliminative subsystem, and the theory concept is Women's Toileting Behavior Related to Urinary Elimination and its four dimensions—behaviors related to voiding place, behaviors related to voiding time, behaviors related to voiding position, and behaviors related to voiding style. This theory concept and its dimensions were discovered in word data extracted from the English-language literature published between January 1960 and May 2009, including book chapters and journal articles focused on adult women's toileting and micturition behaviors.

The eliminative subsystem dimension of Behavioral System guided the selection of the empirical indicators and the analysis of the qualitative data.

Analysis of these qualitative data indicated that the eliminative subsystem dimension of Behavioral System is represented by Women's Toileting Behavior Related to Urinary Elimination and its dimensions.

The CTE structure constructed for Wang and Palmer's (2010) study is illustrated in Figure 2.7. The non-relational propositions for each component of the CTE structure are listed in Box 2.10.

BOX 2.10   An Example of a Conceptual–Theoretical–Empirical Structure for Johnson's Behavioral System Model Descriptive Qualitative Research

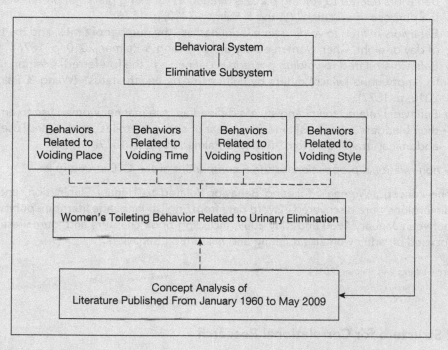

FIGURE 2.7 Conceptual–theoretical–empirical structure (CTE) for Johnson's Behavioral System Model descriptive qualitative research—theory of women's toileting behavior related to urinary elimination.

The *non-relational propositions* for the *C component* of the conceptual–theoretical–empirical (CTE) structure for this study are:

- *Behavioral System* is defined as the whole person.
- The relevant dimension of Behavioral System is eliminative subsystem.
  - o *Eliminative subsystem* is defined as elimination behaviors, with regard to when, how, and under what conditions the person urinates within the context of socially accepted behaviors.

(continued)

BOX 2.10   An Example of a Conceptual–Theoretical–Empirical Structure for Johnson's Behavioral System Model Descriptive Qualitative Research   *(continued)*

The *non-relational propositions* for the *T component* of the CTE structure are:

- *Women's Toileting Behavior Related to Urinary Elimination* is defined as "voluntary actions related to the physiological event of emptying the bladder" (Wang & Palmer, 2010, p. 1881).
- The dimensions of the concept, Women's Toileting Behavior Related to Urinary Elimination, are behaviors related to voiding place, behaviors related to voiding time, behaviors related to voiding position, and behaviors related to voiding style.
  - o *Behaviors related to voiding place* is defined as "seeking places of preference for the purpose of urinating" (Wang & Palmer, 2010, p. 1876).
  - o *Behaviors related to voiding time* is defined as "the number of times, and the time of day or night, when women empty urine" (Wang & Palmer, 2010, p. 1876).
  - o *Behaviors related to voiding position* is defined as "the [preferred] position used to empty urine [which] differs by cultures or by health status" (Wang & Palmer, 2010, p. 1877).
  - o *Behaviors related to voiding style* is defined as "the manner women use to empty their bladders...[such as] time spent near or sitting on toilet seats...[and] use [of] abdominal straining to void" (Wang & Palmer, 2010, p. 1879).

The *non-relational proposition* for the *E component* of the CTE structure is:

- The concept, Women's Toileting Behavior Related to Urinary Elimination, and its dimensions were discovered in word data from English-language literature published between January 1960 and May 2009, including book chapters and journal articles focused on adult women's toileting and micturition behaviors.

Source: Wang and Palmer (2010).

A CTE Structure for Correlational Research

The research report by Wilkie, Lovejoy, Dodd, and Tesler (1988) is an example of Johnson's Behavioral System Model correlational research. The purpose of their study was to examine the relation between pain intensity and pain control behaviors.

The theory of the relation between pain intensity and pain control behaviors was tested by means of a longitudinal correlational research design (see Appendix A), with data collected twice on each of days 2 and 3 of hospitalization. The study sample included 13 hospitalized adults who had a medical diagnosis of Stage III or Stage IV solid tumor cancer.

One conceptual model concept is Behavioral System; the relevant dimension is aggressive-protective subsystem. The other conceptual model concepts are Structural Components–set and Structural Components–choice. The two theory concepts are Pain Intensity and Pain Control Behaviors. The seven dimensions of Pain Control Behaviors are positioning behaviors; distractive behaviors; pressure manipulative behaviors; immobilizing/guarding behaviors; analgesic use behaviors; apply heat/after attitude; and other behaviors, including sleep, food/drink, and moaning.

The Behavioral System dimension of the aggressive–protective subsystem is represented by Pain Intensity, which is measured by the Visual Analog Scale (VAS)-Pain Intensity (Wilkie et al., 1988). Structural Components–set and Structural Components–choice are represented by Pain Control Behaviors and its dimensions, which are measured by the investigator-developed Demographic Pain Data Form (Wilkie et al., 1988), the Behavioral Observation-Validation Form (Wilkie et al., 1988), and a medical record review. The Kendall Correlation Coefficient (see Appendix B) was used to examine the relation between pain intensity and pain control behaviors at each data collection point.

A CTE structure for Wilkie et al.'s (1988) study, which was constructed from the content of their journal article, is illustrated in Figure 2.8. The non-relational and relational propositions for each component of the CTE structure are listed in Box 2.11.

BOX 2.11   An Example of a Conceptual–Theoretical–Empirical Structure for Johnson's Behavioral System Model Correlational Research

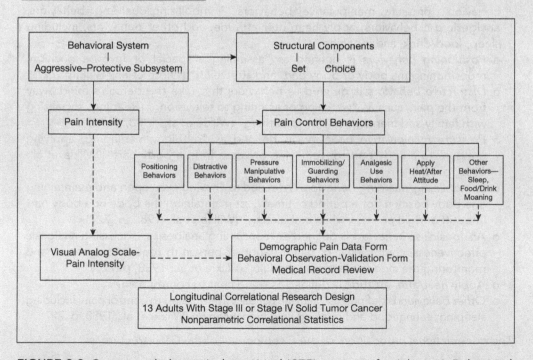

FIGURE 2.8 Conceptual–theoretical–empirical (CTE) structure for Johnson's Behavioral System Model correlational research—theory of the relation between pain intensity and pain control behaviors.

(continued)

BOX 2.11 An Example of a Conceptual–Theoretical–Empirical Structure for Johnson's Behavioral System Model Correlational Research *(continued)*

The *non-relational propositions* for the *C component* of the conceptual–theoretical–empirical (CTE) structure are:

- *Behavioral System* is defined as the whole person.
- The relevant dimension of the Behavioral System is aggressive–protective subsystem.
  o *Aggressive–protective subsystem* is defined as protection and preservation of self and society behaviors.
- *Structural Components–set* is defined as a person's predisposition to act in certain ways, rather than in other ways, to fulfill the function of the aggressive–protective subsystem for protection from pain.
- *Structural Components–choice* is defined as the person's total behavioral repertoire for fulfilling aggressive–protective subsystem functions and achieving particular goals, including the person's recognition of alternatives for behavior for protection from pain.

The *non-relational propositions* for the *T component* of the CTE structure are:

- *Pain Intensity* is defined as amount of pain experienced at a certain time.
- *Pain Control Behaviors* is defined as behaviors that prevent, improve, or intensify pain.
- The dimensions of Pain Control Behaviors are positioning behaviors, distractive behaviors, pressure manipulative behaviors, immobilizing/guarding behaviors, analgesic use behaviors, apply heat/after attitude, and other behaviors, including sleep, food/drink, and moaning.
  o *Positioning behaviors* is defined as "assuming a special or favorite position, repositioning the body or body part, and stretching" (Wilkie et al., 1988, p. 727).
  o *Distractive behaviors* is defined as behaviors that take the person's mind away from the pain, such as "watching or listening to television.... Reading, socializing with family and friends, and slow breathing" (Wilkie et al., 1988, p. 727).
  o *Pressure manipulative behaviors* is defined as "rubbing, massaging, applying pressure to a body part, or removing pressure from a body part" (Wilkie et al., 1988, p. 727).
  o *Immobilizing/guarding behaviors* is defined as "having eyes open and maintaining one body position [for a period of time]... or maintaining the body or a body part in a stiff or rigid position while ambulating" (Wilkie et al., 1988, p. 727).
  o *Analgesic use behaviors* is defined as "consuming analgesics, discussing analgesic effectiveness, complaining of pain to another person to request analgesics, and monitoring the medication time schedule" (Wilkie et al., 1988, p. 727).
  o *Apply heat/after attitude* is defined as using heat to control pain.
  o *Other behaviors* is defined as "activities of daily living" used to control pain, including sleeping, eating food and drinking fluid, and moaning (Wilkie et al., 1988, p. 727).

The *non-relational proposition* for the *E component* of the CTE structure is:

- Pain Intensity is measured by the Visual Analog Scale (VAS)-Pain Intensity. The VAS is a horizontal 100-mm line, "anchored on the left with 'no pain' and on the right with 'pain as bad as it could be'" (Wilkie et al., 1988, p. 725).

(continued)

BOX 2.11   An Example of a Conceptual–Theoretical–Empirical Structure for Johnson's Behavioral System Model Correlational Research *(continued)*

- Pain Control Behaviors and its dimensions, specifically report of subjective pain, are measured by the investigator-developed Demographic Pain Data Form (DPDF; Wilkie et al., 1988). The investigators modified items from McGuire's Pain Assessment Tool (McGuire, 1981) and the McGill Pain Questionnaire (MPQ; Melzack, 1983) for the DPDF. "Subjective pain report included McGuire's questions related to pain quality, onset, and duration; behaviors which improve or intensify pain and behaviors which the pain prevents. The MPQ body outline was included as a measure of pain location" (Wilkie et al., 1988, p. 725).
- Pain Control Behaviors and its dimensions, specifically pain-related behaviors, are measured by the investigator-developed Behavioral Observation-Validation Form (BO-VF; Wilkie et al., 1988). "The BO-VF [is] a two-column *recording* tool…[that] allows the researcher to record verbal and nonverbal behaviors (using a narrative form) and, subsequently, to be validated or denied by the patient" (Wilkie et al., 1988, p. 725).
- Pain Control Behaviors and its dimensions, specifically analgesic use, are measured by a medical record review (Wilkie et al., 1988).

Source: Wilkie, Lovejoy, Dodd, and Tesler (1998).

A CTE Structure for Experimental Research

A research report by Colling, Owen, McCreedy, and Newman (2003) is an example of Johnson's Behavioral System Model experimental research. One purpose of their study was to examine the effects of an experimental Patterned Urge-Response Toileting (PURT) nursing intervention on the frequency of involuntary urination and the volume of urine eliminated during involuntary urination.

The theory of the effects of PURT on urinary incontinence was tested by means of a quasi-experimental longitudinal research design with an experimental (immediate treatment) group and a control (delayed treatment) group (see Appendix A). The study sample included 78 community-dwelling older adults. Data were collected prior to implementation of the PURT intervention and at 3, 6, 9, 12, and 18 weeks after implementation of the intervention protocol.

One conceptual model concept is External Regulatory Control; the relevant dimension is change structure units-set. The other conceptual model concept is Behavioral System; the relevant dimension is eliminative subsystem. The theory concepts are the PURT nursing intervention and Urge/Functional Urinary Incontinence. The two dimensions of Urge/Functional Urinary Incontinence are frequency of involuntary urination and urine volume from involuntary urination.

The External Regulatory Control dimension of change structural units–set is represented by the PURT Nursing Intervention, which was operationalized by the PURT Nursing Intervention protocol (Colling, Ouslander, Hadley, Eisch, & Campbell, 1992; Colling et al., 2003). The Behavioral System concept dimension of eliminative subsystem is represented by Urge/Functional Urinary Incontinence and its two dimensions. The frequency of involuntary urination dimension was measured by caregivers' diary entries and electronic recordings during a period of 24 hours. The urine volume from involuntary urination dimension was measured by the weight of absorbent products during a 24-hour period. Differences in changes in scores for the research instruments for the experimental and control groups were examined using repeated measures analysis of variance statistics (see Appendix B).

A CTE structure for Colling et al.'s (2003) study was constructed from the content of their journal article (see Figure 2.9). The non-relational and relational propositions for each component of the CTE structure are listed in Box 2.12.

A CTE Structure for Mixed-Methods Research

A research report by Coward and Wilkie (2000) is an example of mixed-methods Johnson's Behavioral System Model nursing research. The purposes of their study were to describe the meanings of the pain experiences, self-disclosure of pain, and pain management strategies reported by women and men who had cancer with metastatic bone pain, as well as to quantify the intensity and location of their pain.

The theory of the meaning of metastatic cancer bone pain was generated by means of a mixed-methods research design (QUAL + QUAN; see Appendix A) with a simple descriptive qualitative design used for the QUAL portion of the study and a simple descriptive quantitative design used for the QUAN portion. Ten women and 10 men with metastatic bone pain participated in the study. The conceptual model concept is Behavioral System; the relevant dimension is aggressive–protective subsystem. One theory concept is Meaning of Metastatic Cancer Bone Pain and its four dimensions—thoughts and feelings about pain, impact of pain, reporting pain to others, and self-medication decision making. The other theory concept is Pain Characteristics and its four dimensions—pain location, pain quality, pain pattern, and pain intensity.

The Behavioral System aggressive–protective dimension guided the selection of empirical indicators and the analysis of the qualitative and quantitative data. For the qualitative portion of the study, an investigator-developed Interview Form that included open-ended questions is used to collect the word data (Coward & Wilkie, 2000). These data were analyzed using content analysis (see Appendix B) to discover themes.

For the quantitative portion of the study, the four dimensions of Pain Characteristics represent the Behavioral System concept dimension of aggressive–protective subsystem. The McGill Pain Questionnaire (MPQ; Melzack, 1975) measures the four dimensions of Pain Characteristics—pain location, pain quality, pain pattern, and pain intensity. The pain intensity dimension is also measured by the VAS-Pain Intensity (Paice & Cohen, 1997). Descriptive statistics (numbers, percents, means, and standard deviations; see Appendix B) were used to analyze the scores for the MPQ and the VAS.

BOX 2.12   An Example of a Conceptual–Theoretical–Empirical Structure for Johnson's Behavioral System Model Experimental Research

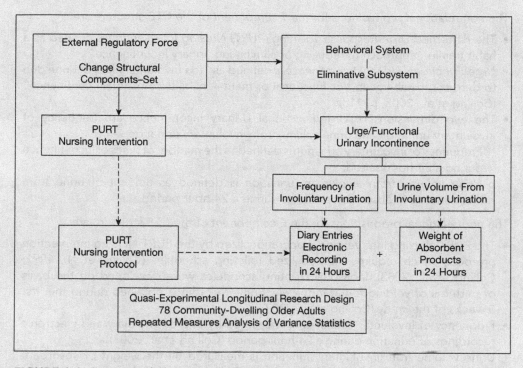

FIGURE 2.9 Conceptual–theoretical–empirical (CTE) structure for Johnson's Behavioral System Model experimental research—theory of the effects of PURT on urinary incontinence.

PURT, Patterned Urge-Response Toileting.

The *non-relational propositions* for the *C component* of the conceptual–theoretical–empirical (CTE) structure are:

- *External Regulatory Force* is defined as nursing activities that preserve Behavioral System balance and stability or overcome Behavioral System imbalance and instability.
- The relevant dimension of External Regulatory Force is change structural components–set.
  - o *Change structural components–set* is defined as nursing activities that change a person's predisposition to act in certain ways, rather than in other ways, to fulfill the function of the eliminative system for urination.
- *Behavioral System* is defined as the whole person.
- The relevant dimension of Behavioral System is eliminative subsystem.
  - o *Eliminative subsystem* is defined as elimination behaviors, with regard to when, how, and under what conditions the person urinates within the context of socially accepted behaviors.

(continued)

BOX 2.12   An Example of a Conceptual–Theoretical–Empirical Structure for Johnson's Behavioral System Model Experimental Research   *(continued)*

The *non-relational propositions* for the *T component* of the CTE structure are:

- The *Patterned Urge-Response Toileting (PURT) Nursing Intervention* is defined as a habit training approach to reducing or eliminating urinary incontinence.
- *Urge/Functional Urinary Incontinence* is defined as "the involuntary loss of urine due to detrusor instability and/or functional or mental inability to maintain continence" (Colling et al., 2003, p. 118).
- The two dimensions of Urge/Functional Urinary Incontinence are frequency of involuntary urination and urine volume from involuntary urination.
  o *Frequency of involuntary urination* is defined as the number of times of incontinence during a 24-hour period.
  o *Urine volume from involuntary urination* is defined as amount of urine from incontinence in absorbent products during a 24-hour period.

The *non-relational propositions* for the *E component* of the CTE structure are:

- The PURT Nursing Intervention is operationalized by the PURT Nursing Intervention protocol, which requires individualized toileting schedules (Colling et al., 1992; Colling et al., 2003). Individual toileting schedules were developed on the basis of patterns of voiding found in the electronic recordings obtained during the first 3 weeks of the study (Colling et al., 2003).
- Frequency of involuntary urination is measured by entries in a diary and electronic recordings of urination during a 24-hour period (Colling et al., 2003).
- Urine volume from involuntary urination is measured by the weight of absorbent products collected during a 24-hour period (Colling et al., 2003).

The *relational propositions* for the *C and T components* of the CTE structure are:

- The External Regulatory Force concept dimension of change structural components-set has a positive effect on the balance and stability of the Behavioral System concept dimension of eliminative subsystem.
- Therefore, the PURT Nursing Intervention has a negative effect on Urge/Functional Urinary Incontinence, such that implementation of the PURT Nursing Intervention will prevent or reduce Urge/Functional Urinary Incontinence.

The *relational proposition* for the *E component* of the CTE structure is:

- Implementation of the PURT Nursing Intervention protocol will reduce or prevent diary entries and electronic recordings of involuntary urination during a 24-hour period.
- Implementation of the PURT Nursing Intervention protocol will reduce the weight of urine in absorbent products or eliminate presence of any urine in absorbent products during a 24-hour period.

Source: Colling, Owen, McCreedy, and Newman (2003).

A CTE structure for Coward and Wilkie's (2000) study, which was constructed from the content of their journal article, is illustrated in Figure 2.10. The non-relational and relational propositions for each component of the CTE structure are listed in Box 2.13.

BOX 2.13 An Example of a Conceptual–Theoretical– Empirical Structure for Johnson's Behavioral System Model Mixed-Methods Research

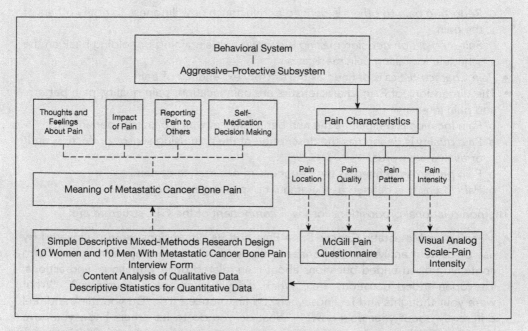

FIGURE 2.10 Conceptual–theoretical–empirical (CTE) structure for Johnson's Behavioral System Model mixed-methods research—theory of the meaning of metastatic cancer bone pain—qualitative and quantitative portions.

The *non-relational propositions* for the *C component* of the conceptual–theoretical– empirical (CTE) structure for the study are:

- *Behavioral System* is defined as the whole person.
- The relevant dimension of the Behavioral System is aggressive–protective subsystem.
  - *Aggressive–protective subsystem* is defined as protection and preservation of self and society behaviors.

The *non-relational propositions* for the *T component* of the CTE structure are:

- *Meaning of Metastatic Cancer Bone Pain* is defined as beliefs and feelings about pain and actions taken to control pain.
- The dimensions of Meaning of Metastatic Cancer Bone Pain are thoughts and feelings about pain, impact of pain, reporting pain to others, and self-medication decision making.
  - *Thoughts and feelings about pain* is defined as beliefs about the origin of the pain and emotional reactions to the lack of effectiveness of cancer treatment.
  - *Impact of pain* is defined as the ways in which pain interfered with work and leisure activities and family relationships.

(continued)

BOX 2.13   An Example of a Conceptual–Theoretical–
Empirical Structure for Johnson's Behavioral System Model
Mixed-Methods Research   *(continued)*

- o *Reporting pain to others* is defined as reluctance or willingness to notify others of the pain.
- o *Self-medication decision making* is defined as maintaining or holding back on the schedule for taking pain medication.
- *Pain Characteristics* is defined as the sensory experience of pain.
- The dimensions of Pain Characteristics are pain location, pain quality, pain pattern, and pain intensity.
  - o *Pain location* is defined as the number of sites at which pain is experienced.
  - o *Pain quality* is defined as the description of the pain using sensory, affective, and/or evaluative words.
  - o *Pain pattern* is defined as the frequency of occurrence of pain.
  - o *Pain intensity* is defined as the amount of pain experienced.

The *non-relational propositions* for the E *component* of the CTE structure are:

- Meaning of Metastatic Cancer Bone Pain and its dimensions were discovered by use of content analysis of responses to the investigator-developed Interview Form containing open-ended questions about pain-related beliefs, feelings, and actions. The open-ended questions are: "When did you first notice your pain?" "What were your thoughts and feelings when you first noticed it?" "Do you think and feel differently about your pain now?" "What do you do to let others know you have pain?" "How do you go about deciding to take your pain medication?" (Coward & Wilkie, 2000).
- The pain location, pain quality, pain pattern, and pain intensity dimensions of Pain Characteristics are measured by the McGill Pain Questionnaire (Melzack, 1975). Pain location is the number of sites at which pain is experienced, marked on a body outline. Pain quality items are rated on a pain rating index by categorizing words about pain as a sensory score with a maximum of 42; an affective score with a maximum of 14; an evaluative score with a maximum of 5; a miscellaneous score with a maximum of 17; and a total score with a maximum of 78. Pain pattern is a categorization of words about pain as constant, intermittent, brief/transient, or a combination. Pain intensity items are rated on a scale of 0 = none, 1 = mild, 2 = discomforting, 3 = distressing, 4 = horrible, and 5 = excruciating.
- The pain intensity dimension of Pain Characteristics is also measured by the Visual Analog Scale-Pain Intensity (VAS-Pain Intensity; Paice & Cohen, 1997). The VAS-Pain Intensity is a horizontal 100-mm (10 cm) line with anchors for no pain and worst pain imaginable.

Source: Coward and Wilkie (2000).

CONCLUSION

Johnson's Behavioral System Model makes a substantial contribution to nursing knowledge by focusing on behavior, rather than on health state or disease condition. This focus clearly distinguishes nursing from medicine, although Johnson acknowledged boundary overlaps. She stated:

> [T]his model attempts to specify [the goal of nursing] in keeping with our historical concerns, and to reclarify nursing's mission and area of responsibility. In doing so, no denial of nursing's old relationship with medicine is intended. Nursing has, and undoubtedly always will play an important role in assisting medicine to fulfill its mission. We do this directly by taking on activities delegated by medicine, but also, and perhaps more importantly, we may contribute to the achievement of medicine's goals by fulfilling our own mission. (Johnson, 1968, p. 9)

In summarizing the contributions of the Behavioral System Model to the discipline of nursing, Johnson (1992) explained that "the body of knowledge about the behavioral system and its subsystems is sufficiently substantial to allow pertinent observations and useful interpretations in practice. It also points to many possibilities for intervention as well as avenues for research" (p. 26). The broad utility of Johnson's Behavioral System Model is evident in the examples of its use as a guide for practice, QI projects, and research given in this chapter.

NOTE

1. Portions of this chapter are from Fawcett, J., & DeSanto-Madeya, S. (2013). *Contemporary nursing knowledge: Analysis and evaluation of nursing models and theories* (3rd ed., Chapter 4). Philadelphia, PA: F. A. Davis, with permission.

REFERENCES

Colling, J., Ouslander, J. Hadley, B. J., Eisch, J., & Campbell, E. (1992). The effects of patterned urge-response toileting (PURT) on urinary incontinence among nursing home residents. *Journal of the American Geriatrics Society, 39*, 135–141.

Colling, J., Owen, T. R., McCreedy, M., & Newman, D. (2003). The effects of a continence program on frail community-dwelling elderly. *Urologic Nursing, 23*, 117–122, 127–131.

Coward, D. D., & Wilkie, D. J. (2000). Metastatic bone pain: Meanings associated with self-report and self-management decision making. *Cancer Nursing, 23*, 101–108.

Dee, V., van Servellen, G., & Brecht, M. (1998). Managed behavioral health care patients and their nursing care problems, level of functioning, and impairment on discharge. *Journal of the American Psychiatric Nurses Association, 4*, 57–66.

Fawcett, J., & DeSanto-Madeya, S. (2013). *Contemporary nursing knowledge: Analysis and evaluation of nursing models and theories* (3rd ed.). Philadelphia, PA: F. A. Davis.

Figueiredo, B., Bifulco, A. Pecheco, A., Costa, R., & Magarinho, R. (2006). Teenage pregnancy, attachment style, and depression: A comparison of teenage and adult pregnant women in a Portuguese series. *Attachment and Human Development, 8*, 123–138.

Grubbs, J. (1974). An interpretation of the Johnson Behavioral System Model. In J. P. Riehl & C. Roy (Eds.), *Conceptual models for nursing practice* (pp. 160–197). New York, NY: Appleton-Century-Crofts.

Johnson, D. E. (1968). *One conceptual model of nursing.* Unpublished paper presented at Vanderbilt University, Nashville, TN.

Johnson, D. E. (1980). The behavioral system model for nursing. In J. P. Riehl & C. Roy (Eds.), *Conceptual models for nursing practice* (2nd ed., pp. 207–216). New York, NY: Appleton-Century-Crofts.

Johnson, D. E. (1990). The behavioral system model for nursing. In M. E. Parker (Ed.), *Nursing theories in practice* (pp. 23–32). New York, NY: National League for Nursing.

Johnson, D. E. (1992). The origins of the behavioral system model. In F. N. Nightingale (Ed.), *Notes on nursing: What it is, and what it is not* (Commemorative ed., pp. 23–27). Philadelphia, PA: Lippincott.

Ma, T., & Gaudet, D. (1997). Assessing the quality of life of our end-stage renal disease client population. *Journal of the Canadian Association of Nephrology Nurses and Technicians, 7*(2), 13–16.

Maxwell, A., Proctor, J., & Hammond, L. (2011). "Me and my child": Parenting experiences of young mothers leaving care. *Adoption and Fostering, 35*(4), 29–40.

McGuire, L. (1981). A short simple tool for assessing your patient's pain. *Nursing 81, 11*(3), 48–49.

Melzack, R. (1975). The McGill Pain Questionnaire: Major properties and scoring methods. *Pain, 1,* 277–299.

Melzack, R. (1983). Concepts of pain management. In R. Melzack (Ed.), *Pain measurement and assessment* (pp. 1–5). New York, NY: Raven Press.

Oyedele, O. A., Wright, S. C. D., & Maja, T. M. M. (2013). Prevention of teenage pregnancies in Soshanguve, South Africa: Using the Johnson Behavioral System Model. *Africa Journal of Nursing and Midwifery, 15,* 95–108.

Paice, J. A., & Cohen, F. L. (1997). Validity of a verbally administered numeric rating scale to measure cancer pain intensity. *Cancer Nursing, 20,* 88–93.

Rogers, E. M. (2003). *Diffusion of innovations* (5th ed.) New York, NY: Free Press.

Schreck, C. J., & Fisher, B. S. (2004). Specifying the influence of family and peers on violent victimization: Extending routine activities and lifestyle theories. *Journal of Interpersonal Violence, 19,* 1021–1041.

Smith, C. A. (1997). Factors associated with early sexual activity among urban adolescents. *Social Work, 42,* 334–346.

Walker, L. O., & Avant, K. C. (2005). *Strategies for theory construction in nursing* (4th ed.). Upper Saddle River, NJ: Pearson/Prentice Hall.

Wang, K., & Palmer, M.H. (2010). Women's toileting behavior related to urinary elimination: Concept analysis. *Journal of Advanced Nursing, 66,* 1874–1884.

White, K. (2010). Practice exemplar. In M. E. Parker & M. C. Smith (Eds.), *Nursing theories and nursing practice* (3rd ed., pp. 117–118). Philadelphia, PA: F. A. Davis.

Wilkie, D., Lovejoy, N., Dodd, M., & Tesler, M. (1988). Cancer pain control behaviors: Description and correlation with pain intensity. *Oncology Nursing Forum, 15,* 723–731.

Wilmoth, M.C., & Tingle, L.R. (2001). Development and psychometric testing of the Wilmoth Sexual Behaviors Questionnaire—Female. *Canadian Journal of Nursing Research, 32,* 135–151.

Yi, C., Pan, E., Chang, Y., & Chan, C. (2006). Grandparents, adolescents, and parents: Intergenerational relations of Taiwanese youth. *Journal of Family Issues, 27,* 1042–2067.

CHAPTER 3

KING'S CONCEPTUAL SYSTEM[1]

Imogene M. King's Conceptual System focuses on the continuing ability of people to meet their basic needs so that they may function in their socially defined roles, as well as on their interactions within three open, dynamic, interacting systems (King, 2007). The goal of nursing is to help individuals, families, groups, and communities attain, maintain, and restore health, so that they can function in their respective roles, and to help people die with dignity (King, 1981, 1986a, 1986b, 1992, 1995, 1997).

KING'S CONCEPTUAL SYSTEM: CONCEPTS AND NON-RELATIONAL PROPOSITIONS

This section of the chapter includes the concepts of King's Conceptual System and the definitions (non-relational propositions) of the concepts and dimensions of the multidimensional concepts.

Personal System is defined as "a unified, complex whole self who perceives, thinks, desires, imagines, decides, identifies goals, and selects means to achieve them" (King, 1981, p. 27). The seven dimensions of the concept are perception, self, growth and development, body image, time, personal space, and learning.

Perception is defined as each person's awareness of what is real in his or her life and the environment.

Self is defined as a unified, complex whole person who perceives, thinks, desires, imagines, decides, identifies goals, selects means to achieve them, and is synonymous with I and me.

Growth and development is defined as constant changes that occur within each person at the cellular, molecular, and behavioral levels of existence.

Body image is defined as a person's perceptions of his or her own body, which may reflect others' reactions to the person's physical body.

Time is defined as the interval between events in the past, present, and future.

Personal space is defined as the territory identified by each person as the boundary between self and others or the environment that provides a sense of identity and security.

Learning is defined as a process of perceiving, conceptualizing, and thinking critically.

Interpersonal System is defined as being made up of two or more personal systems that are engaged in interaction. The six dimensions of the concept are interaction, communication, transaction, role, stress, and coping.

Interaction is defined as a process of perception and communication between two or more personal systems and/or the environment that includes a sequence of verbal and nonverbal goal-directed behaviors.

Communication is defined as the way in which personal systems develop and maintain relationships. The two subdimensions of communication are verbal communication and nonverbal communication.

Verbal communication, which is both intrapersonal and interpersonal in nature, encompasses verbal signs and symbols, including spoken and written words, used by personal systems to express goals and values.

Nonverbal communication, which also is both intrapersonal and interpersonal in nature, encompasses nonverbal signs and symbols, including gestures and touch, used by personal systems to express goals and values.

Transaction is defined as an observable goal-directed interaction with the environment.

Role is defined as expected behaviors that are associated with the position of each personal system in a social system.

Stress is defined as a dynamic state of personal system–environment interaction that involves an exchange of energy and information for the purpose of regulating and controlling the environment. Stress may be negative or positive, or constructive or destructive.

Coping is regarded as an essential area of knowledge related to the interpersonal system that refers to coping with stress and stressors.

Social System is defined as a group, such as a family, a school, a hospital, an industry, a religious organization, or a community, that forms to carry out particular purposes needed to maintain a society. The six dimensions of the concept are organization, authority, power, status, decision making, and control.

Organization is defined as personal systems who have specific positions and roles and who utilize certain resources to accomplish personal and organizational goals.

Authority is defined as a process that is characterized by active, reciprocal relations that reflect how one personal system influences others.

Power is defined as a process that involves a situation in which a personal system accepts the dictates of another even if he or she does not agree with those dictates.

Status is defined as the ascribed or achieved position of a personal system within a group or the ascribed or achieved position of a group within an organization.

Decision making in organizations is defined as a dynamic, systematic process that involves choices among alternatives to attain goals.

Control is defined as exerting influence on personal or interpersonal systems.

Internal Environment is defined as source of stressors and energy that enables a personal system to adjust to continuous external environmental changes.

External Environment is defined as a source of stressors and continuous changes within which a personal system grows, develops, and performs activities of daily living.

Health is defined as the dynamic life experiences of a personal system that involve continuous adjustment to internal and external environmental stressors and that support the ability of the personal system to function in social roles.

Illness, which may also be referred to as disability, is defined as a deviation from normal that results from an imbalance or disturbance in the biologic structure or psychological makeup of a personal system, or a conflict in a social relationship. Disease is one kind of illness.

Interaction–Transaction Process is defined as a dynamic process during which a nurse and a client share their perceptions about a nursing situation, communicate to identify specific problems and goals, explore the means by which goals can be attained, agree on those means, implement the means to attain the goals, and identify the outcomes. The 10 dimensions of the concept are perception, judgment, action, reaction, disturbance, mutual goal setting, exploration of means to achieve goals, agreement on means to achieve goals, transaction, and attainment of goals.

Perception is defined as the nurse and the client meeting in some nursing situation and becoming aware of each other.

Judgment is defined as the nurse and the client making mental judgments about each other.

Action is defined as a sequence of nurse and client behaviors in interaction, including recognition of the situation, activities related to the situation, and motivation to control the situation to attain goals.

Reaction is defined as the nurse and the client mentally reacting to each other's perceptions of each other.

Disturbance is defined as the nurse and the client communicating and interacting as the nurse identifies the client's concerns, problems, and disturbances in health.

Mutual goal setting is defined as the nurse and the client purposefully interacting to set mutually agreed on goals.

Exploration of means to attain goals is defined as the nurse and the client purposefully interacting to explore the means to achieve the mutually set goals.

Agreement on Means to Attain Goals is defined as the nurse and the client purposefully interacting to agree on the means to achieve the mutually set goals.

Transaction is defined as the nurse and the client carrying out measures agreed on to attain the mutually set goals.

Attainment of Goals is defined as the nurse and the client identifying the outcome of the Interaction–Transaction Process, expressed in terms of the client's ability to function in social roles.

KING'S CONCEPTUAL SYSTEM: RELATIONAL PROPOSITIONS

The statements of associations (relational propositions) among concepts of King's Conceptual System are listed here.

- The Personal System, Interpersonal System, and Social System are interrelated.
- The dimensions of each system—Personal, Interpersonal, and Social—are interrelated.
- The manifestations of each dimension of each system—Personal, Interpersonal, and Social—are interrelated.
- The extent of Health is related to the extent to which the person adjusts to Internal and External Environmental stressors.
- The extent of Illness is related to the extent of disturbance in a person's biologic structure or psychological makeup or a conflict in a social relationship.
- The Interaction–Transaction Process has a positive effect on all dimensions of the Personal System, the Interpersonal System, and the Social System.
- The extent to which the nurse and the client mutually set goals, explore means to achieve goals, and agree on the means to achieve those goals is positively related to transaction.
- Transaction has a positive effect on attainment of goals.

KING'S CONCEPTUAL SYSTEM: APPLICATION TO NURSING PRACTICE

The guidelines for King's Conceptual System nursing practice are listed in Box 3.1. A diagram of the practice methodology for King's Conceptual System, which is called the Interaction–Transaction Process, is illustrated in Figure 3.1.

A practice tool that includes all parts of the practice methodology is given in Box 3.2.

A Conceptual–Theoretical–Empirical Structure for Assessment

King's (1981) description of the use of the Goal-Oriented Nursing Record (GONR), which she developed, includes an example of King's Conceptual System–guided nursing practice focused on assessment of a young girl who

BOX 3.1 Guidelines for King's Conceptual System Nursing Practice

The purpose of nursing practice is to help individuals attain and maintain their health, and if there is some disturbance such as illness or disability, nurses' actions are goal directed to help individuals regain health or live with a chronic illness or a disability.

Practice problems encompass the client's activities of daily living related to the performance of social roles.

Nursing practice can occur in acute and chronic care settings, as well as those appropriate to delivery of care for the maintenance of health. Opportunities for health promotion exist wherever people are in their communities, regardless of their age and health state.

Legitimate participants in nursing are people who can actively participate in decisions that influence their care, as well as clients who have family members with whom nurses can make transactions until the clients can participate.

The nursing process is King's Interaction–Transaction Process.

King's Conceptual System–based nursing practice contributes to the well-being of clients by enhancing their abilities to function in the activities of daily living associated with their social roles.

Adapted from Fawcett and DeSanto-Madeya (2013).

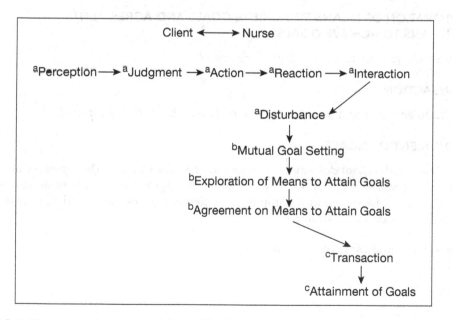

FIGURE 3.1 King's practice methodology: The Interaction–Transaction Process.
[a]Identify the client's problem; [b]set goals; [c]implement and evaluate interventions.

was comatose following an automobile accident. The girl had sustained head, chest, and abdominal injuries.

The theory used to guide practice is assessment of neurological status. The conceptual model concept is Personal System and its dimensions—perception,

BOX 3.2   The King's Conceptual System Practice Methodology Tool

PERCEPTION, JUDGMENT, ACTION, AND REACTION

Personal System

Please tell me about yourself.

Interpersonal System

Please tell me about your relationships and interactions with family, friends, and other people.

Social System

Who makes the decisions in your family?

DISTURBANCE

What problems do you have at this time?

MUTUAL GOAL SETTING

What are your goals with regard to those problems?

EXPLORATION OF MEANS TO ACHIEVE GOALS AND AGREEMENT ON MEANS TO ACHIEVE GOALS

What would you like to do to attain those goals?

TRANSACTION

The nurse and the client agree on a plan to achieve the mutually set goal.

ATTAINMENT OF GOALS

The nurse and the client determine whether the goal was attained. They review whether the client was able to successfully implement the agreed on means to achieve the goal, discuss barriers and facilitators to attainment of the goal, and, if necessary, implement additional strategies.

Adapted from Fawcett and DeSanto-Madeya (2013).

self, growth and development, body image, time, personal space, and learning. Personal System and its dimensions are represented by the theory concept, Neurological Status, which is assessed using the GONR.

The conceptual–theoretical–empirical (CTE) structure that was constructed from King's (1981) example is illustrated in Figure 3.2. The non-relational propositions for each component of the CTE structure are listed in Box 3.3.

BOX 3.3 An Example of a Conceptual–Theoretical–Empirical Structure for King's Conceptual System Nursing Practice: Assessment

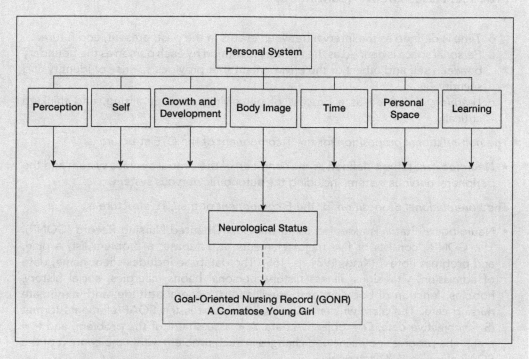

FIGURE 3.2 Conceptual–theoretical–empirical (CTE) structure for King's Conceptual System nursing practice: Assessment—theory of assessment of neurological status.

The *non-relational propositions* for the *C component* of the conceptual–theoretical–empirical (CTE) structure are:

- *Personal System* is defined as "a unified, complex whole self who perceives, thinks, desires, imagines, decides, identifies goals, and selects means to achieve them" (King, 1981, p. 27).
- The seven dimensions of Personal System are perception, self, growth and development, body image, time, personal space, and learning.
  - o *Perception* is defined as each person's awareness of what is real in his or her life and the environment.
  - o *Self* is defined as a unified, complex, whole person who perceives, thinks, desires, imagines, decides, identifies goals, selects means to achieve them, and is synonymous with I and me.
  - o *Growth and development* is defined as constant changes that occur within each person at the cellular, molecular, and behavioral levels of existence.
  - o *Body image* is defined as a person's perceptions of his or her own body, which may reflect others' reactions to the person's physical body.

(continued)

BOX 3.3 An Example of a Conceptual–Theoretical–
Empirical Structure for King's Conceptual System Nursing
Practice: Assessment *(continued)*

- o *Time* is defined as the interval between events in the past, present, and future.
- o *Personal space* is defined as the territory identified by each person as the boundary between self and others or the environment that provides a sense of identity and security.
- o *Learning* is defined as a process of perceiving, conceptualizing, and thinking critically.

The *non-relational proposition* for the *T component* of the CTE structure is:

- *Neurological Status* is defined as the condition of the central nervous system and the peripheral nervous system, including the autonomic nervous system.

The *non-relational proposition* for the *E component* of the CTE structure is:

- Neurological Status is assessed using the Goal-Oriented Nursing Record (GONR). The GONR "consists of five major elements: a database, a problem list, a plan, and progress notes" (King, 1981, p. 165). The database includes client name, date of admission, vital signs, illness history, personal habits, allergies, social history, hobbies, function of body systems, medications, general attitude, and immediate nursing care. The plan, written as goals, incorporates the SOAP elements format (S = subjective data, O = objective data, A = assessment of the problem, and P = plan). The progress notes include changes in each problem within the context of the SOAP elements for each goal.

Source: King (1981).

A CTE Structure for Intervention

An example of King's Conceptual System–guided nursing practice that includes a focus on intervention was extracted from an example of nursing care of a critically ill infant (Gunther, 2014). The theory used to guide practice is the effect of a parental care intervention on parental ability. The conceptual model concept is Interaction–Transaction Process. Two dimensions of this concept are relevant—transaction and attainment of goals. The theory concepts are Parental Care Nursing Intervention and Parental Ability.

The transaction dimension of Interaction-Transaction Process is represented by Parental Care Nursing Intervention, which is operationalized by a protocol for Parental Care Nursing Intervention. The attainment of goals dimension of Interaction-Transaction Process is represented by Parental Ability, which is measured by observation of parents' care of their critically ill infant in a neonatal intensive care unit.

The CTE structure constructed from the content of Gunther's (2014) practice example is illustrated in Figure 3.3. The non-relational and relational propositions for each component of the CTE structure are listed in Box 3.4.

BOX 3.4 An Example of a Conceptual–Theoretical–Empirical Structure for King's Conceptual System Nursing Practice: Intervention

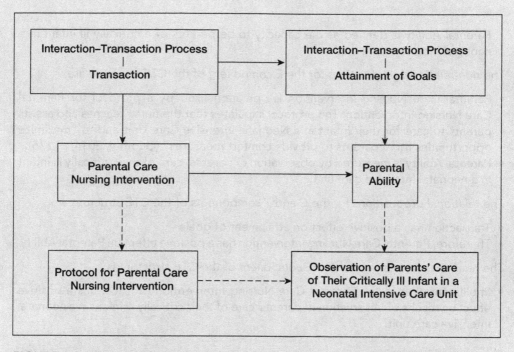

FIGURE 3.3 Conceptual–theoretical–empirical (CTE) structure for King's Conceptual System nursing practice: Intervention—theory of the effect of a parental care nursing intervention on parental ability.

The *non-relational propositions* for the C *component* of the conceptual–theoretical–empirical (CTE) structure are:

- *The Interaction–Transaction Process* is defined as a dynamic process during which a nurse and a client share their perceptions about a nursing situation, communicate to identify specific problems and goals, explore the means by which goals can be attained, agree on those means, implement the means to attain the goals, and identify the outcomes.
- The relevant dimensions of the Interaction–Transaction Process are transaction and attainment of goals.
  - o *Transaction* is defined as the nurse and the client carrying out measures agreed on to attain the mutually set goals.
  - o *Attainment of goals* is defined as the nurse and the client identifying the outcome of the Interaction–Transaction Process, expressed in terms of the client's ability to function in social roles.

The *non-relational propositions* for the T *component* of the CTE structure are:

- *Parental Care Nursing Intervention* is defined as teaching parents how to care for their critically ill infant in the neonatal intensive care unit.

(continued)

BOX 3.4   An Example of a Conceptual–Theoretical–Empirical Structure for King's Conceptual System Nursing Practice: Intervention   *(continued)*

- *Parental Ability* is defined as the capacity to be parents of a critically ill infant in a neonatal intensive care unit.

The *non-relational propositions* for the *E component* of the CTE structure are:

- Parental Care Nursing Intervention is operationalized by a protocol for Parental Care Nursing Intervention. The protocol stipulates that the nurse teaches and assists parents to care for their infant in a Neonatal Intensive Care Unit and to "maximize opportunities for…parents to provide comfort measures" (Gunther, 2014, p. 176).
- Parental Ability is measured by observation of parents' care of their critically ill infant in a neonatal intensive care unit.

The *relational propositions* for the *C* and *T components* of the CTE structure are:

- Transaction has a positive effect on attainment of goals.
- Therefore, Parental Care Nursing Intervention has a positive effect on Parental Ability.

The *relational proposition* for the *E component* of the CTE structure is:

- Implementation of the Parental Care Nursing Intervention protocol has a positive effect on results of observation of parents' care of their critically ill infant in a neonatal intensive care unit.

Source: Gunther (2014).

KING'S CONCEPTUAL SYSTEM: APPLICATION TO QUALITY IMPROVEMENT

The guidelines for King's Conceptual System quality improvement (QI) projects are listed in Box 3.5.

A CTE Structure for a QI Project

A journal article by Mann (2011) is an example of a QI project guided by King's Conceptual System. The purpose of the QI project was "to enhance the current system of providing information to patients newly diagnosed with cancer and their families" (p. 55). Mann explained that inasmuch as the goal of the project "was to improve the existing system of providing new patient education…it was a quality improvement intervention rather than a research project" (p. 58).

The theory is the effects of individualized patient education on anxiety, quality of life, and satisfaction. The two conceptual model concepts are Interaction–Transaction Process and Personal System. The relevant dimensions of Personal System are self and learning. The four theory concepts are QI Individualized

> ## BOX 3.5 Guidelines for King's Conceptual System Quality Improvement Projects
>
> The purpose of quality improvement (QI) projects is to test the effectiveness of nurses' use of King's practice methodology (the Interaction–Transaction Process).
> The phenomenon of interest for QI projects is nurses' use of the Interaction–Transaction Process.
> Data for QI projects are to be collected from clients and/or nurses in various settings, such as clients' homes, practitioners' private offices, ambulatory clinics, hospitals, and communities.
> Any methodological theory of change or QI may be used to guide the design of the QI project and the times for data collection. Checklists, rating scales, and responses to open-ended questions may be used to determine the extent to which nurses actually implement one or more dimensions of the Interaction–Transaction Process. Descriptive statistics may be used to analyze data obtained from checklists or rating scales, and content analysis may be used to identify categories or themes found in responses to open-ended questions.
> The results of King's Conceptual System-based QI projects enhance understanding of the effectiveness of nurses' use of the Interaction–Transaction Process.

Patient Education, Anxiety, Quality of Life, and Satisfaction. The two dimensions of Satisfaction are education content and time for and location of education.

Interaction–Transaction Process is represented by QI Individualized Patient Education. The self dimension of Personal System is represented by Anxiety and by Quality of Life; the learning dimension is represented by Satisfaction and its two dimensions—education content and time for and location of education.

QI Individualized Patient Education is operationalized by a QI Individualized Patient Education protocol that is guided by Doran and Sidani's (2007) outcomes-focused knowledge translational intervention framework (OFKTIF; see Appendix A). Anxiety, Quality of Life, and the two dimensions of Satisfaction—education content and time for and location of education—are measured by the project manager–developed Evaluation Form.

Mann (2011) used descriptive statistics (numbers and percents) to analyze the data for the QI project (see Appendix B). Specifically, she provided a narrative comparison of the number and percent of 32 patients newly diagnosed with cancer who received QI Individualized Patient Education from oncology nurses and who reported a reduction in anxiety, improvement in quality of life, and satisfaction with education content and the time allotted for and location of education delivery with the number and percent of 40 patients who had received general education and had been treated for cancer within the past 2 years who reported a reduction in anxiety, improvement in quality of life, and satisfaction with education content and the time and location of education delivery.

The CTE structure constructed from an interpretation of Mann's (2011) report of her QI project is illustrated in Figure 3.4. The non-relational and relational propositions for each component of the CTE structure are listed in Box 3.6.

BOX 3.6 An Example of a Conceptual–Theoretical–Empirical Structure for King's Conceptual System Quality Improvement Projects

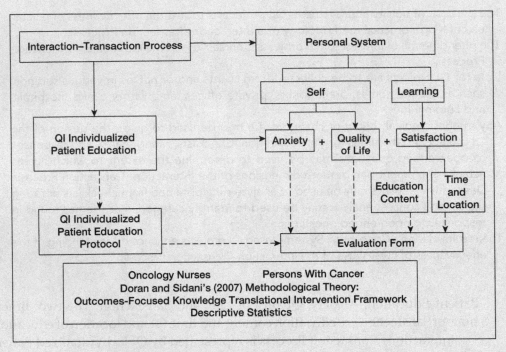

FIGURE 3.4 Conceptual–theoretical–empirical (CTE) structure for a King's Conceptual System quality improvement project—theory of the effects of individualized patient education on anxiety, quality of life, and satisfaction.

QI, quality improvement.

The *non-relational propositions* for the *C component* of the conceptual–theoretical–empirical (CTE) structure are:

- *Personal System* is defined as "a unified, complex whole self who perceives, thinks, desires, imagines, decides, identifies goals, and selects means to achieve them" (King, 1981, p. 27).
- The two relevant dimensions of Personal System are self and learning.
  o *Self* is defined as a unified, complex whole person who perceives, thinks, desires, imagines, decides, identifies goals, selects means to achieve them, and is synonymous with I and me.
  o *Learning* is defined as a process of perceiving, conceptualizing, and thinking critically.

The *non-relational propositions* for the *T component* of the CTE structure are:

- *Quality Improvement (QI) Individualized Patient Education* is defined as amount and type of information preferred by a person and provided by a nurse.

(continued)

BOX 3.6   An Example of a Conceptual–Theoretical–Empirical Structure for King's Conceptual System Quality Improvement Projects   (continued)

- *Anxiety* is defined as a person's feelings of discomfort, dread, and uneasiness, which can be a barrier to learning.
- *Quality of Life* is defined as the person's overall subjective satisfaction with his or her life.
- *Satisfaction* is defined as gratification with or fulfillment of something that is desired.
- The two dimensions of Satisfaction are education content and time for and location of education.
  - o *Education content* is defined as satisfaction with the content of the individualized patient education.
  - o *Time for and location of education* is defined as satisfaction with the time allocated for the individualized patient education and with the environment in which the education was delivered.

The *non-relational propositions* for the *E component* of the CTE structure are:

- QI Individualized Patient Education is operationalized as the QI Individualized Patient Education protocol, which identifies content selected from teaching material available at the clinical facility for each patient, including "tapes, booklets, chemotherapy information sheets, and a new patient brochure. Included in the brochure were areas for documenting current treatment regimens and medications, calendar pages for scheduling appointments, basic facility information, and other vital facts such as local and national support groups, home health agencies, hospices, and pharmacies. The information presentation was scheduled prior to chemotherapy, allowing an hour of instruction for the patient and family in an environment conducive to learning. The instruction was provided on a one-on-one basis" (Mann, 2011, p. 58). The protocol is based on Doran and Sidani's (2007) outcomes-focused knowledge translational intervention framework (OFKTIF). This methodological theory includes four components—measurement of patient outcomes and feedback about achievement of outcomes, guidelines for best practices that are reflected in tools for delivery of messages identified from patient assessment, identification of patients' care preferences, and facilitation by practice leaders and advanced practice nurses. "The four areas of concentration included facilitation, content, patient preference, and sources of evidence. Facilitation occurs as nurses help patients adjust to a cancer diagnosis by providing valuable information in relation to personal preferences.... Positive coping skills were encouraged along with self-care, therapeutic actions, and functional abilities in the model, and individual needs were identified. Patient preference of learning materials is important for the oncology nurse to determine to achieve the best possible outcome. Some patients may prefer written materials, whereas others may benefit from audiotapes or websites for information. Although content of new patient education varies greatly from center to center, common areas usually are addressed, such as chemotherapy drugs and associated side effects, treatment schedule, care of venous access device, nutrition, routine laboratory tests, and clinic regulations regarding telephone calls and

(continued)

BOX 3.6   An Example of a Conceptual–Theoretical–Empirical Structure for King's Conceptual System Quality Improvement Projects   (continued)

emergencies. Sources of evidence should be closely evaluated and used to provide the most accurate up-to-date information to the patient. Using reputable websites and [high] quality educational material will prevent confusion and misinformation" (Mann, 2011, p. 56).

- Anxiety, quality of life, and satisfaction are measured by a project manager–developed Evaluation Form. This form consists of six questions that ask patients to record their "feelings of satisfaction about the education experience, including timing, environment, and content. In addition, questions concerning anxiety and quality of life also were included" (Mann, 2011, p. 58).

The *relational propositions* for the *C and T components* of the CTE structure are:

- The Interaction–Transaction Process has a positive effect on the Personal System dimensions of self and learning.
- Therefore, QI Individualized Patient Education has a positive effect on Quality of Life and the two dimensions of Satisfaction, and a negative effect on Anxiety.

The *relational proposition* for the *E component* of the CTE structure is:

- A greater number and percent of patients newly diagnosed with cancer who receive the QI Individualized Patient Education protocol report improved quality of life, greater satisfaction with education content and time and location of education delivery, and reduced anxiety on the Evaluation Form than patients with a diagnosis of cancer who did not receive the QI Individualized Patient Education protocol.

Source: Mann (2011).

KING'S CONCEPTUAL SYSTEM: APPLICATION TO NURSING RESEARCH

The guidelines for King's Conceptual System nursing research are listed in Box 3.7.

A CTE Structure for a Systematic Literature Review

Ryle's (2008) journal article is an example of a report of a literature review guided by King's Conceptual System. The purpose of her integrative literature review was to identify options for anticoagulant management and the outcomes for patients who had a colonoscopy and possible removal of polyps.

Ryle (2008) limited the search of literature to reports of research published from 1991 to 2005. She searched three electronic databases: the Cumulative Index of Nursing and Allied Health Literature (CINAHL), MEDLINE, and PubMed. The search terms were "anticoagulant management," "periprocedural

BOX 3.7 Guidelines for King's Conceptual System Research

The ultimate purpose of King's Conceptual System–based research is to determine the effects of transactions on goal attainment.

The phenomena of interest are transactions and goal attainment.

The precise problems to be studied are actual or potential disturbances in the client's ability to function in social roles.

Study participants include individuals; dyads, triads, and other groups; families; social organizations; and health care systems.

Data may be collected using instruments derived from or consistent with King's Conceptual System. Research designs may be qualitative, quantitative, and/or mixed methods. The method used must relate to the problem to be studied. The objective of qualitative, descriptive studies would be to gather information that is not already available. The qualitative methodology selected must adhere to the problem to be studied and the focus of the Conceptual System. Quantitative experimental studies measuring goal attainment can view goal attainment as a dichotomy—the goal is attained or not attained—a rank order, or a continuous score. Data may be gathered in health care systems, the home of the individual, a school, an industry or a business, or another social setting.

Qualitative and quantitative data analysis techniques may be used.

King's Conceptual System–based research findings enhance understanding of factors that affect goal attainment.

Adapted from Fawcett and DeSanto-Madeya (2013).

management," "bleeding," "warfarin," "complications," "colonoscopy," "endoscopy," and "polypectomy." She used Ganong's (1987) method for coding and integration (see Appendix A) of a sample of 10 research reports selected from a total of 25 research reports identified in the databases.

The theory of the effects of anticoagulant management on outcomes following colonoscopy was generated from the results of the literature review. The conceptual model concept that guided the literature review is Interpersonal System; the relevant dimension is communication. Inasmuch as the goal of Ryle's (2008) literature review was to generate evidence that could be used by nurses to educate clients about anticoagulants when they are scheduled for colonoscopy, she selected the Interpersonal System dimension of communication as the guide for her literature review. She explained, "Each interaction [between nurse and client] is characterized by values, experiences, present needs, expectations, and goals that influence perceptions in the interactions. Education provided must be evidence based and clearly communicated [by the nurse] to each individual client, with consideration given to that client's values, experiences, need, and current expectations" (p. 355).

The two theory concepts that emerged from the literature review are Anticoagulant Management and Outcomes. The three dimensions of Outcomes are postprocedure bleeding, thromboembolism, and stroke.

The CTE structure constructed for Ryle's (2008) literature review is illustrated in Figure 3.5. The non-relational propositions for each component of the CTE structure are listed in Box 3.8, along with a relational proposition for the T component that was generated from the results of the literature review.

A CTE Structure for Instrument Development

Sieloff and Bularzik's (2011) report of the development and psychometric testing of the Sieloff–King Assessment of Group Outcome Attainment Within Organizations (SKAGOAO) instrument provides a source for construction of a King's Conceptual System CTE structure for instrument development.

The theory is Group Outcome Attainment Within Organizations (GOAO). This theory, originally called the theory of departmental power and then the theory of group power within organizations, became the theory of GOAO as Sieloff discovered that nurses were concerned about the negative connotation of the term *power*, that goal attainment pertained to the entire organization rather than only to a department, and that goals are frequently referred to in the literature as outcomes (Sieloff, 2007; Sieloff & Bularzik, 2011).

The conceptual model concepts are Personal System, Interpersonal System, and Social System. The relevant dimensions of Personal System are perception and self. The relevant dimensions of Interpersonal System are communication and role. The relevant dimensions of Social System are organization, status, decision making, and power. The theory concept, GOAO, has eight dimensions— outcome attainment capacity perspective, group leader's outcome attainment competency, communication competency, role, controlling the effects of environmental forces, resources, position, and goals/outcomes competency.

The Personal System perception dimension is represented by the GOAO outcome attainment capacity perspective dimension, and the self dimension is represented by the GOAO group leader's outcome attainment competency dimension. The Interpersonal System communication dimension is represented by the GOAO communication competency dimension, and the role dimension is represented by the GOAO role dimension. The Social System organization dimension is represented by the GOAO controlling the effects of environmental forces and resources dimensions, the status dimension is represented by the GOAO position dimension, and the decision-making dimension is represented by the GOAO goals/outcomes competency dimension. The Social System power dimension is represented by GOAO.

GOAO is measured by the SKAGOAO. The eight subscales of the SKAGOAO are measures of the theory concept, GOAO.

The SKAGOAO has adequate estimates of psychometric properties. Internal consistency reliability was estimated with Cronbach's alpha and split-half reliability statistics. Content validity was estimated with the Content Validity Index applied to item relevance ratings by a panel of eight experts in King's Conceptual System. Construct validity was estimated using exploratory factor analysis, and criterion-related validity was estimated by calculating a correlational coefficient (r) between SKAGOAO and the abbreviated form of the About Your

BOX 3.8 An Example of a Conceptual–Theoretical–Empirical Structure for King's Conceptual System Systematic Literature Reviews

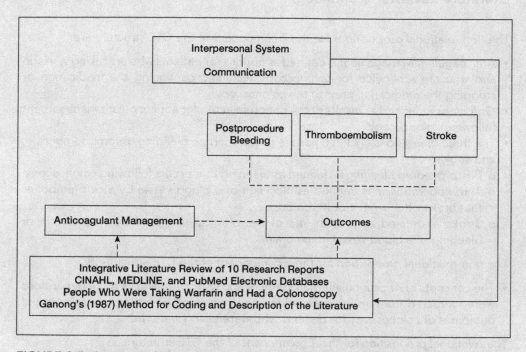

FIGURE 3.5 Conceptual–theoretical–empirical (CTE) structure for King's Conceptual System literature review—theory of effects of anticoagulant management on outcomes following colonoscopy.

The *non-relational propositions* for the *C component* of the conceptual–theoretical–empirical (CTE) structure are:

- *Interpersonal System* is defined as being made up of two or more personal systems who are engaged in interaction.
- The relevant dimension of Interpersonal System is communication.
  - *Communication* is defined as the way in which personal systems develop and maintain relationships.
  - The two subdimensions of communication are verbal communication and nonverbal communication.
    - *Verbal communication*, which is both intrapersonal and interpersonal in nature, encompasses verbal signs and symbols, including spoken and written words, used by personal systems to express their goals and values.
    - *Nonverbal communication*, which also is both intrapersonal and interpersonal in nature, encompasses nonverbal signs and symbols, including gestures and touch, used by personal systems to express their goals and values.

(continued)

BOX 3.8   An Example of a Conceptual–Theoretical–Empirical Structure for King's Conceptual System Systematic Literature Reviews   *(continued)*

The *non-relational propositions* for the *T component* of the CTE structure are:

- *Anticoagulant Management* is defined as options for patients who are taking warfarin and who are scheduled for colonoscopy, including continuing the medication or stopping the medication prior to the colonoscopy.
- *Outcomes* is defined as results of the option selected for anticoagulant management following colonoscopy.
- The three dimensions of Outcomes are postprocedure bleeding, thromboembolism, and stroke.
  - o *Postprocedure bleeding* is defined as bleeding that occurs following colonoscopy.
  - o *Thromboembolism* is defined as blockage of a blood vessel by a clot (embolus) that broke off a larger clot (thrombus).
  - o *Stroke* is defined as sudden loss of neurological function due to a clot in or bleeding of a blood vessel in the brain.

The *non-relational proposition* for the *E component* of the CTE structure is:

- The concepts of Anticoagulant Management and Outcomes and its three dimensions were extracted from an integrative literature review of 10 research reports about outcomes of colonoscopy for patients who were taking warfarin.

The *relational proposition* for the *T component* of the CTE structure is:

- Anticoagulant Management is related to the presence or absence of the three dimensions of Outcomes—postprocedure bleeding, thromboembolism, and stroke.

Source: Ryle (2008).

Own and Other Departments instrument (Hickson, Hinings, Lee, Schneck, & Pennings, as cited in Sieloff, 2003, 2007) (see Appendix B).

The SKAGOAO is the fourth version of the Sieloff–King Assessment instrument. The Sieloff–King Assessment of Departmental Power (SKADP) was designed to test the original theory of departmental power. As the theory was modified, the instrument was revised and became the Sieloff–King Assessment of Group Power within Organizations (SKAGPO). Semantic refinements of the theory led to semantic revisions of the instrument, which was referred to as the Sieloff–King Assessment of Group Goal Attainment Capacity within Organizations (SKAG²ACO); additional semantic refinements of the theory led to more semantic revisions of the instrument, which currently is referred to as the SKAGOAO.

The CTE structure constructed for Sieloff and Bularzik's (2011) instrument development study is illustrated in Figure 3.6. The non-relational propositions for each component of the CTE structure are listed in Box 3.9.

BOX 3.9 An Example of a Conceptual–Theoretical–Empirical Structure for King's Conceptual System Instrument Development

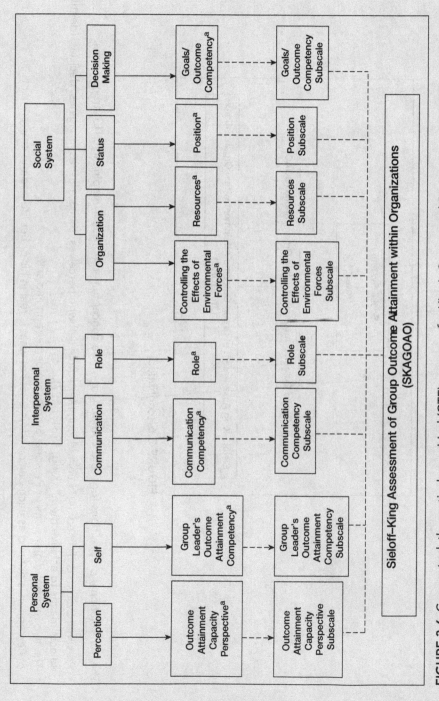

FIGURE 3.6 Conceptual–theoretical–empirical (CTE) structure for King's Conceptual System instrument development research—theory of Group Outcome Attainment Within Organizations.

[a]Dimensions of Group Outcome Attainment within Organizations (GOAO).

(continued)

BOX 3.9 An Example of a Conceptual–Theoretical–Empirical Structure for King's Conceptual System Instrument Development (continued)

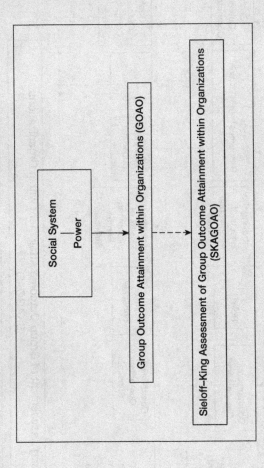

Social System

Power

Group Outcome Attainment within Organizations (GOAO)

Sieloff–King Assessment of Group Outcome Attainment within Organizations (SKAGOAO)

FIGURE 3.6 (continued)

The *non-relational propositions* for the C component of the conceptual–theoretical–empirical (CTE) structure are:

- *Personal System* is defined as "a unified, complex whole self who perceives, thinks, desires, imagines, decides, identifies goals, and selects means to achieve them" (King, 1981, p. 27).
- The two relevant dimensions of Personal System are perception and self.
  o *Perception* is defined as each person's awareness of what is real in his or her life and the environment.

(continued)

BOX 3.9 An Example of a Conceptual–Theoretical–Empirical Structure for King's Conceptual System Instrument Development (continued)

o *Self* is defined as a unified, complex whole person who perceives, thinks, desires, imagines, decides, identifies goals, selects means to achieve them, and is synonymous with I and me.

- *Interpersonal System* is defined as being made up of two or more personal systems who are engaged in interaction.
- The two relevant dimensions of Interpersonal System are communication and role.
  o *Communication* is defined as the way in which personal systems develop and maintain relationships.
  o *Role* is defined as expected behaviors that are associated with each personal system's position in a social system.
- *Social System* is defined as a group, such as a family, a school, a hospital, an industry, a religious organization, or a community, that forms to carry out particular purposes needed to maintain a society.
- The four relevant dimensions of Social System are decision making, organization, status, and power.
  o *Organization* is defined as personal systems who have specific positions and roles and who utilize certain resources to accomplish personal and organizational goals.
  o *Status* is defined as the ascribed or achieved position of a personal system within a group or the ascribed or achieved position of a group within an organization.
  o *Decision making* is defined as a dynamic, systematic process that involves choices among alternatives to attain goals.
  o *Power* is defined as a process that involves a situation in which one group accepts the dictates of another group even if they do not agree with those dictates.

The *non-relational propositions* for the T component of the CTE structure are:

- *Group Outcome Attainment within Organizations* is defined as "the group's outcome attainment capability or the implementation of a group's outcome attainment capacity… [which may be considered] a group's level of empowerment" (Sieloff & Bularzik, 2011, p. 1024).
- The eight dimensions of Group Outcome Attainment within Organizations are outcome attainment capacity perspective, group leader's outcome attainment competency, communication competency, role, controlling the effects of environmental forces, resources, position, and goals/outcomes competency.
  o *Outcome attainment capacity perspective* is defined as "The perception and value regarding the achievement of goals" (Sieloff, 2007, p. 208).

(continued)

BOX 3.9 An Example of a Conceptual–Theoretical–Empirical Structure for King's Conceptual System Instrument Development *(continued)*

o *Group leader's outcome attainment competency* is defined as "The knowledge and skills of the nurse leader in relation to the achievement of group goals" (Sieloff, 2007, p. 208).

o *Communication competency* is defined as "The knowledge and skill related to the giving of information from one group to another group" (Sieloff, 2007, p. 208).

o *Role* is defined as the "Degree to which the work of [an organization] is accomplished through the efforts of the [group]" (Sieloff, 2007, p. 208).

o *Controlling the effects of environmental forces* is defined as "Effectively managing the potential negative consequences that result from the effect of changing health care trends on the ability of [an organization] to achieve its goals" (Sieloff, 2007, p. 208).

o *Resources* is defined as "Any commodity that the [organization] can use for goal achievement" (Sieloff, 2007, p. 208).

o *Position* is defined as the "centrality of . . . nursing . . . within the communication network of [an organization]" (Sieloff, 2007, p. 208).

o *Goals/outcomes competency* is defined as "The knowledge and skill of a group in relation to the process of achieving [desired outcomes] by [the] group" (Sieloff, 2007, p. 208).

The non-relational proposition for the E component of the CTE structure is:

• Group Outcome Attainment within Organizations and its dimensions are measured by the Sieloff–King Assessment of Group Outcome Attainment within Organizations (SKAGOAO). The 36 items of the SKAGOAO are arranged in eight subscales—outcome attainment capacity perspective (five items), group leader's outcome attainment competency (four items), communication competency (three items), role (three items), controlling the effects of environmental forces (seven items), resources (six items), position (four items), and goals/outcomes competency (four items)—that are measures of the dimensions of GOAO.

Source: Sieloff and Bularzik (2011).

A CTE Structure for Descriptive Qualitative Research

A journal article by Batson and Yoder (2012) is an example of a report of descriptive qualitative research guided by King's Conceptual System. The purpose of their research was to analyze the concept of managerial coaching.

The theory of correlates of managerial coaching was generated from their concept analysis, which is a type of descriptive qualitative research. Batson and Yoder (2012) modified Walker and Avant's (2005) approach to concept analysis by using King's Conceptual System as the conceptual model guide for their selection and analysis of the literature (see Appendix A).

The conceptual model concepts are Personal System, Interpersonal System, and Social System. The relevant dimensions of Personal System are self and growth and development. The relevant dimensions of Interpersonal System are interaction and transaction. The relevant dimension of Social System is organization. These concept dimensions guided the analysis of the literature reviewed.

One theory concept is Managerial Coaching and its nine dimensions—developing an interpersonal relationship of mutual trust and respect, setting clear expectations for performance, providing and soliciting feedback, setting goals, providing training and/or resources, role modeling, promoting a sense of positive accountability for actions, removing obstacles, and challenging/broadening perspectives. Two other theory concepts are Antecedents and its two dimensions—manager (coach) and employee—and Consequences and its three dimensions—staff nurse/employee, nurse manager/coach, and organization.

All of the theory concepts and their dimensions were discovered in word data extracted from English-language journal articles and texts published from 1980 through 2009 that were located through a search of the CINAHL, ProQuest, Business Source Complete, and PsychINFO electronic databases. The search terms were "coaching," "managerial coaching," "nurse manager support," "job satisfaction," and "nursing work environment."

Following the concept analysis, the Interpersonal System dimensions of interaction and communication and the Social System dimension of organization could be represented by Managerial Coaching and its nine dimensions. The Personal System dimensions of self and growth and development could be represented by Antecedents and its two dimensions—manager (coach) and employee, and by Consequences and two of its dimensions—nurse manager/coach and staff nurse/employee. The Social System dimension of organization could be represented by the Consequences dimension of organization.

The CTE structure, constructed for an interpretation of Batson and Yoder's (2012) study, is illustrated in Figure 3.7. The non-relational propositions for each component of the CTE structure are listed in Box 3.10, along with the relational propositions for the T component that were generated from the results of the concept analysis.

A CTE Structure for Correlational Research

The research report by Hobdell (2004) is an example of correlational research guided by King's Conceptual System. The purpose of her study was "to

BOX 3.10   An Example of a Conceptual–Theoretical–
Empirical Structure for King's Conceptual System Descriptive
Qualitative Research

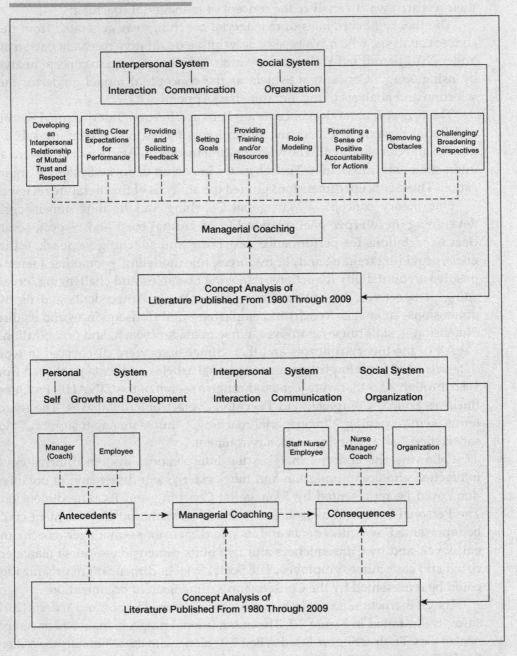

FIGURE 3.7 Conceptual–theoretical–empirical (CTE) structure for King's Conceptual System descriptive qualitative research—theory of correlates of managerial coaching.

(continued)

BOX 3.10 An Example of a Conceptual–Theoretical–Empirical Structure for King's Conceptual System Descriptive Qualitative Research (continued)

The *non-relational propositions* for the *C component* of the conceptual–theoretical–empirical (CTE) structure are:

- *Personal System* is defined as "a unified, complex whole self who perceives, thinks, desires, imagines, decides, identifies goals, and selects means to achieve them" (King, 1981, p. 27).
- The two relevant dimensions of Personal System are self and growth and development.
  - *Self* is defined as a unified, complex whole person who perceives, thinks, desires, imagines, decides, identifies goals, selects means to achieve them, and is synonymous with I and me.
  - *Growth and development* is defined as constant changes that occur within each person at the cellular, molecular, and behavioral levels of existence.
- *Interpersonal System* is defined as being made up of two or more persons who are engaged in interaction.
- The two relevant dimensions of Interpersonal System are interaction and communication.
  - *Interaction* is defined as a process of perception and communication between two or more personal systems and/or the environment that includes a sequence of verbal and nonverbal goal-directed behaviors.
  - *Communication* is defined as the way in which personal systems develop and maintain relationships.
- *Social System* is defined as a group, such as a family, a school, a hospital, an industry, a religious organization, or a community that forms to carry out particular purposes needed to maintain a society.
- The relevant dimension of Social System is organization.
  - *Organization* is defined as personal systems who have specific positions and roles and who utilize certain resources to accomplish personal and organizational goals

The *non-relational propositions* for the *T component* of the CTE structure are:

- *Managerial Coaching* is defined as "a specific dyadic relationship between the nurse manager and staff nurse intended to improve skills and knowledge as they relate to expected job performance" (Batson & Yoder, 2012, 1658). More specifically, Managerial Coaching "is an ongoing, face-to-face process of influencing behavior by which the manager (superior, supervisor) and employee (subordinate) collaborate to achieve increased job knowledge, improved skills in carrying out job responsibilities, a stronger and more positive working relationship, and opportunities for personal and professional growth of the employee" (Yoder as cited in Baton & Yoder, 2012, p. 1661).
- The nine dimensions of Managerial Coaching are developing an interpersonal relationship of mutual trust and respect, setting clear expectations for performance, providing and soliciting feedback, setting goals, providing training and/or resources, role modeling, promoting a sense of positive accountability for actions, removing obstacles, and challenging/broadening perspectives.
  - *Developing an interpersonal relationship of mutual trust and respect* is defined as a facilitating attribute of Managerial Coaching that "requires the manager to see the employee as an individual with unique beliefs, values, knowledge and skills and the innate ability to grow and learn" (Batson & Yoder, 2012, p. 1661).

(continued)

BOX 3.10   An Example of a Conceptual–Theoretical–Empirical Structure for King's Conceptual System Descriptive Qualitative Research   *(continued)*

- o *Setting clear expectations for performance* is defined as a facilitating attribute of Managerial Coaching that involves "helping the employee link personal and professional desires for growth and development to the mission, vision, values and goals of the organization [and]...promoting an environment of excellence and commitment to continual improvement by the manager" (Batson & Yoder, 2012, p. 1661).
- o *Providing and soliciting feedback* is defined as a facilitating attribute of Managerial Coaching; feedback is "data that are evaluated through a filter of values, beliefs and experiences on the part of manager" (Batson & Yoder, 2012, p. 1661).
- o *Setting goals* is defined as a facilitating attribute of Managerial Coaching that "is a mutual process that ensures alignment between the employee's personal desires and organizational needs...[and that] increases motivation and accountability by the employee for completing the development plan" (Batson & Yoder, 2012, p. 1662).
- o *Providing training and/or resources* is defined as a facilitating attribute of Managerial Coaching; training and resources are given either directly by the manager or by identifying resources for training (Batson & Yoder, 2012).
- o *Role modeling* is defined as an empowering attribute that is "perhaps the most critical empowering behaviour for leadership" (Batson & Yoder, 2012, p. 1662).
- o *Promoting a sense of positive accountability for actions* is defined as an empowering attribute that involves "helping employees continue to work through issues, and practice and incorporate new skills to move through change and growth" (Batson & Yoder, 2012, p. 1662).
- o *Removing obstacles* is defined as an empowering attribute that involves "behaviours by the manager to give resources, information and facilitate learning" (Batson & Yoder, 2012, p. 1662).
- o *Challenging/broadening perspectives* is defined as an empowering attribute that involves "behaviour by the manager aimed at assisting employees to incorporate multiple perspectives in viewing issues and problems" (Batson & Yoder, 2012, p. 1662).
- *Antecedents* is defined as "events or incidents that must be present for [Managerial Coaching] to occur" (Batson & Yoder, 2013, p. 1663).
- The two dimensions of Antecedents are manager (coach) and employee.
  - o *Manager (coach)* is defined as a nurse leader who provides coaching and who is characterized by age, education, coaching skill, and positive intent.
  - o *Employee* is defined as a staff nurse who is the recipient of coaching and who is characterized by age, education, experience, motivation, and receptivity.
- *Consequences* is defined as "the outcomes produced by occurrence of [Managerial Coaching]" (Batson & Yoder, 2013, p. 1663).
- The three dimensions of Consequences are staff nurse/employee, nurse manager/coach, and organization.
  - o *Staff nurse/employee* is defined as a nurse who experiences growth ("increased technical competence, clinical decision-making, ability for autonomous practice,

(continued)

BOX 3.10   An Example of a Conceptual–Theoretical–Empirical Structure for King's Conceptual System Descriptive Qualitative Research   *(continued)*

and alignment with organizational values and goals"), self-efficacy ("confidence in one's ability to accomplish both routine and complex tasks...[and willingness] to persevere in the face of obstacles"), empowerment ("the ability of nurses to accomplish their work in meaningful ways"), and job satisfaction ("the extent to which the staff nurse believes the work environment enables nurses to give [high] quality patient care") as a result of receiving coaching (Batson & Yoder, 2013, pp. 1663–1664).

o *Nurse manager/coach* is defined as a nurse leader who demonstrates greater ability to delegate, increased ability to balance work priorities, greater attainment of departmental goals, and greater professional work satisfaction as a result of providing coaching.

o *Organization* is defined as the clinical agency that experiences improved ability to meet goals, improved high-quality outcomes, and a greater reputation as a preferred workplace as a result of Managerial Coaching.

The *non-relational propositions* for the *E component* of the CTE structure are:

• Managerial Coaching and its dimensions were discovered in word data from English-language literature published between 1980 and 2009, including texts and journal articles focused on coaching and managers.

• Dimensions of Antecedents were discovered in word data from English-language literature published between 1980 and 2009, including texts and journal articles focused on coaching and managers.

• Dimensions of Consequences were discovered in word data from English-language literature published between 1980 and 2009, including texts and journal articles focused on coaching and managers.

The *relational propositions* for the *T component* of the CTE structure are:

• Antecedents are related to Managerial Coaching.
• Managerial Coaching is related to Consequences.

Source: Batson and Yoder (2012).

describe parental chronic sorrow following the birth of a child with [a neural tube defect] and explore the relation between chronic sorrow and depression" (p. 82).

The theory of the relation between parental chronic sorrow and depression was tested by means of a cross-sectional bivariate correlational research design (see Appendix A). The study sample included 68 mothers and 64 fathers of children with neural tube defects.

The conceptual model concept is Personal System; the relevant dimensions are self and perception. The theory concepts are Parental Gender, Chronic

Sorrow, and Depression. The two dimensions of Parental Gender are mother and father. The three dimensions of Chronic Sorrow are mood state, intensity, and cyclical.

The Personal System self dimension is represented by Parental Gender and its two dimensions, which are measured by self-reports of parents of children with neural tube defects. The Personal System perception dimension is represented by Chronic Sorrow and by Depression. The Chronic Sorrow mood state and intensity dimensions are measured by the Adapted Burke Questionnaire (ABQ; Burke, 1989), the intensity dimension also is measured by the Direct Question (DQ; Damrosch & Perry, 1989), and the cyclical dimension is measured by the Adjustment Graph (AG; Damrosch & Perry, 1989). Depression is measured by the Brief Symptom Inventory (BSI; Derogatis & Spencer, 1982). The Pearson product moment coefficient of correlation (r; see Appendix B) is used to examine the relations between scores for the research instruments.

A CTE structure for Hobell's (2004) study, which was constructed from the content of her journal article, is illustrated in Figure 3.8. The non-relational and relational propositions for each component of the CTE structure are listed in Box 3.11.

A CTE Structure for Experimental Research

Cho's (2013) journal article is an example of a report of experimental research guided by King's Conceptual System. The purpose of the randomized controlled trial, which is a type of experimental research (see Appendix A), was "to examine the effect of the [health contract intervention (HCI)] on the self-care behavior of renal dialysis patients and physiological indices ([serum phosphorus, serum potassium, and] mean weight gain)" (p. 87).

The theory of the effects of health contract information on self-care behaviors and physiological indices was tested by means of an experimental pretest–posttest design with random assignment of research participants to the experimental treatment group and the control treatment group. The research participants were Korean adult men and women who were receiving outpatient renal dialysis. The experimental treatment group ($n = 21$) received health contract information, and the control treatment group ($n = 22$) received routine care.

The conceptual model concept is Interaction–Transaction Process; the dimensions are mutual goal setting, exploration of means to achieve goals, agree on means to achieve goals, transaction, and attainment of goals. The theory concepts are Type of Nursing Invention, Self-Care Behaviors, and Physiological Indices. The two dimensions of Type of Nursing Intervention are health contract information and routine care. The three dimensions of Physiological Indices are serum phosphorus, serum potassium, and mean weight gain.

The mutual goal setting, exploration of means to achieve goals, agree on means to achieve goals, and transaction dimensions of the Interaction–Transaction Process are represented by Type of Nursing Intervention, and the

BOX 3.11 An Example of a Conceptual–Theoretical–Empirical Structure for King's Conceptual System Correlational Research

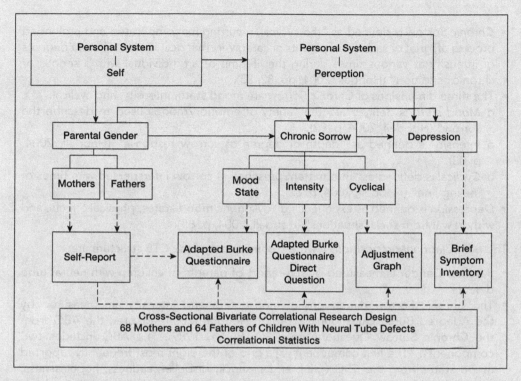

FIGURE 3.8 Conceptual–theoretical–empirical (CTE) structure for King's Conceptual System correlational research—theory of the relation between parental chronic sorrow and depression.

The *non-relational propositions* for the *C component* of the conceptual–theoretical–empirical (CTE) structure are:

- *Personal System* is defined as "a unified, complex whole self who perceives, thinks, desires, imagines, decides, identifies goals, and selects means to achieve them" (King, 1981, p. 27).
- The two relevant dimensions of Personal System are self and perception.
  - *Self* is defined as a unified, complex whole person who perceives, thinks, desires, imagines, decides, identifies goals, selects means to achieve them, and is synonymous with I and me.
  - *Perception* is defined as each person's awareness of what is real in his or her life and the environment.

The *non-relational propositions* for the *T component* of the CTE structure are:

- *Parental Gender* is defined as a mother or a father of a child with a neural tube defect.

(continued)

BOX 3.11   An Example of a Conceptual–Theoretical–Empirical Structure for King's Conceptual System Correlational Research *(continued)*

- *Chronic Sorrow* is defined as "the cyclical, recurring [uncomplicated and prolonged process of] grief or sadness of parents or caregivers that occurs with different degrees of intensity at various times during the lifetime of an individual with a serious or chronic condition" (Hobdell, 2004, pp. 82, 85).
- The three dimensions of Chronic Sorrow are mood state, intensity, and cyclical.
  o *Mood state* is defined as "the variety of emotion/moods used to describe the sorrow" (Hobdell, 2004, p. 82).
  o *Intensity* is defined as "depth or degree of sorrow response" (Hobdell, 2004, p. 82).
  o *Cyclical* is defined as "intermittent presence of sorrow interspersed with times of feeling fine" (Hobdell, 2004, p. 82).
- *Depression* is defined as experiencing "dysphoric mood states, physical effects, and withdrawal from social situations" (Hobdell, 2004, p. 85).

The *non-relational propositions* for the *E component* of the CTE structure are:

- Parental Gender is measured by self-report of parents of children with neural tube defects.
- The Chronic Sorrow dimensions of mood state and intensity are measured by the Adapted Burke Questionnaire (ABQ). Hobdell (2004) adapted the ABQ from the Chronic Sorrow Questionnaire (CSQ; Burke, 1989). The ABQ includes two components. "The first component [is] a grid of the eight most frequently reported mood states from the CSQ (grief, anger, shock, disbelief, sadness, hopelessness, fear, and guilt). More specifically, both parents were asked to indicate the intensity of these mood states on a 4-point Likert scale (3 = very intense, 2 = somewhat intense, 1 = not intense, 0 = absent)....[The second component is five questions, which] "were asked to measure the mood state, cyclical nature, and intensity dimension(s) of chronic sorrow. 1. What other feelings did you have that are not listed here? 2. Has there been a time when the feelings from the time of birth returned? 3. How do those feelings compare to the first time you had them? 4. Are there events that bring up these feelings? 5. Was the intensity for these events the same, less, or more intense than the first time you had them?" (p. 85).
- The Chronic Sorrow dimension of intensity is also measured by the Direct Question (DQ). The DQ about chronic sorrow is rated on a 4-point scale of 0 = never to 4 = most of the time (Hobdell, 2004). The question is: "In the field of handicapped children, there's a phrase that's often used to describe how the parents of handicapped children feel—chronic sorrow. Things can be going along just fine, and suddenly out of the blue you might begin to feel sad again. Sometimes it may be little things that set off those feelings—those moments may be trimming the Christmas tree, hearing a special piece of music, seeing your child outside playing—or it may be the big life changes that bring back strong feelings of sadness such as the beginning of school. To what extent do you experience chronic sorrow?" (Damrosch & Perry, as cited in Hobdell, 2004, p. 86).

(continued)

BOX 3.11 An Example of a Conceptual–Theoretical–Empirical Structure for King's Conceptual System Correlational Research *(continued)*

- The Chronic Sorrow dimension of cyclical is measured by the Adjustment Graph (AG; Damrosch & Perry, 1989). The AG is made up of "two contrasting graphs, one representing a gradual adjustment and lessening of sorrow, and one representing a cyclical recurrence or chronic sorrow. Scoring was based on 1 = recovery graph, 2 = chronic sorrow" (Hobdell, 2004, p. 86).
- Depression is measured by the Brief Symptom Inventory (BSI; Derogatis & Spencer, 1982). The BSI is made up of 53 items that are rated on a 5-point scale of 0 = not at all, 1 = a little bit, 2 = moderately, 3 = quite a bit, and 4 = extremely; depression is one of the nine subscales of the BSI (Hobdell, 2004).

The *relational propositions* for the C and T components of the CTE structure are:

- The self and perception dimensions of Personal Self are interrelated.
- Therefore, there is a relation between Parental Gender and Chronic Sorrow, such that mothers experience greater Chronic Sorrow than fathers, and there is a relation between Parental Gender and Depression.
- Different manifestations of the perception dimension of Personal Self are interrelated.
- Therefore, there is a relation between Chronic Sorrow and Depression, such that the greater the Chronic Sorrow, the greater the Depression.

The *relational propositions* for the E component of the CTE structure are:

- Self-report of Parental Gender is related to scores on the Adapted Burke Questionnaire (ABQ), the Adjustment Graph (AG), the Direct Question (DQ), and the Brief Symptom Inventory (BSI).
- Scores on the ABQ, AG, and DQ are positively related to scores on the BSI.

Source: Hobdell (2004).

---

attainment of goals dimension of the Interaction–Transaction Process is represented by Self-Care Behaviors and by Physiological Indices. The two dimensions of Type of Nursing Intervention are operationalized by the experimental HCI protocol and the control routine care protocol. Self-Care Behaviors is measured by the Self-Care Behaviors Inventory (SCBI; adapted from Song, 2000). The Physiological Indices serum phosphorus and serum potassium dimensions are measured by medical record laboratory autoanalyzer reports. The Physiological Indices mean weight gain dimension is determined by a mathematical calculation of previous dialysis session and current session weights. Weight is measured by a scale. Analysis of covariance (ANCOVA) statistics (see Appendix B) are used to examine the differences between the scores for the research instruments for the experimental treatment group and the control treatment group, with the pretest scores as the covariates.

A CTE structure for Cho's (2013) study, which was constructed from an interpretation of the content of her journal article, is illustrated in Figure 3.9. The non-relational and relational propositions for each component of the CTE structure are listed in Box 3.12.

A CTE Structure for Mixed-Methods Research

Mwangi's (2013) doctoral dissertation is an example of mixed-methods research guided by King's Conceptual System. The purposes of her study were:

1. To determine the factors that predispose Kenyan women to higher HIV vulnerability; 2. To measure the social structural perspectives of stigma among Kenyan women living with HIV/AIDS; 3. To understand the lived experiences of Kenyan women with HIV/AIDS in rural and urban settings. (p. 11)

The theory of Kenyan rural and urban women's experiences of living with the stigma of HIV/AIDS, which includes the relation between sociodemographic characteristics and perceived stigma (quantitative portion) and life experiences of HIV/AIDS (qualitative portion), was the result of the conduct of a concurrent mixed-methods design (QUAN + QUAL; see Appendix A), with collection of "both quantitative and qualitative data...during a single session with quantitative data preceding the qualitative" (Mwangi, 2013, p. 63). A descriptive comparative research design was used for the quantitative portion of the study, and a phenomenological research design was used for the qualitative portion. The sample for the quantitative portion of the study was 200 women living in either rural or urban areas of Kenya; the sample for the qualitative portion was 28 women selected from the 200 women who participated in the quantitative portion.

The conceptual model concepts for both portions of the study are Personal System, Interpersonal System, and Social System. The theory concepts are Sociodemographic Characteristics (QUAN), Perceived Stigma (QUAN), and Life Experiences of HIV/AIDS (QUAL). The six dimensions of Perceived Stigma are fear of contagion, health care neglect, negative self-perception, social isolation, verbal abuse, and workplace stigma. The four dimensions of Life Experiences of HIV/AIDS are discovering HIV/AIDS, societal responses, societal support/ God's grace or divine intervention, and self-process.

Personal System, Interpersonal System, and Social System are represented by Sociodemographic Characteristics (QUAN), Perceived Stigma. Mwangi (2013) provided more specific linkages for the dimensions of Perceived Stigma: Personal System is represented by fear of contagion and negative self-perception; Interpersonal System and/or Social System are represented by health care neglect, social isolation, and verbal abuse; and Social System is represented by workplace stigma. The conceptual model concepts, Personal System, Interpersonal System, and Social System guided selection of the empirical indicator for the qualitative portion of the study and guided the analysis of the word data.

BOX 3.12 An Example of a Conceptual–Theoretical–Empirical Structure for King's Conceptual System Experimental Research

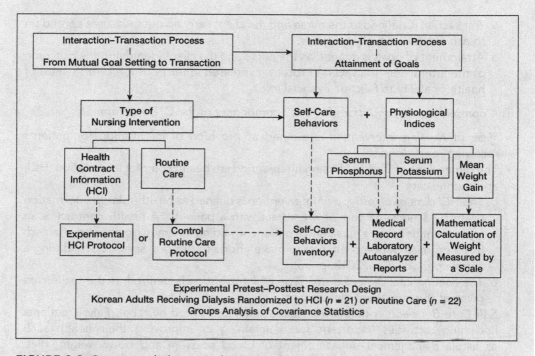

FIGURE 3.9 Conceptual–theoretical–empirical (CTE) structure for King's Conceptual System experimental research—theory of the effects of health contract information on self-care behaviors and physiological indices.

The *non-relational propositions* for the *C component* of the conceptual–theoretical–empirical (CTE) structure are:

- *The Interaction–Transaction Process* is defined as a dynamic process during which a nurse and a client share their perceptions about a nursing situation, communicate to identify specific problems and goals, explore the means by which goals can be attained, agree on those means, implement the means to attain the goals, and identify the outcomes.
- The relevant dimensions of Interaction–Transaction Process are mutual goal setting, exploration of means to attain goals, agreement on means to attain goals, transactions, and attainment of goals.
  - o *Mutual goal setting* is defined as the nurse and the client purposefully interacting to set mutually agreed on goals.
  - o *Exploration of means to achieve goals* is defined as the nurse and the client purposefully interacting to explore the means to achieve the mutually set goals.
  - o *Agreement on means to achieve goals* is defined as the nurse and the client purposefully interacting to agree on the means to achieve the mutually set goals.

(continued)

BOX 3.12   An Example of a Conceptual–Theoretical–Empirical Structure for King's Conceptual System Experimental Research   (continued)

   o *Transaction* is defined as the nurse and the client carrying out measures agreed on to achieve the mutually set goals.

   o *Attainment of goals* is defined as the nurse and the client identifying the outcome of the Interaction–Transaction Process, expressed in terms of the client's state of health or ability to function in social roles.

The *non-relational propositions* for the *T component* of the CTE structure are:

• *Type of Nursing Intervention* is defined as provision of information for patients receiving renal dialysis.

• The dimensions of Type of Nursing Intervention are health contract information (HCI) and routine care.

   o *The HCI dimension of Type of Intervention* is defined as health-related information given by a nurse as part of a contract with a patient. "A health contract is an agreement between a nurse and a patient regarding common goals to be attained. It is a promise between the two to make efforts to perform specific acts during a certain period" (Cho, 2013, p. 86).

   o *The routine care dimension of Type of Intervention* is defined as the usual care given at the outpatient dialysis unit.

• *Self-Care Behaviors* is defined as "behavior[s] performed by renal dialysis patients [including] activities important for maintaining or improving their health such as fistula management, measurement of blood pressure and body weight, diet, medication, exercise and rest, physical problem management, and social adjustment by themselves" (Cho, 2013, p. 88).

• *Physiological Indices* is defined as "objective data that are affected by the performance of self-care behaviors, such as medication, diet, and weight control" (Cho, 2013, p. 87).

• The three dimensions of Physiological Indices are serum phosphorus (P), serum potassium (K), and mean weight gain.

   o *Serum P* is defined as the concentration of phosphorus in blood.

   o *Serum K* is defined as the concentration of potassium in blood.

   o *Mean weight gain* is defined as the average difference between body weight immediately after previous dialysis sessions and body weight immediately prior to current dialysis sessions.

The *non-relational propositions* for the *E component* of the CTE structure are:

• The HCI dimension of Type of Nursing Intervention is operationalized by the experimental HCI protocol. "The [experimental treatment] HCI was used once a week for 4 weeks...Each session lasted between 30 and 60 minutes. The first 5 to 10 minutes of each session consisted of introduction, followed by mutual goal setting for 20 to 40 minutes and finally by contracting/recontracting for 5 to 10 minutes. The self-care behavior performance of the participants was reinforced through praise, encouragement, and support for 5 to 10 minutes at each time of dialysis. A week

(continued)

BOX 3.12   An Example of a Conceptual–Theoretical–Empirical Structure for King's Conceptual System Experimental Research   (continued)

prior to each session, participants were provided with, and requested to complete a self-care log, which covered fistula management, blood pressure and body weight measurement, exercise, and a dietary intake diary. At the introduction stage, the participants were permitted to talk freely about their self-care behavior, based on their self-care logs. At the mutual goal setting stage, the self-care performance of the participants was assessed using the self-care logs and laboratory test results. Knowledge and background of self-care behavior were assessed. Moreover, the researcher and each participant selected together the self-care items for which goals would be set. Each participant also set the goals that [he or she] felt would be achievable in a week, and looked for specific methods to achieve them. From the second week onwards, goal achievement was measured on the basis of self-care logs and a checklist, and the participants were requested to talk about the difficulties and benefits in their goal achievement. At this time, goals were reset and specific methods and resources for goal achievement were discussed. At the contracting/recontracting stage, participants were instructed to state their expected reward for goal achievement, to write the goals and goal achievement methods set at the mutual goal setting stage on the contract, and then to read them aloud. After that, each participant signed, and thereby the researcher completed the contract. Checking to ascertain whether participants had performed the set goals correctly was done at the reinforcement stage, which occurred during each session of dialysis, within the first 2 h[ours] of initiation" (Cho, 2013, pp. 87–88).

- The routine care dimension of Type of Nursing Intervention is operationalized by the control routine care protocol. "The control group received routine care, which entailed checking the self-care behaviors of the participants monthly and informing them of the results. From these results, the participants were advised regarding changes in medication and their diet, educated about diet and fluid restriction, given guidance on blood pressure level based on weight gain, provided with adequate self-care methods, and encouraged to practice these methods. At the end of the study, the researcher explained to the participants the methods and advantages of the HCI for ethical reasons, and provided this intervention to those who wanted the HCI" (Cho, 2013, p. 88).
- Self-Care Behaviors is measured by the Self-Care Behaviors Inventory (SCBI; adapted from Song, 2000). The SCBI contains 35 items about self-care behaviors, with each item rated on a 5-point scale of 1 = low performance of the self-care behavior and 5 = high performance of the self-care behavior (Cho, 2013).
- The serum phosphorus and serum potassium dimensions of Physiological Indices are measured by medical record laboratory autoanalyzer reports (Cho, 2013).
- The mean weight gain dimension of Physiological Indices is measured by a mathematical calculation of weight between dialysis sessions "obtained by subtracting weight measured right after the previous dialysis from that measured right before the current dialysis. Weight was measured by a digital autoplatform scale . . . or a wheelchair scale" (Cho, 2013, p. 88).

(continued)

BOX 3.12   An Example of a Conceptual–Theoretical–Empirical Structure for King's Conceptual System Experimental Research   *(continued)*

The *relational propositions* for the C and T components of the CTE structure are:

- The mutual goal setting, exploration of means to attain goals, agree on means to attain goals, and transaction dimensions of Interaction–Transaction Process have a positive effect on the attainment of goals dimension of Interaction–Transaction Process.
- Therefore, Type of Nursing Intervention has a positive effect on Self-Care Behaviors and on the three dimensions of Physiological Indices, such that the group that receives HCI will perform more Self-Care Behaviors and will have lower serum P, lower serum K, and less mean weight gain than the group that receives routine care.

The *relational propositions* for the E component of the CTE structure are:

- Self-Care Behavior Inventory scores will be higher in the experimental group that receives the HCI protocol than in the control group that receives the routine care protocol.
- Serum P levels will be lower in the experimental group that receives the HCI protocol than in the control group that receives the routine care protocol.
- Serum K levels will be lower in the experimental group that receives the HCI protocol than in the control group that receives the routine care protocol.
- There will be less mean weight gain in the experimental group that receives the HCI protocol than in the control group that receives the routine care protocol.

Source: Cho (2013).

Sociodemographic Characteristics is measured by the Sociodemographic Characteristics Survey (Mwangi, 2013). Perceived Stigma and its dimensions are measured by the HIV/AIDS Stigma Instrument-PLWA (HASI-P) and its six subscales—fear of contagion, health care neglect, negative self-perception, social isolation, verbal abuse, and workplace stigma (Holzemer et al., 2007). These quantitative data were analyzed using descriptive statistics (numbers, percents, means, standard deviations), *t*-tests, and Chi-square statistics (see Appendix B) to determine differences in scores for the research instruments between rural and urban research participants, and correlational statistics (*r*; see Appendix B) to examine relations between scores for items on the Sociodemographic Characteristics Survey and the HASI-P scores.

The theory concept, Life Experiences of HIV/AIDS and its dimensions, emerged from interpretive phenomenological analysis (see Appendix B) of the women's individual responses to open-ended questions on a Semi-Structured Interview Form (Mwangi, 2013). The four dimensions of Life Experiences of

HIV/AIDS—discovering HIV/AIDS, societal responses, societal support/ God's grace or divine intervention, and self-process—which Mwangi (2013) referred to as superordinate themes—are a synthesis of 10 categories of themes. The 10 thematic categories are feelings of living with HIV/AIDS; common challenges and experiences of living with HIV/AIDS; experiences with husband; relationships with extended family; health care experiences; work experiences; social issues or concerns and stigmas; sources of personal strength; current experiences; taking charge; and message to others.

The CTE structure for the quantitative and qualitative portions of Mwangi's (2013) study, which was constructed from the content of her dissertation, is illustrated in Figure 3.10. The non-relational and relational propositions for each component of the CTE structure are listed in Box 3.13.

BOX 3.13   An Example of a Conceptual–Theoretical–Empirical Structure for King's Conceptual System Mixed-Methods Research

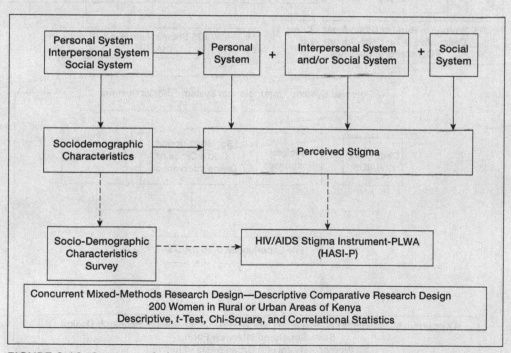

FIGURE 3.10 Conceptual–theoretical–empirical (CTE) structure for King's Conceptual System mixed-methods research—theory of the Kenyan rural and urban women's experiences of living with the stigma of HIV/AIDS.

(continued)

BOX 3.13   An Example of a Conceptual–Theoretical–Empirical Structure for King's Conceptual System Mixed-Methods Research *(continued)*

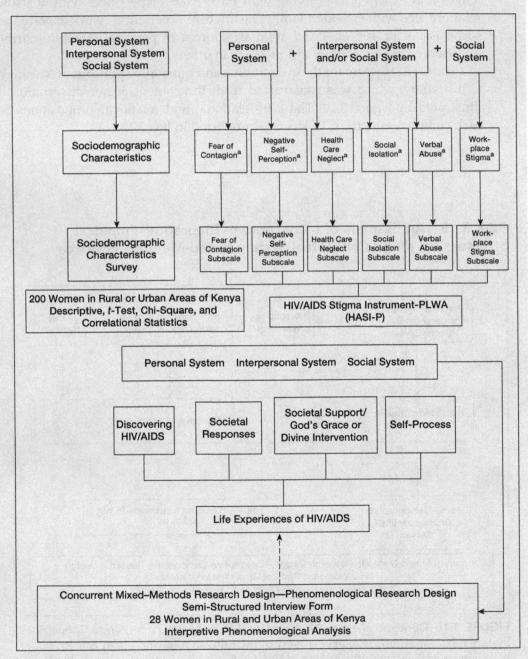

FIGURE 3.10 *(continued)*

[a]Dimensions of Perceived Stigma.

BOX 3.13 An Example of a Conceptual–Theoretical–Empirical Structure for King's Conceptual System Mixed-Methods Research *(continued)*

The *non-relational propositions* for the *C component* of the conceptual–theoretical–empirical (CTE) structure are:

- *Personal System* is defined as "a unified, complex whole self who perceives, thinks, desires, imagines, decides, identifies goals, and selects means to achieve them" (King, 1981, p. 27).
- *Interpersonal System* is defined as being made up of two or more personal systems who are engaged in interaction.
- *Social System* is defined as a group, such as a family, a school, a hospital, an industry, a religious organization, or a community, that forms to carry out particular purposes needed to maintain a society.

The *non-relational propositions* for the *T component* of the CTE structure are:

- *Sociodemographic Characteristics* is defined as self-reported age, primary language spoken, marital status and length of marriage, present state of health, school attendance, educational level, source of income, employment status, monthly income, number of people living with the woman, number of years living with HIV/AIDS, level of activity, placed on HIV/AIDS medications [currently taking medications], knowledge of CD4 count and date of last count, knowledge of viral load, viral load, how HIV medication obtained, HIV medication provider, support group involvement and support group, and place of residence (rural or urban) (Mwangi, 2013).
- *Perceived Stigma* is defined as awareness of "discredit and shame to [self] in acceptance to societal stereotype" (Mwangi, 2013, p. 362), as well as awareness of "[a] powerful discrediting and tainting social label that radically changes the way individuals view themselves and are viewed as persons" (Alonso & Reynolds as cited in Mwangi, 2013, p. 32).
- The six dimensions of Perceived Stigma are fear of contagion, health care neglect, negative self-perception, social isolation, verbal abuse, and workplace stigma.
  - o *Fear of contagion* is defined as "Any behavior [that] shows fear of close or direct contact with the women living with HIV/AIDS or with things she has used for fear of being infected (e.g., not wanting close proximity; not wanting to touch; not wanting to touch/share an object; not wanting to eat together)" (Mwangi, 2013, p. 75).
  - o *Health care neglect* is defined as "Offering a patient less care in a healthcare setting; less care than is expected in the situation or than is given by others or disallowing access to services based on HIV status of the women" (Mwangi, 2013, p. 75).
  - o *Negative self-perception* is defined as "Negative evaluation of self-based on HIV/AIDS status" (Mwangi, 2013, p. 75).
  - o *Social isolation* is defined as "Deliberately limiting social contact with women living with HIV/AIDS and/or breaking off relationships, based on their HIV/AIDS status" (Mwangi, 2013, p. 75).
  - o *Verbal abuse* is defined as "Verbal behavior (e.g., ridicule, insult, blame) intended to harm the women living with HIV/AIDS" (Mwangi, 2013, p. 75).

(continued)

BOX 3.13 An Example of a Conceptual–Theoretical– Empirical Structure for King's Conceptual System Mixed-Methods Research *(continued)*

    o *Workplace stigma* is defined as "Disallowing access to employment/work opportunities, based on one's HIV/AIDS status" (Mwangi, 2013, p. 75).

- *Life Experiences of HIV/AIDS* is defined as the participants' "suffering, injustice, and frustrations as well as their triumphs, joys, and successes" (Mwangi, 2013, p. 296).
- The four dimensions of Life Experiences of HIV/AIDS are discovering HIV/AIDS, societal responses, societal support/God's grace or divine intervention, and self-process.

    o *Discovering HIV/AIDS* is defined as participants' descriptions of "their experiences, briefly beginning with their lives before diagnosis and how they discovered their HIV/AIDS diagnosis" (Mwangi, 2013, p. 232). "Feelings of shock and fear, rejection and abandonment, worthlessness, being alone with the added responsibility of caring for the children, and fear of social stigmatization were common among participants, likely stemming from the reported experiences of death associated with HIV/AIDS, betrayal and information kept secret, abandonment and rejection (even by family), and overall social stigmatization and discrimination" (Mwangi, 2013, p. 282).

    o *Societal responses* is defined as participants' descriptions of their supportive or stigmatizing relationships with family, friends, employers, hospitals, and social support groups that were associated with participants' experiences. "Primary social concerns and issues related to ignorance and inaccurate perceptions of HIV/AIDS and assumptions of promiscuity, which fuel the public stigmatization, ridicule, humiliation, discrimination, and societal fear of association. The social concerns also included dichotomous nature of healthcare settings dependent on the individuals and organizations behind the facility, with instances of reported discrimination and neglect among healthcare providers as well as reports of quality and supportive care received" (Mwangi, 2013, p. 282).

    o *Societal support/God's grace or divine intervention* is defined as "unsolicited acts of kindness extended to the participants at critical times in their transition of living the HIV diagnosis [including] social, instrumental, and spiritual support" (Mwangi, 2013, p. 265). "Care and support received from a third party or individual's or organization (frequent religious affiliation) are often responsible for providing or obtaining medical care, medications, and support group intervention and often seen as a lifeline and source of strength along with the belief and faith in God" (Mwangi, 2013, p. 282).

    o *Self-process* is defined as a "panoramic picture of how the participants described their lived experiences from the initial time of their diagnosis to where they were at the time of the interview" as a transition (Mwangi, 2013, p. 273). "Participants highlighted the importance of self-acceptance and self-care, managing one's health particularly in terms of continuing to take the medication, eating a healthy diet, and reducing stress, toward the achievement of health and well-being. This self-process allowed the women to pursue work/career to support the family and volunteer opportunities to affect positive change and promote awareness for other HIV/AIDS positive women in Kenya" (Mwangi, 2013, p. 283).

(continued)

BOX 3.13 An Example of a Conceptual–Theoretical–Empirical Structure for King's Conceptual System Mixed-Methods Research *(continued)*

The *non-relational propositions* for the *E component* of the CTE structure are:

- Sociodemographic Characteristics is measured by the Socio-Demographic Characteristics Survey (SDCS; Mwangi, 2013). The SDCS includes 23 items addressing demographic and HIV/AIDS-related data.
- Perceived Stigma and its dimensions are measured by the HIV/AIDS Stigma Instrument-PLWA (HASI-P) and its subscales. The HASI-P is made up of 33 items that are arranged in six subscales—"verbal abuse (8 items), negative self-perception (5 items), health care neglect (7 items), social isolation (5 items), fear of contagion (6 items), and workplace stigma (2 items)" (Holzemer et al., as cited in Mwangi, 2013, p. 75). The items are rated on a 4-point scale of frequency of the item occurring, with choices of "never," "once or twice," "several times," or "most of the time."
- Life Experiences of HIV/AIDS and its dimensions were generated from interpretive phenomenological analysis of the women's responses to several open-ended items on an investigator-developed Semi-Structured Interview Form (Mwangi, 2013). The items are: "What is it like for you to live every day with HIV/AIDS? How does it make you feel?" "How do people in your neighborhood treat you? How does it make you feel?" "Have you been to a clinic for treatment or admitted to the hospital. Tell me about a time that you were very sick. What happened? Who helped you? How did you get better?" "If you were admitted to the hospital for something related to your HIV/AIDS, what happened? How did that make you feel?" "When you think about living with HIV/AIDS every day, what things do you find the hardest? What worries you the most?" "Tell me about what has helped you to live with HIV/AIDS (e.g., faith, support, church, coping)" (Mwangi, 2013, pp. 90–91).

The *relational proposition* for the quantitative phase of the *C and T components* of the CTE structure is:

- Sociodemographic Characteristics are related to Perceived Stigma.

The *relational proposition* for the quantitative phase of the *E component* of the CTE structure is:

- Scores for the items on the Sociodemographic Characteristics Survey are related to the subscale scores on the HIV/AIDS Stigma Instrument-PLWA (HASI-P).

Source: Mwangi (2013), with permission of Rosemary Mwangi.

CONCLUSION

King's Conceptual System has made a substantial contribution to the discipline of nursing. The emphasis that King placed on client participation, including mutual goal setting and exploration of means to achieve goals, is completely in keeping with the patient (or client)-centered care mandate of contemporary nursing practice. For example, the Quality and Safety Education for Nurses initiative stipulates that the client or his or her designee is recognized as "the source of control and full partner in providing compassionate and coordinated care based on respect for [the client's] preferences, values, and needs" (Cronenwett et al., 2007, p. 123; 2009, p. 339).

King (1995) summarized the contributions of her Conceptual System, stating that it is:

> A holistic view of the complexity in nursing, within various groups, [and] in different types of health care systems...[that] provides a way of thinking about the "real world" of nursing practice..., suggests one approach for selecting concepts from the literature that represent fundamental knowledge for the practice of professional nursing..., [and] shows a process for developing concepts that symbolize experiences within various environments in which nursing is practiced. (pp. 17, 21)

The comprehensive utility of King's Conceptual System is evident in the examples of its use as a guide for practice, QI projects, and research given in this chapter.

NOTE

1. Portions of this chapter are adapted from Fawcett, J., & DeSanto-Madeya, S. (2013). *Contemporary nursing knowledge: Analysis and evaluation of nursing models and theories* (3rd ed., Chapter 5). Philadelphia, PA: F. A. Davis, with permission.

REFERENCES

Batson, V. D., & Yoder, L. H. (2012). Managerial coaching: A concept analysis. *Journal of Advanced Nursing, 68*, 1658–1669.

Burke, M. L. (1989). Chronic sorrow in mothers of school-age children with myelomeningocele disability. *Dissertations Abstract International, 50*, 2334B.

Cho, M-K. (2013). Effect of health contract intervention on renal dialysis patients in Korea. *Nursing and Health Sciences, 15*, 86–93.

Cronenwett, L, Sherwood, G., Barnsteiner, J., Disch, J., Johnson, J., Mitchell, P.,...Warren, J. (2007). Quality and safety education for nurses. *Nursing Outlook, 55*, 122–131.

Cronenwett, L, Sherwood, G., Pohl, J., Barnsteiner, J., Moore, S., Sullivan, D. T., & Warren, J. (2009). Quality and safety education for advanced practice nursing. *Nursing Outlook, 57*, 338–348.

Damrosch, S. P., & Perry, L. A. (1989). Self-reported adjustment, chronic sorrow, and coping of parents of children with Down syndrome. *Nursing Research, 38*, 25–30.

Derogatis, L. R., & Spencer, P. M. (1982). *Administration procedures: BSI manual—I.* Baltimore, MD: Clinical Psychometric Research.

Doran, D., & Sidani, S. (2007). Outcomes-focused knowledge translation: A framework for knowledge translation and patient outcomes improvement. *Worldviews on Evidence-Based Nursing, 4*, 3–13.

Fawcett, J., & DeSanto-Madeya, S. (2013). *Contemporary nursing knowledge: Analysis and evaluation of nursing models and theories* (3rd ed.). Philadelphia, PA: F. A. Davis.

Ganong, L. H. (1987). Integrative reviews of nursing research. *Research in Nursing and Health, 10,* 1–11.

Gunther, M. (2014). King's conceptual system and theory of goal attainment in nursing practice. In M. R. Alligood (Ed.), *Nursing theory: Utilization and application* (5th ed., pp. 160–280). Maryland Heights, MO: Mosby Elsevier.

Hobdell, E. (2004). Chronic sorrow and depression in parents of children with neural tube defects. *Journal of Neuroscience Nursing, 36,* 82–88, 94.

Holzemer, W. L., Uys, L. R., Chirwa, M. L., Greeff, M., Makoae, L. N., Kohi, T. W.,… Durrheim, K. (2007). Validation of the HIV/AIDS Stigma Instrument-PLWA. *AIDS Care, 19,* 1002–1012.

King, I. M. (1981). *A theory for nursing: Systems, concepts, process.* New York, NY: Wiley. [Reissued 1990. Albany, NY: Delmar.]

King, I. M. (1986a). *Curriculum and instruction in nursing.* Norwalk, CT: Appleton-Century-Crofts.

King, I. M. (1986b). King's theory of goal attainment. In P. Winstead-Fry (Ed.), *Case studies in nursing theory* (pp. 197–213). New York, NY: National League for Nursing.

King, I.M. (1992). King's theory of goal attainment. *Nursing Science Quarterly, 5,* 19–26.

King, I. M. (1995). A systems framework for nursing. In M.A. Frey & C.L. Sieloff (Eds.), *Advancing King's systems framework and theory of nursing* (pp. 14–22). Thousand Oaks, CA: Sage.

King, I. M. (1997). Knowledge development for nursing: A process. In I. M. King & J. Fawcett (Eds.), *The language of nursing theory and metatheory* (pp. 19–25). Indianapolis, IN: Sigma Theta Tau International Center Nursing Press.

King, I. M. (2007). King's conceptual system, theory of goal attainment, and transaction process in the 21st century. *Nursing Science Quarterly, 20,* 109–111.

Mann, K.S. (2011). Education and health promotion for new patients with cancer: A quality improvement model. *Clinical Journal of Oncology Nursing, 15,* 55–61.

Mwangi, R. N. (2013). *Kenyan women living with HIV/AIDS: A mixed methods study.* (Doctoral dissertation). Retrieved from ProQuest Dissertations and Theses Full Text (Dissertation Number 3589554; ProQuest Document ID 1430545502).

Ryle, S. (2008). Current evidence on anticoagulant management and outcomes for post-polypectomy: An integrative literature review to assist advanced practice nurses. *Gastroenterology Nursing, 31,* 354–364.

Sieloff, C. L. (2003). Measuring nurse power within organizations. *Journal of Nursing Scholarship, 35,* 183–187.

Sieloff, C. L. (2007). The theory of group power within organizations—Evolving conceptualization within King's conceptual system. In C. L. Sieloff & M. A. Frey (Eds.), *Middle range theory development using King's conceptual system* (pp. 196–214). New York, NY: Springer Publishing.

Sieloff, C. L., & Bularzik, A. M. (2011). Group power through the lens of the 21st century and beyond: Further validation of the Sieloff–King Assessment of Group Power within Organizations. *Journal of Nursing Management, 19,* 1020–1027.

Song, M. R. (2000). The development and test of self-efficacy promotion program on self-care of hemodialysis patients. *Journal of the Korean Academy of Nursing, 30,* 1066–1077.

Walker, L. O., & Avant, K. C. (2005). *Strategies for theory construction in nursing* (4th ed.). Upper Saddle River, NJ: Pearson/Prentice Hall.

CHAPTER 4

LEVINE'S CONSERVATION MODEL[1]

Myra E. Levine's Conservation Model focuses on conservation of human beings' wholeness or integrity (Levine, 1969, 1973, 1989, 1990, 1991, 1996). The goal of nursing guided by Levine's Conservation Model is the promotion of wholeness for all people, well or sick.

LEVINE'S CONSERVATION MODEL: CONCEPTS AND NON-RELATIONAL PROPOSITIONS

This section of the chapter includes the concepts of Levine's Conservation Model and the definitions (non-relational propositions) of the concepts and dimensions of the multidimensional concepts.

Holistic Being is defined as an individual. The three dimensions of the concept are system of systems, wholeness, and integrity.
> *System of systems* is defined as the human being.
> *Wholeness* is defined as "a sound, organic, progressive mutuality between diversified functions and parts within an entirety, the boundaries of which are fluid and open" (Erikson as cited in Levine, 1996, p. 39). Parts of holistic beings have meaning only when considered within the context of the whole being.
> *Integrity* is defined as the equivalent of wholeness.

Internal Environment is defined as the *milieu interne*, which is susceptible to constant change. The two dimensions of the concept are homeostasis and homeorrhesis.
> *Homeostasis* is defined as a stable state that reflects congruence of human beings with the environment.
> *Homeorrhesis* is defined as a stabilized flow that reflects the fluidity of change within a holistic being.

External Environment is defined as more than a stage setting against which holistic beings play out their lives. The three dimensions of the concept are perceptual environment, operational environment, and conceptual environment.

Perceptual environment is defined as the part of the external environment to which holistic beings respond through their visual, auditory, touch, smell, taste, thermal, and kinesthetic senses.

Operational environment is defined as the part of the external environment of which holistic beings are not aware through their senses, such as radiation, microorganisms, and odorless and colorless pollutants.

Conceptual environment is defined as "the environment of language, ideas, symbols, concepts, and invention" (Bates as cited in Levine, 1989, p. 326), including "emotions, values, religious beliefs, and ethnic and cultural traditions" (Levine, 1973, p. 12).

Adaptation is defined as the process of continual change throughout life that may be more or less successful. The three dimensions of the concept are historicity, specificity, and redundancy.

Historicity is defined "a consequence of a historical progression: the evolution of the species through time, reflecting the sequence of change in the genetic patterns that have recorded the change in the historical environments" (Levine, 1989, p. 327).

Specificity is defined as the synchronized tasks of body systems that serve the holistic being.

Redundancy is defined as responses that are available to holistic beings, such as anatomical, physiological, and psychological fail-safe options, when they encounter environmental challenges,

Organismic Responses is defined as physiological and behavioral responses to environmental challenges. The four dimensions of the concept are fight or flight response, inflammatory immune response, stress response, and perceptual awareness.

Fight or flight response is defined as an adrenocortical-sympathetic reaction that is an instantaneous response to a real or imagined threat.

Inflammatory immune response is defined as a response to injury that is important for maintenance of structural continuity and promotion of healing.

Stress response is defined as a response that is "recorded over time and is influenced by the accumulated experience of the individual" (Selye, as cited in Levine, 1989, p. 330).

Perceptual awareness is defined as the response that is mediated through the sense organs and is concerned with gathering information from the environment and converting it to meaningful experience. The perceptual awareness dimension has five subdimensions—basic orienting system, visual system, auditory system, haptic system, and taste–smell system.

Basic orienting system is defined as the balancing portion of the inner ear, which responds to changes in gravity, acceleration, and movement, and provides a general orientation to the environment that is essential to the function of the other perceptual systems.

Visual system is defined as that which permits the human being to look.

Auditory system is defined as that which permits listening to sounds as well as identifying the direction from which sounds are coming.

Haptic system is defined as that which permits responses to touch through reception of sensations by the skin, joints, and muscles.

Taste–smell system is defined as that which provides information about chemical stimuli and facilitates safe nourishment.

Conservation is defined as "keeping together" (Levine, 1989, p. 331). The four dimensions of the concept are energy, structural integrity, personal integrity, and social integrity.

Energy is defined as "balancing energy output and energy input to avoid excessive fatigue, that is, adequate rest, nutrition, and exercise" (Levine, 1988, p. 227).

Structural integrity is defined as "maintaining or restoring the structure of the body, that is, preventing physical breakdown and promoting healing" (Levine, 1988, p. 227).

Personal integrity is defined as "the maintenance or restoration of the patient's sense of identity, self-worth, and acknowledgment of uniqueness" (Levine, 1988, p. 227).

Social integrity is defined as "acknowledgment of the patient as a social being" (Levine, 1988, p. 227).

Change is defined as the life process, which is characterized as unceasing change that has direction, purpose, and meaningfulness.

Health is defined as a pattern of adaptive change that is identified as such by each holistic being.

Disease is defined as a pattern of adaptive change that is undisciplined and unregulated change, a disruption in the orderly sequential pattern of change that is characteristic of life.

Nursing Process as Conservation is defined as a "scientific approach in the determination of nursing care" (Levine, 1966, p. 57). The three dimensions of the concept are trophicognosis, intervention/action, and evaluation of intervention/action.

Trophicognosis is defined as "the scientific approach in the determination of nursing care" (Levine, 1966, p. 57); a method to label problems of conservation of wholeness. The trophicognosis dimension has three subdimensions—observation, awareness of provocative facts, and construction of a testable hypothesis.

Observation is defined as a collection of data about the conditions of the internal and external environments; the status of organismic responses; and the extent of conservation of energy, structural integrity, personal integrity, and social integrity, all of which influence nursing intervention.

Awareness of provocative facts is defined as data that provoke the nurse's attention on the basis of observations and knowledge of the situation.

Construction of a testable hypothesis is defined as the trophicognosis that is deduced from the provocative facts.

Intervention/action is defined as a test of the hypothesis formulated by trophicognosis. The dimension of intervention/action has six subdimensions—conservation of energy, conservation of structural integrity, conservation of personal integrity, conservation of social integrity, therapeutic nursing intervention, and supportive nursing intervention.

Conservation of energy is defined as therapeutic or supportive nursing intervention that is targeted to the patient's energy through an adequate deposit of energy resources and regulation of the expenditure of energy.

Conservation of structural integrity is defined as therapeutic or supportive nursing intervention that is targeted to the patient's structural integrity through maintenance or restoration of the structure of the body cells, tissues, and organs.

Conservation of personal integrity is defined as therapeutic or supportive nursing intervention that is targeted to the patient's personal integrity through maintenance or restoration of his or her sense of identity, self-worth, and acknowledgment of uniqueness.

Conservation of social integrity is defined as therapeutic or supportive nursing intervention that is targeted to the patient's social integrity through acknowledging him or her as a social being.

Therapeutic nursing intervention is defined as nursing intervention directed toward conservation of energy and/or structural integrity and/or personal integrity and/or social integrity that influences adaptation favorably, or toward renewed social well-being.

Supportive nursing intervention is defined as nursing intervention directed toward conservation of energy and/or structural integrity and/or personal integrity and/or social integrity that cannot alter the course of the adaptation, that can only maintain the status quo, or that fails to halt a downward course.

Evaluation of Intervention/Action is defined as a judgment about the effects of nursing intervention based on the patient's organismic responses.

LEVINE'S CONSERVATION MODEL: RELATIONAL PROPOSITIONS

The statements of associations (relational propositions) among concepts of Levine's Conservation Model are listed here.

- Conservation and Adaptation are related, such that conservation is the product of adaptation.
- The four dimensions of Conservation—energy, structural integrity, personal integrity, and social integrity—are interrelated.
- Conservation and its four dimensions are related to Health.
- Conservation and its four dimensions are related to the two dimensions of Internal Environment—homeostasis and homeorrhesis—and the three dimensions of External Environment—perceptual, operational, and conceptual.
- The two dimensions of Internal Environment and the three dimensions of External Environment and related to the three dimensions of Adaptation—historicity, specificity, and redundancy.

- The four dimensions of Organismic Responses—fight or flight response, inflammatory immune response, stress response, and perceptual awareness—are interrelated.
- The dimensions of Nursing Process as Conservation are positively related, such that trophicognosis is positively related to intervention/action, which is positively related to evaluation of intervention/action.
- Nursing Process as Conservation has a positive effect on Organismic Responses.
- Nursing Process as Conservation has a positive effect on Health.
- Conservation and its four dimensions are related to each dimension of Nursing Process as Conservation.
- Nursing Process as Conservation and its dimensions have a positive effect on each dimension of Conservation.

LEVINE'S CONSERVATION MODEL: APPLICATION TO NURSING PRACTICE

The guidelines for Levine's Conservation Model nursing practice are listed in Box 4.1. A diagram of the practice methodology for Levine's Conservation Model, which is called Nursing Process as Conservation, is illustrated in Figure 4.1.

A practice tool that includes all parts of the practice methodology is given in Box 4.2.

BOX 4.1 Guidelines for Levine's Conservation Model Nursing Practice

The purpose of Conservation Model–based nursing practice is conservation of the patient's wholeness.

Practice problems encompass conditions of health and disability reflected in the four conservation principles. "Concerns for energy conservation and structural, personal, and social integrity are always present—though one area may present a more demanding problem than another. These areas can be explored individually, but they cannot be separated from the person" (Levine, 1990, p. 199).

Nursing practice occurs in virtually any setting, ranging from patients' homes to shelters for the homeless to ambulatory clinics to emergency departments to critical care units.

Legitimate participants of nursing are those individuals who become patients when they require the expert services that members of the health care team can provide for wellness or sick care. Individuals are no longer patients when they are no longer dependent on members of the health care team for care.

The nursing process is Nursing Process as Conservation.

Levine's Conservation Model–based nursing practice contributes to the well-being of individuals by promoting wholeness.

Adapted from Fawcett and DeSanto-Madeya (2013, p. 125), with permission.

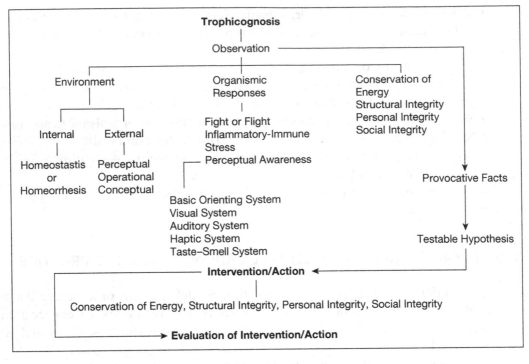

FIGURE 4.1 Levine's practice methodology: Nursing process as conservation.

BOX 4.2 The Levine's Conservation Model Practice Methodology Tool

TROPHICOGNOSIS

The nurse observes and collects data that will influence nursing practice rather than medical practice.

The nurse conducts a nursing history with specific reference to aspects that will influence the nursing care plan.

OBSERVATION

Assessment of internal environment
Is homeostasis or homeorrhesis evident?

Assessment of the external environment
What do you think is happening to you? (perceptual environment)
How much time do you spend outside? With or without sun screen? (operational environment)
To what extent and how does the quality of the air affect you? (operational environment)
What are your and your family's cultural traditions? (conceptual environment)

Assessment of organismic responses
What do you usually do when upset? (fight or flight responses)

(continued)

BOX 4.2 The Levine's Conservation Model Practice Methodology Tool (*continued*)

Please describe your reactions to infections or injuries. (inflammatory and immune responses)

What situations are stressful for you? (stress response)

Please describe any difficulties you have with balance, seeing, hearing, feeling things, taste, or smell. (perceptual awareness)

Assessment of conservation of personal integrity
Please tell me about yourself and what is important to you.

Assessment of conservation of social integrity
Please tell me about your family and friends.

Assessment of conservation of structural integrity
How do you feel physically right now? Do you have a medical diagnosis?

Assessment of conservation of energy
Have you maintained your usual level of physical energy recently? Please answer using a scale of 1 = not at all, 2 = partially, and 3 = fully.

AWARENESS OF PROVOCATIVE FACTS

The nurse identifies the provocative facts within the data collected, that is, the data that provoke attention on the basis of knowledge of the situation.

TESTABLE HYPOTHESES

The provocative facts provide the basis for a hypothesis, or trophicognosis.
Examples of testable hypotheses:

The patient will regain conservation of…through…
The patient will follow recommendations carefully and maintain…

INTERVENTION/ACTION

The nurse implements the nursing care plan within the context of the four conservation principles and within the structure of administrative policy, availability of equipment, and established standards of nursing.

Therapeutic nursing intervention is nursing intervention that influences adaptation favorably, or toward renewed social well-being.

Supportive nursing intervention is nursing intervention that cannot alter the course of the adaptation, that can only maintain the status quo, or that fails to halt a downward course.

EVALUATION OF INTERVENTION/ACTION

The nurse evaluates the effects of intervention and revises the trophicognosis as necessary.

Adapted from Fawcett and DeSanto-Madeya (2013).

A CONCEPTUAL–THEORETICAL–EMPIRICAL STRUCTURE FOR ASSESSMENT

McCall's (1991) book chapter is an example of use of Levine's Conservation Model for assessment. She developed the Neurological Intensive Monitoring System Unit Assessment Tool for use with patients experiencing epilepsy with refractory seizures. McCall explained that the tool "was designed to obtain data crucial to meeting the physical and psychosocial needs of [the patient population with epileptic refractory seizures] and facilitating successful adaptation" (p. 86).

The theory is assessment of the experience of epilepsy with refractory seizures. The conceptual model concept is Conservation with its four dimensions—energy, structural integrity, personal integrity, and social integrity. The theory concept is Experience of Epileptic Refractory Seizures. The four dimensions of Experience of Epileptic Refractory Seizures are seizure description and other medical history, safety measures, personal history, and social history.

The energy dimension of Conservation is represented by the seizure description and other medical history dimension of Experience of Epileptic Refractory Seizures, the structural integrity dimension of Conservation is represented by the safety measures dimension of Experience of Epileptic Refractory Seizures, the personal integrity dimension of Conservation is represented by the personal history dimension of Experience of Epileptic Refractory Seizures, and the social integrity dimension of Conservation is represented by the social history dimension of Experience of Epileptic Refractory Seizures. All four dimensions of Experience of Epileptic Refractory Seizures are measured by the data recorded in the semi-structured Neurological Intensive Monitoring System Unit Assessment Tool (McCall, 1991).

The conceptual–theoretical–empirical (CTE) structure constructed from the content of McCall's (1991) book chapter is illustrated in Figure 4.2. The non-relational propositions for each component of the CTE structure are listed in Box 4.3.

A CTE STRUCTURE FOR INTERVENTION

An example of Levine's Conservation Model nursing practice focused on intervention was extracted from a practice exemplar of nursing care of a pregnant woman who had a medical diagnosis of fibromyalgia (FM; Schaefer, 2010). Assessment of the four dimensions of Conservation revealed six trophicognoses—inadequate nutrition, poor sleep quality, lower back pain, poor self-esteem, anxiety about delivery, and inadequate social support.

The theory used to guide practice is effects of therapeutic conservation interventions on nutrition, sleep quality, lower back pain, self-esteem, anxiety, and social support. One conceptual model concept is Nursing Process as Conservation. The relevant dimension of Nursing Process as Conservation is intervention/action. The relevant four subdimensions of interaction/action are

BOX 4.3 An Example of a Conceptual–Theoretical–Empirical Structure for Levine's Conservation Model Nursing Practice: Assessment

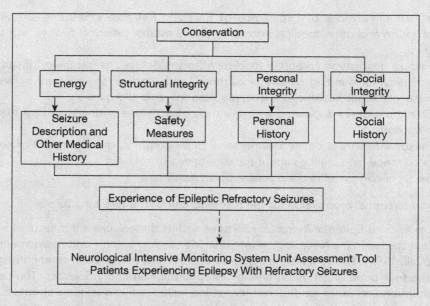

FIGURE 4.2 Conceptual–theoretical–empirical (CTE) structure for Levine's Conservation Model nursing practice: Assessment—theory of assessment of the experience of epilepsy with refractory seizures.

The *non-relational propositions* for the *C component* of the conceptual–theoretical–empirical (CTE) structure are:

- *Conservation* is defined as "keeping together" (Levine, 1989, p. 331).
- The four dimensions of the concept are energy, structural integrity, personal integrity, and social integrity.
  - o *Energy* is defined as "balancing energy output and energy input to avoid excessive fatigue, that is, adequate rest, nutrition, and exercise" (Levine, 1988, p. 227).
  - o *Structural integrity* is defined as "maintaining or restoring the structure of the body, that is, preventing physical breakdown and promoting healing" (Levine, 1988, p. 227).
  - o *Personal integrity* is defined as "the maintenance or restoration of the patient's sense of identity, self-worth, and acknowledgment of uniqueness" (Levine, 1988, p. 227).
  - o *Social integrity* is defined as "acknowledgment of the patient as a social being" (Levine, 1988, p. 227).

The *non-relational propositions* for the *T component* of the CTE structure are:

- *Experience of Epileptic Refractory Seizures* is defined as convulsions or other detectable clinical events that result from sudden electrical activity in the brain that is resistant to medication and occurs at least once each month for 2 or more years in people with epilepsy (McCall, 1991; Venes, 2013).

(continued)

BOX 4.3   An Example of a Conceptual–Theoretical–Empirical Structure for Levine's Conservation Model Nursing Practice: Assessment   (continued)

- The four dimensions of Experience of Epileptic Refractory Seizures are seizure description and other medical history, safety measures, personal history, and social history.
  - o *Seizure description and other medical history* is defined as frequency of seizures, activities surrounding seizure occurrence, and medication regimen, as well as history of other health conditions, medications, and allergies.
  - o *Safety measures* is defined as prevention of activities during a seizure that are hazardous.
  - o *Personal history* is defined as personal demographics, demographics of seizure occurrence, and feelings about the experience of seizures.
  - o *Social history* is defined as social support resources.

The *non-relational proposition* for the *E component* of the CTE structure is:

- Experience of Epileptic Refractory Seizures and its dimensions are measured by the data recorded in the Neurological Intensive Monitoring System Unit Assessment Tool (McCall, 1991). This tool includes questions in each of four sections that correspond to the four dimensions of Experience of Epileptic Refractory Seizures. The seizure description and other medical history section includes five questions about seizures and three questions about other medical conditions, medications, and allergies. Six questions make up the safety measures section. Another six questions make up the personal history section. Five questions are included in the social history section.

Source: McCall (1991).

conservation of energy, conservation of structural integrity, conservation of personal integrity, and conservation of social integrity. The other conceptual model concept is Conservation and its four dimensions—energy, structural integrity, personal integrity, and social integrity. The theory concepts are Therapeutic Conservation Interventions, Nutrition, Sleep Quality, Lower Back Pain, Self-Esteem, Anxiety, and Social Support.

The four subdimensions of the Nursing Process as Conservation dimension of intervention/action are represented by Therapeutic Conservation Interventions. The energy dimension of Conservation is represented by Nutrition and Sleep Quality; the structural integrity dimension is represented by Lower Back Pain; the personal integrity dimension is represented by Self-Esteem and Anxiety; and the social integrity dimension is represented by Social Support.

Therapeutic Conservation Interventions is operationalized by the Therapeutic Conservation Interventions protocol. Nutrition, Sleep Quality, Lower Back Pain, Self-Esteem, Anxiety, and Social Support are measured by observations of organismic responses (Schaefer, 2010).

The CTE structure constructed from the content of Schaefer's (2010) practice exemplar is illustrated in Figure 4.3. The non-relational and relational propositions for each component of the CTE structure are listed in Box 4.4.

BOX 4.4 An Example of a Conceptual–Theoretical–Empirical Structure for Levine's Conservation Model Nursing Practice: Intervention

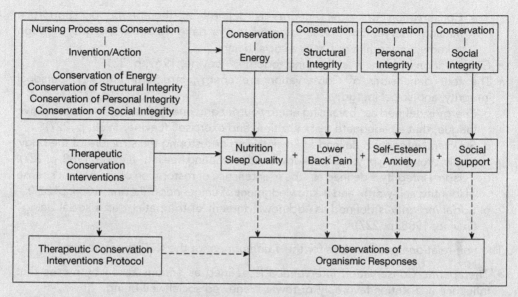

FIGURE 4.3 Conceptual–theoretical–empirical (CTE) structure for Levine's Conservation Model nursing practice: Intervention—theory of the effects of Therapeutic Conservation Interventions on nutrition, sleep quality, lower back pain, self-esteem, anxiety, and social support.

The *non-relational propositions* for the *C component* of the conceptual–theoretical–empirical (CTE) structure are:

- *Nursing Process as Conservation* is defined as a "scientific approach in the determination of nursing care" (Levine, 1966, p. 57).
- The relevant dimension of Nursing Process as Conservation is interaction/action.
  - o *Intervention/action* is defined as a test of the hypothesis formulated by trophicognosis.
  - o The four relevant subdimensions of intervention/action are conservation of energy, conservation of structural integrity, conservation of personal integrity, and conservation of social integrity.
    - *Conservation of energy* is defined as therapeutic or supportive nursing intervention that is targeted to the patient's energy through an adequate deposit of energy resources and regulation of the expenditure of energy.
    - *Conservation of structural integrity* is defined as therapeutic or supportive nursing intervention that is targeted to the patient's structural integrity through maintenance or restoration of the structure of the body cells, tissues, and organs.
    - *Conservation of personal integrity* is defined as therapeutic or supportive nursing intervention that is targeted to the patient's personal integrity through maintenance or restoration of his or her sense of identity, self-worth, and acknowledgment of uniqueness.

(continued)

BOX 4.4   An Example of a Conceptual–Theoretical–Empirical Structure for Levine's Conservation Model Nursing Practice: Intervention   *(continued)*

- ■ *Conservation of social integrity* is defined as therapeutic or supportive nursing intervention that is targeted to the patient's social integrity through acknowledging him or her as a social being.
- *Conservation* is defined as "keeping together" (Levine, 1989, p. 331).
- The four dimensions of Conservation are energy, structural integrity, personal integrity, and social integrity.
  - o *Energy* is defined as "balancing energy output and energy input to avoid excessive fatigue, that is, adequate rest, nutrition, and exercise" (Levine, 1988, p. 227).
  - o *Structural integrity* is defined as "maintaining or restoring the structure of the body, that is, preventing physical breakdown and promoting healing" (Levine, 1988, p. 227).
  - o *Personal integrity* is defined as "the maintenance or restoration of the patient's sense of identity, self-worth, and acknowledgment of uniqueness" (Levine, 1988, p. 227).
  - o *Social integrity* is defined as "acknowledgment of the patient as a social being" (Levine, 1988, p. 227).

The *non-relational propositions* for the *T component* of the CTE structure are:

- *Therapeutic Conservation Intervention* is defined as actions taken by nurses that influence adaptation favorably, or toward renewed social well-being.
- *Nutrition* is defined as selection of healthy fast foods, eating small frequent meals throughout the day, preparing food in sufficiently large quantities to avoid constant cooking, and avoiding gas-forming foods (Schaefer, 2010).
- *Sleep Quality* is defined as restful, comfortable sleep (Schaefer, 2010).
- *Lower Back Pain* is defined as discomfort felt in the lower back.
- *Self-Esteem* is defined as personal evaluation of one's self.
- *Anxiety* is defined as feelings of dread and apprehension from an unknown source.
- *Social Support* is defined as information and encouragement from family, friends, and health care providers.

The *non-relational propositions* for the *E component* of the CTE structure are:

- Therapeutic Conservation Intervention is operationalized by the Therapeutic Conservation Interventions protocol, which stipulates specific interventions for conservation of energy, structural integrity, personal integrity, and social integrity (Schaefer, 2010).
- Nutrition is measured by observations of the organismic response of dietary intake.
- Sleep Quality is measured by observations of the organismic response of restful, comfortable sleep using soft pillows for support.
- Lower Back Pain is measured by observations of the organismic response of reduced discomfort in the lower back.
- Self-Esteem is measured by observations of the organismic response of "excitement about becoming a mother" (Schaefer, 2010, p. 100).
- Anxiety is measured by observations of the organismic response of "successful delivery of a healthy child" (Schaefer, 2010, p. 100).
- Social Support is measured by observations of the organismic responses of help from family members following delivery and consultation with a lactation consultant (Schaefer, 2010).

(continued)

> **BOX 4.4   An Example of a Conceptual–Theoretical–Empirical Structure for Levine's Conservation Model Nursing Practice: Intervention   *(continued)***
>
> The *relational propositions* for the C and T components of the CTE structure are:
>
> - Nursing Process as Conservation and its dimensions have a positive effect on each dimension of Conservation.
> - Therefore, Therapeutic Conservation Interventions have a positive effect on Nutrition, Sleep Quality, Self-Esteem, Anxiety, and Social Support, and a negative effect on Lower Back Pain.
>
> The *relational proposition* for the E component of the CTE structure is:
>
> - There is a positive effect of implementation of the Therapeutic Conservation Interventions protocol on results of observations of organismic responses, such that the patient experiences better nutrition, restful and comfortable sleep, reduced lower back pain, improved self-esteem, less anxiety, and greater social support than before the implementation of the protocol.
>
> *Source:* Schaefer (2010).

LEVINE'S CONSERVATION MODEL: APPLICATION TO QUALITY IMPROVEMENT

The guidelines for Levine's Conservation Model quality improvement (QI) projects are listed in Box 4.5.

A CTE STRUCTURE FOR A QI PROJECT

A journal article by Odesina et al. (2010) is an example of a report of a quality improvement project guided by Levine's Conservation Model. The purpose of their project was to examine "the current [sickle cell disease] SCD pain management practice patterns, [explore] evidence-based SCD pain management clinical guidelines, and [develop] and [implement] an adapted [emergency department] ED sickle cell pain management clinical pathway" (p. 104). The QI project participants were nurses working in an ED and patients with a diagnosis of SCD.

The theory is implementation of a sickle cell pain management clinical pathway. The conceptual model concept is Nursing Process as Conservation. The three dimensions are trophicognosis, intervention/action, and evaluation of intervention/action. The theory concepts are Sickle Cell Pain Management, Pharmacologic Pain Management Intervention, and Nonparmacologic Pain Management Intervention. The trophicognosis and intervention/action dimensions of Nursing Process as Conservation are represented by Sickle Cell Pain Management. The evaluation of intervention/action dimension of Nursing

BOX 4.5   Guidelines for Levine's Conservation Model Quality
Improvement Projects

The purpose of quality improvement projects is to test the effectiveness of nurses' use
    of Levine's practice methodology (Nursing Process as Conservation) on nurses' and/
    or patients' wholeness.
The phenomenon of interest for a quality improvement projects is the extent of nurses'
    use of Nursing Process as Conservation on nurses' and/or patients' conservation of
    energy, structural integrity, personal integrity, and/or social integrity.
Data for quality improvement projects are to be collected from patients and/or nurses
    in various settings, such as patients' homes, practitioners' private offices, ambulatory
    clinics, hospitals, and communities.
Any methodological theory of change or quality improvement may be used to guide
    the design of the quality improvement project and the times for data collection.
    Checklists, rating scales, and responses to open-ended questions may be used
    to determine the extent to which nurses actually implement Nursing Process as
    Conservation. Descriptive statistics may be used to analyze data obtained from
    checklists or rating scales, and content analysis may be used to identify categories
    or themes found in responses to open-ended questions.
The results of Levine's Conservation Model-based quality improvement projects
    enhance understanding of how using Nursing Process as Conservation influences
    maintenance of wholeness.

Process as Conservation is represented by Pharmacologic Pain Management
Intervention and Nonpharmacologic Pain Management Intervention.

Sickle Cell Pain Management is operationalized by the Sickle Cell Pain
Management Clinical Pathway, which was guided by Melnyk and Fineout-
Overholt's (2005) methodological theory of advancing research and clinical practice through close collaboration (ARCC) model for QI (see Appendix A). Data
abstracted from a retrospective medical record review, which are recorded on a
Sickle Cell Disease Form (Odesina et al., 2010), are used to measure the extent
of use of pharmacologic pain management interventions and the extent of use
of nonpharmacologic pain management interventions. The data were analyzed
using descriptive statistics (numbers, percents, means, standard deviations)
and the Pearson product moment coefficient of correlation (r) (see Appendix B).

The CTE structure constructed from an interpretation of Odesina et al.'s
(2010) QI project is illustrated in Figure 4.4. The non-relational and relational
propositions for each component of the CTE structure are listed in Box 4.6.

LEVINE'S CONSERVATION MODEL: APPLICATION TO NURSING RESEARCH

The guidelines for Levine's Conservation Model System nursing research are
listed in Box 4.7.

BOX 4.6 An Example of a Conceptual–Theoretical–Empirical Structure for a Levine's Conservation Model Quality Improvement Project

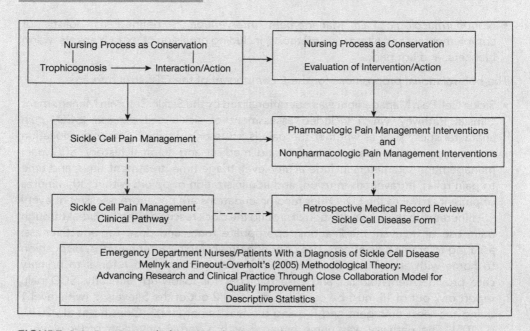

FIGURE 4.4 Conceptual–theoretical–empirical (CTE) structure for a Levine's Conservation Model quality improvement project—theory of implementation of a sickle cell pain management clinical pathway.

The *non-relational propositions* for the *C component* of the conceptual–theoretical–empirical (CTE) structure are:

- *Nursing Process as Conservation* is defined as a "scientific approach in the determination of nursing care" (Levine, 1966, p. 57).
- The three dimensions of the concept are trophicognosis, intervention/action, and evaluation of intervention/action.
  - o *Trophicognosis* is defined as "the scientific approach in the determination of nursing care" (Levine, 1966, p. 57); a method to label problems of conservation of wholeness.
  - o *Intervention/action* is defined as a test of the hypothesis formulated by trophicognosis.
  - o *Evaluation of intervention/action* is defined as a judgment about the effects of nursing intervention based on the patient's organismic responses.

The *non-relational propositions* for the *T component* of the CTE structure are:

- *Sickle Cell Disease Pain Management* is defined as identification of ways to treat pain from sickle cell disease.
- *Pharmacologic Pain Management Intervention* is defined as administration of opioids, including hydromorphone, morphine, fentanyl, oxycodone, or oxycodone with acetaminophen, as well as adjunct medications, including promethazine, diphenhydramine, ondansetron, diazepam, enoxaparin, metoclopramide, and acetaminophen.

(continued)

BOX 4.6 An Example of a Conceptual–Theoretical–Empirical Structure for a Levine's Conservation Model Quality Improvement Project *(continued)*

- *Nonpharmacologic Pain Management Intervention* is defined as holistic or complementary and alternative methods, including provision of extra blankets, warm blankets, and hot packs.

The *non-relational propositions* for the *E component* of the CTE structure are:

- Sickle Cell Pain Management was operationalized by the Sickle Cell Pain Management Clinical Pathway, which included assessment of sickle cell disease (SCD) pain characteristics "such as whether the pain is acute or chronic; the intensity, location and quality of pain; past treatment; and medical and surgical history. SCD pain management parameters include acuity level, triage time, treatment time, and time to pain relief, intravenous infusion, and administration of opioid within [30] minutes of patient arrival to the ED. Other recommendations are patient reassessment every 15 minutes with the administration of around the clock rescue dosing for breakthrough pain, use of adjuvant medications, appropriate route and dose for effectiveness, assuring tolerable side effects, use of nonpharmacological interventions, disposition to home with enough medications for pain management, and referral to primary care provider/hematologist and case manager for follow-up. Similarly, SCD pain report of 7 out of 10 must be considered a level 2 out of the 5 levels...(with level 1 being the most emergent and 5 being the least emergent)" (Odesina et al., 2010, p. 105). The pathway was nurse initiated with a verbal physician order when a physician was not available. The pathway implementation was guided by Melnyk and Fineout-Overholt's (2005) methodological theory of advancing research and clinical practice through close collaboration (ARCC) model for quality improvement. "The focus of ARCC model is to evaluate the effectiveness of evidence-based practice implementation strategies and outcomes of clinical care, as well as to disseminate and facilitate use of best evidence from well-designed studies to advance an evidence-based approach through clinical care studies" (Odesina et al., 2010, p. 105). The five phases of the ARCC model are: assessment of organizational culture and readiness for evidence-based practice (EBP); identification of major strengths and barriers to EBP implementation; development and use of EBP mentors; EBP implementation; and nurse, patient, and organization outcomes.
- Pharmacologic Pain Management Intervention and Nonpharmacologic Pain Management Intervention are measured using the SCD Form for abstraction of data from a retrospective medical record review to determine extent of use of the interventions by nurses. Odesina et al. (2010) explained that the SCD Form was adapted from Tanabe et al.'s (2007) form.

The *relational propositions* for the *C* and *T components* of the CTE structure are:

- The trophicognosis dimension of Nursing Process as Conservation is related to the intervention/action dimension, which is related to the evaluation of intervention/action dimension.
- Therefore, Sickle Cell Pain Management is positively related to Pharmacologic Pain Management Intervention and Nonpharmacologic Pain Management Intervention

(continued)

BOX 4.6   An Example of a Conceptual–Theoretical–Empirical Structure for a Levine's Conservation Model Quality Improvement Project   *(continued)*

The *relational proposition* for the *E component* of the CTE structure is:

- Implementation of the Sickle Cell Pain Management Clinical Pathway is positively related to data abstracted from a retrospective medical record review using the SCD Form for extent of use of Pharmacologic Pain Management Intervention and Nonpharmacologic Pain Management Intervention.

Source: Odesina et al. (2010).

BOX 4.7   Guidelines for Levine's Conservation Model Research

The purpose of Conservation Model–based nursing research is to identify nursing interventions derived from the conservation of energy, structural integrity, personal integrity, and social integrity that will maintain wholeness and support adaptation, within the context of the unique predicament of the individual, the family, or both.

The phenomena of interest are the conservation of energy, structural integrity, personal integrity, and social integrity. Studies may address just one dimension of conservation, but ultimately all four dimensions must be considered. "Research and scholarly study must focus on discrete issues. But the integrity of the whole person cannot be violated. However narrow the study problem may be, the influence of all four conservation principles must be acknowledged, and the wholeness of the person sustained" (Levine, 1991, p. 10). Other relevant phenomena are the levels of organismic responses and the perceptual, operational, and conceptual environments.

The precise problems to be studied are those dealing with the maintenance of the individual's wholeness and the interface between the internal and external environments of the person.

Study participants may be healthy or sick individuals of all ages in virtually any setting.

Qualitative, quantitative, and/or mixed-method designs are appropriate. Qualitative research designs should focus on discovering how patients experience challenges to their internal and external environments. Quantitative designs should focus on testing relations among study concepts and testing the effects of interventions on conservation of energy, structural integrity, personal integrity, and social integrity, as well as on organismic responses. Ideally, research designs should combine qualitative and quantitative methodologies for mixed-methods research. Practice tools derived from the Conservation Model may be used to collect data for research purposes. A question that can be used to identify aspects of nursing directed toward the whole person is: "How has this predicament (illness, lifestyle change, new baby, marriage, change in job) affected your normal lifestyle?" (Schaefer, 1991, p. 52).

Techniques for data analysis should be appropriate for the particular qualitative, quantitative, and/or mixed-methods design used.

Conservation Model–based research findings enhance understanding of factors and nursing interventions that promote adaptation and the maintenance of wholeness.

Adapted from Fawcett and DeSanto-Madeya (2013), with permission.

A CTE STRUCTURE FOR A SYSTEMATIC LITERATURE REVIEW

Review of the comprehensive list of research guided by Levine's Conservation Model published by Fawcett and DeSanto-Madeya (2013) and updated by Fawcett (2014) revealed several studies constituting a program of research about the prevalence and incidence of pressure ulcers conducted by Langemo and her colleagues. Langemo et al. (1993) explained, "Since 1987, Langemo and her colleagues have conducted a series of studies on pressure ulcers" guided by Levine's Conservation Model (p. 13). A description of their program of research provides an example of a systematic literature review explicitly guided by Levine's Conservation Model.

Eight journal articles were retrieved from a search of a comprehensive bibliography of Levine's Conservation Model publications (Fawcett & DeSanto-Madeya, 2013) and a more recent updated bibliography (Fawcett, 2014), using the search term, "pressure ulcers" (Burd et al., 1992; Burd et al., 1994; Hanson et al., 1991; Hanson, Langemo, Olson, Hunter, & Burd, 1994; Hunter et al., 1992; Hunter et al., 1995; Langemo et al., 1991; Langemo et al., 1993).

This search was augmented by a search of the Complete Comprehensive Index to Nursing and Allied Health Literature (CINAHL Complete) electronic database from 1937 to September 2014, using the search terms, "Levine's Conservation Model" and "pressure ulcer." This search yielded three journal articles already included in the Fawcett and DeSanto-Madeya (2013) bibliography (Burd et al., 1994; Hanson et al., 1991; Langemo et al., 1993).

Inasmuch as these two searches revealed that Langemo is the lead researcher for the studies, a separate search of CINAHL Complete using the search terms "Langemo [AU]" and "pressure ulcer" was done. This search yielded 67 journal articles, including all of those in the Fawcett and DeSanto-Madeya (2013) and Fawcett (2014) bibliographies. However, none of the other articles included an explicit citation to Levine's Conservation Model.

A review of the content of one article (Langemo et al., 1993) yielded three other articles that the researchers indicated were guided by Levine's Conservation Model, although the model was not cited in those articles. These three articles are included in the literature review (Langemo et al., 1989; Langemo et al., 1990; Olson et al., 1996).

The research reports included in this example of a literature review are limited to the 11 journal articles that included an explicit citation to Levine's Conservation Model ($n = 8$) or were reported to be guided by the model ($n = 3$). The results of the literature review were entered into a coding sheet (see Table 4.1) and are written here as a brief narrative.

All 11 research reports were coauthored by members of a research team led by Langemo, with a different research team member assuming the role of first author for each set of articles. Langemo et al. (1989) is the first report of the program of research that could be located. The Langemo et al. (1989) and (1990) articles are reports of the same study; the 1990 article is an expanded version of the 1989 article. The Hanson et al. (1991) and Langemo et al. (1991) articles are the first in which Levine's Conservation Model is explicitly identified as the framework for the research. The Langemo et al.

TABLE 4.1 Coding Sheet for Literature Review for Pressure Ulcer Prevalence and Incidence Research Guided by Levine's Conservation Model

LEVINE'S CONSERVATION MODEL	
LITERATURE REVIEWED	**CONCEPTUAL MODEL CONCEPT:** **CONSERVATION—STRUCTURAL INTEGRITY**
Burd et al., 1992	
Theory concept studied	Pressure ulcers—prevalence and incidence
Sample size and characteristics	Prevalence phase—159 residents, aged 18 years and older, in a skilled nursing home
	Incidence phase—25 residents in the same skilled nursing home as the prevalence phase
Instrument	Skin assessment tool
Results	Prevalence—23% (64 pressure ulcers on 37 residents)
	Incidence—28% (14 pressure ulcers on 7 residents)
Comment	Phases 1 and 2 of a three-phase study (see Burd et al., 1994 for Phase 3)
Burd et al., 1994	
Theory concept studied	Pressure ulcers—prevalence
	Four audits conducted quarterly after implementation of pressure ulcer prevention and treatment interventions (skin care protocols)
Sample size and characteristics	151–157 residents of a skilled nursing home (same nursing home as Burd et al., 1992)
	Total of 621 skin assessments
Instrument	Skin assessment tool
Results	Prevalence—17%, averaged over the four audits (134 pressure ulcers on 103 residents)
Comment	Phase 3 of a three-phase study (see Burd et al., 1992 for phases 1 and 2)
Hanson et al., 1991	
Theory concept studied	Pressure ulcers—prevalence and incidence
Sample size and characteristics	Prevalence phase—eight patients, aged 18 years and older, of a Medicare-certified hospital–affiliated hospice seen by hospice staff in their homes
	Incidence prospective phase—19 newly admitted patients of the same hospice as the prevalence phase; each patient was followed for 4 weeks
	Incidence retrospective phase—61 patients of the same hospice as the prevalence phase; data audit (retrospective chart review) encompassed 9 months

(continued)

TABLE 4.1 Coding Sheet for Literature Review for Pressure Ulcer Prevalence and Incidence Research Guided by Levine's Conservation Model *(continued)*

LEVINE'S CONSERVATION MODEL	
LITERATURE REVIEWED	**CONCEPTUAL MODEL CONCEPT: CONSERVATION—STRUCTURAL INTEGRITY**
Hanson et al., 1991 *(continued)*	
Instrument	Skin assessment tool
Results	Prevalence—13% (1 pressure ulcer on 1 patient)
	Prospective incidence—0% (no pressure ulcers developed during study period)
	Retrospective incidence—13% (13 pressure ulcers on 8 patients)
Comments	Phases 1 and 2 of a three-phase study (see Hanson et al., 1994 for Phase 3)
	One of first two research reports in which Levine is cited (see also Langemo et al., 1991)
Hanson et al., 1994	
Theory concept studied	Pressure ulcers—prevalence
Sample size and characteristics	105 patients, aged 18 years and older, of a Medicare-certified hospital–affiliated hospice seen by hospice staff in their homes
	Four audits conducted quarterly after implementation of skin care protocols
Instrument	Skin assessment tool
Results	Prevalence—14.3%, averaged over the four audits (19 pressure ulcers on 15 patients)
Comment	Phase 3 of a three-phase study (see Hanson et al., 1991 for phases 1 and 2)
Hunter et al., 1992	
Theory concept studied	Pressure ulcers—prevalence and incidence
Sample size and characteristics	Prevalence phase—40 patients, aged 18 years and older, at a rehabilitation hospital
	Incidence phase—40 other patients at the same rehabilitation hospital
Instrument	Skin assessment tool
Results	Prevalence—25% (12 pressure ulcers on 10 patients)
	Incidence—0% (no pressure ulcers developed during study period)
Comment	See Hunter et al. (1995) for follow-up study

(continued)

TABLE 4.1 Coding Sheet for Literature Review for Pressure Ulcer Prevalence and Incidence Research Guided by Levine's Conservation Model *(continued)*

LEVINE'S CONSERVATION MODEL	
LITERATURE REVIEWED	**CONCEPTUAL MODEL CONCEPT: CONSERVATION—STRUCTURAL INTEGRITY**
Hunter et al., 1995	
Theory concept studied	Pressure ulcers—prevalence
Sample size and characteristics	118 patients, aged 18 years and older, at the same rehabilitation hospital as the Hunter et al. (1992) study Quarterly audits for 16 months after implementation of pressure ulcer prevention and treatment (skin care) protocols
Instrument	Skin assessment tool
Results	Prevalence—11% (18 pressure ulcers on 13 patients) Total of 116 skin assessments
Comment	See Hunter et al. (1992) for first study (baseline data)
Langemo et al., 1989, 1990	
Theory concept studied	Pressure ulcers—prevalence
Sample size and characteristics	368 medical and surgical patients, ranging in age from 18 to 95 years, in an acute care hospital (n = 135), a rehabilitation hospital (n = 159), a skilled nursing home (n = 40), a home health care agency (n = 26), or a hospital-affiliated hospice (n = 8), "all located within a large medical complex" (Langemo et al., 1989, p. 42)
Instrument	Skin assessment tool
Results	Overall prevalence rate—20% (110 pressure ulcers on 72 patients) Acute care hospital—14% Skilled nursing home—23% Rehabilitation hospital—25% Home health care agency—19% Hospice—13%
Comments	Langemo et al. (1990) is a more detailed report of the study reported by Langemo et al. (1989) Levine's Conservation Model is not cited but this research is regarded as guided by this conceptual model in Langemo et al. (1993)

(continued)

TABLE 4.1 Coding Sheet for Literature Review for Pressure Ulcer Prevalence and Incidence Research Guided by Levine's Conservation Model   *(continued)*

LEVINE'S CONSERVATION MODEL	
LITERATURE REVIEWED	CONCEPTUAL MODEL CONCEPT: CONSERVATION—STRUCTURAL INTEGRITY
Langemo et al., 1991	
Theory concept studied	Pressure ulcers—incidence
Sample size and characteristics	190 medical and surgical patients, aged 18 years and older, at an acute care hospital (*n* = 74), a rehabilitation hospital (*n* = 25), a skilled nursing home (*n* = 40), a home health agency (*n* = 30), or a hospice (*n* = 20), all affiliated with a health center complex in the Midwestern United States
Instruments	Skin assessment tool
Results	Incidence—acute care setting—14% (14 pressure ulcers on 11 patients)
	Incidence—skilled nursing home—28% (13 pressure ulcers on 7 patients)
	Incidence—rehabilitation hospital, home health care agency, hospice—0% (0 pressure ulcers on 90 patients)
Comment	One of first two research reports in which Levine's Conservation Model is cited (see also Hanson et al., 1991)
Langemo et al., 1993	
Theory concept studied	Pressure ulcers—prevalence and incidence
Sample size and characteristics	Prevalence—368 medical and surgical patients, aged 18 years and older, at an acute care hospital (*n* = 135), a rehabilitation hospital (*n* = 159), a skilled nursing home (*n* = 40), a home health agency (*n* = 26), or a hospice (*n* = 8), all affiliated with a health center complex in the Midwestern United States (see Langemo et al., 1989, 1990)
	Incidence—190 medical and surgical patients, aged 18 years and older, at an acute care hospital, a rehabilitation hospital, a skilled nursing home, a home health agency, or a hospice, all affiliated with a health center complex in the Midwestern United States (see Langemo et al., 1991)
	Total of 621 skin assessments of patients in a skilled nursing home following implementation of skin care protocols (see Burd et al., 1994)
	Total of 116 skin assessments of patients in a skilled nursing home following implementation of skin care protocols (see Hunter et al., 1995)
Instrument	Skin assessment tool

(continued)

TABLE 4.1 Coding Sheet for Literature Review for Pressure Ulcer Prevalence and Incidence Research Guided by Levine's Conservation Model   *(continued)*

LEVINE'S CONSERVATION MODEL	
LITERATURE REVIEWED	CONCEPTUAL MODEL CONCEPT: CONSERVATION—STRUCTURAL INTEGRITY
Langemo et al., 1993 *(continued)*	
Results	Prevalence—acute care setting—14% (see Langemo et al., 1989, 1990)
	Prevalence—skilled nursing home—23% (see Langemo et al., 1989, 1990)
	Prevalence—rehabilitation hospital—25% (see Langemo et al., 1989, 1990)
	Prevalence—home health care agency—19% (see Langemo et al., 1989, 1990)
	Prevalence—hospice—13% (see Langemo et al., 1989, 1990)
	Prevalence—skilled nursing home—16.6% (see Burd et al., 1994)
	Prevalence—rehabilitation hospital—11.2% (see Hunter et al., 1995)
	Incidence—acute care setting—14% (see Langemo et al., 1991)
	Incidence—skilled nursing home—28% (see Langemo et al., 1991)
	Incidence—rehabilitation hospital, home health care agency, hospice—0% (see Langemo et al., 1991)
	Retrospective incidence—hospice—13% (see Hanson et al., 1991)
Comment	A summary of some of the other studies conducted by Langemo and her colleagues
Olson et al., 1996	
Theory concept studied	Pressure ulcers—incidence
Sample size and characteristics	149 medical and surgical patients, aged 18 years and older with no pressure ulcers at admission to an acute care hospital
Instrument	Skin assessment tool
Results	Incidence—13.4% (28 pressure ulcers on 20 patients)
Comment	Levine's Conservation Model is not cited but this research is regarded as guided by this conceptual model in Langemo et al. (1993)

(1993) article is a summary of the results of studies that had been completed—although not all had been published—by the time of writing (Burd et al., 1994; Hanson et al., 1991; Hunter et al., 1995; Langemo et al., 1989, 1990, 1991; Olson et al., 1996).

A total of nine articles are original reports of the prevalence and/or incidence of pressure ulcers found on patients in one or more of five settings—an acute care hospital, a rehabilitation hospital, a skilled nursing home, a home health care agency, and a hospice. All of these settings were affiliated with a health center complex in the Midwestern United States.

Sample sizes ranged from eight to 368 patients. The smaller samples were drawn from populations of patients in the hospice setting, and the larger samples were drawn from populations of medical and surgical patients in the acute care hospital. The number of skin assessments was used for data for two studies—Hunter et al. (1995) performed 116 skin assessments and Burd et al. (1994) performed 621 skin assessments.

The articles by Burd et al. (1992, 1994), Hanson et al. (1991, 1994), and Hunter et al. (1992, 1995) are reports of multiphase studies. The earlier articles are reports of the prevalence and incidence of pressure ulcers before the implementation of skin care protocols (phases 1 and 2), whereas the later articles are reports of pressure ulcer prevalence after the implementation of the protocols (phase 3). Langemo et al. (1989, 1990) reported only the prevalence of pressure ulcers, whereas Langemo et al. (1991) and Olson et al. (1996) reported only the incidence of pressure ulcers.

As can be seen in Table 4.1, prevalence varied within and between studies, ranging from 13% in the hospice setting to 25% in the rehabilitation setting. Incidence also varied within and between studies, ranging from 0% in rehabilitation, home health care, and hospice settings to 28% in a skilled nursing home. Hanson et al. (1991) reported a prospective incidence of 0% in the hospice setting during the study period but a retrospective incidence of 13% when a retrospective chart review was done.

Data were collected for every study using a skin assessment tool developed by the researchers. This tool included a definition for each of four stages (I, II, III, IV) of pressure ulcers and a diagram of pressure point locations on the body where pressure ulcers tend to form. Each site of a pressure ulcer was rated on a scale of 0 (redness) to 4 (stage IV pressure ulcer).

The theory of pressure ulcer prevalence and incidence was generated from the results of the literature review. The conceptual model concept is Conservation, and the relevant dimension is structural integrity; the theory concept is Pressure Ulcer and its two dimensions—prevalence and incidence. The structural integrity dimension of Conservation guided the selection of literature to review and the analysis of the data extracted from the literature review. Analysis of these data indicated that the structural integrity dimension of Conservation is represented by Pressure Ulcer and its two dimensions.

Examination of the 11 research reports reviewed yielded explicit definitions for Pressure Ulcer, prevalence, and incidence (see Box 4.8). These definitions are consistent in all of the research reports.

The CTE structure for the literature review is illustrated in Figure 4.5. The nonrelational propositions for each component of the CTE structure are listed in Box 4.8.

BOX 4.8   An Example of a Conceptual–Theoretical–Empirical Structure for a Levine's Conservation Model Systematic Literature Review

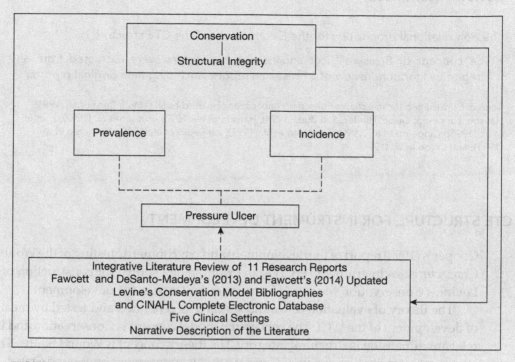

FIGURE 4.5 Conceptual–theoretical–empirical (CTE) structure for Levine's Conservation Model literature review—theory of pressure ulcer prevalence and incidence.

The *non-relational propositions* for the *C component* of the conceptual–theoretical–empirical (CTE) structure are:

- *Conservation* is defined as "keeping together" (Levine, 1989, p. 331).
- The relevant dimension of the concept is structural integrity.
  - o *Structural integrity* is defined as "maintaining or restoring the structure of the body, that is, preventing physical breakdown and promoting healing" (Levine, 1988, p. 227).

The *non-relational propositions* for the *T component* of the CTE structure are:

- *Pressure Ulcer* is defined as "localized areas of tissue necrosis that tend to develop when soft tissue is compressed between a bony prominence and an external surface for a prolonged period" (National Pressure Ulcer Advisory Panel, as cited in Burd et al., 1992, p. 31).
- The two dimensions of Pressure Ulcer are prevalence and incidence.
  - o *Prevalence* is defined as "the number of new and old cases assessed on a cross-sectional one-time basis" (National Pressure Ulcer Advisory Panel, as cited in Burd et al., 1992, p. 31).
  - o *Incidence* is defined as "the number of new cases over a given…period" (National Pressure Ulcer Advisory Panel, as cited in Burd et al., 1992, p. 31).

(continued)

BOX 4.8   An Example of a Conceptual–Theoretical–Empirical
Structure for a Levine's Conservation Model Systematic Literature
Review   *(continued)*

The *non-relational proposition* for the *E component* of the CTE structure is:

• The concept of Pressure Ulcer and its two dimensions were extracted from an integrative literature review of 11 research reports, including nine original reports.

Source: Constructed for this chapter based on publications by Burd et al. (1992); Burd et al. (1994); Hanson, Langemo, Olson, Hunter, and Burd (1994); Hanson et al. (1991); Hunter et al. (1992); Hunter et al. (1995); Langemo et al. (1990); Langemo et al. (1993); Langemo et al. (1989); Langemo et al. (1991); and Olson et al. (1996).

A CTE STRUCTURE FOR INSTRUMENT DEVELOPMENT

Cooper's (1990) report of the development and psychometric testing of the Wound Characteristics Instrument (WCI) is an example of a source for construction of a Levine's Conservation Model CTE structure for instrument development.

The theory of evaluation of wound status was generated and tested by means of development of the WCI. The conceptual model concept is Conservation and its relevant dimension is structural integrity. The theory concept is Wound Status. The structural integrity dimension of Conservation is represented by Wound Status.

The dimensions of Wound Status are architectural structure with the subdimensions of floor, walls, and edge or rim; wound floor and wall tissue with the subdimensions of moisture, color, sheen, and topography; wound floor and wall exudate with the subdimensions of consistency and distribution; new edge with the subdimenions of amount of new edge, color of new edge, and extension of new edge over the wound; and suture material.

Wound Status is measured by the WCI, an instrument that Cooper (1990) developed to evaluate the visual macroscopic characteristics of soft tissue wounds deliberately left open following surgery with the goal of healing by secondary intention. Cooper (1990) reported adequate estimates of internal consistency reliability using coefficient alpha and stability reliability using test–retest reliability for the WCI. She also reported an adequate estimate of face validity, which is a type of content validity, using a panel of two surgeon experts and two registered nurse experts in wound healing by secondary intention, and a more formal content validity procedure using Popham's (1978) average congruency technique with a panel of six experts in soft tissue wound healing. In addition, Cooper reported an adequate estimate of construct validity using the known groups technique with calculations for item discrimination and item difficulty (see Appendix B).

The CTE structure constructed for Cooper's (1990) instrument development research is illustrated in Figure 4.6. The non-relational propositions for each component of the CTE structure are listed in Box 4.9.

BOX 4.9 An Example of a Conceptual–Theoretical–Empirical Structure for Levine's Conservation Model for Instrument Development

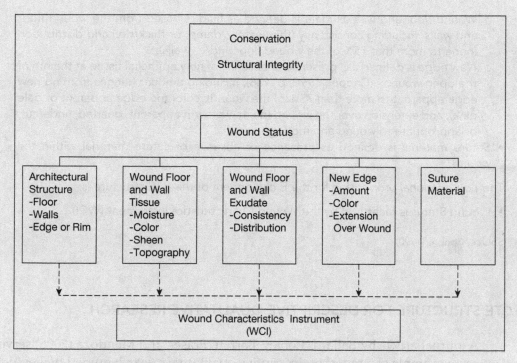

FIGURE 4.6 Conceptual–theoretical–empirical (CTE) structure for Levine's Conservation Model instrument development research—theory of evaluation of wound status.

The *non-relational propositions* for the *C component* of the conceptual–theoretical–empirical (CTE) structure are:

- *Conservation* is defined as "keeping together" (Levine, 1989, p. 331).
- The relevant dimension of Conservation is structural integrity.
  - o *Structural integrity* is defined as "maintaining or restoring the structure of the body, that is, preventing physical breakdown and promoting healing" (Levine, 1988, p. 227).

The *non-relational propositions* for the *T component* of the CTE structure are:

- *Wound Status* is defined as the condition of a soft tissue wound deliberately left open following surgery with the goal of healing by secondary intention.
- The dimensions of Wound Status are architectural structure, wound floor and wall tissue, wound floor and wall exudate, new edge, and suture material.
  - o *Architectural structure* is defined as the physical anatomy of a wound, including its floor (bottom of the wound), walls (sides of the wound), and edge or rim "position on the wound where the open tissue meets the normal hair bearing skin" (Cooper, 1990, p. 134).
  - o *Wound floor and wall tissue* is defined as the condition of wound floor and walls epithelial cells, including moisture (dry, damp, or wet), color (dusky, pink, beefy red), sheen (dull, semi-glossy, or glistening), and topography (large crevices, humps, or flat).

(continued)

BOX 4.9   An Example of a Conceptual–Theoretical–Empirical Structure for Levine's Conservation Model for Instrument Development   (continued)

   o *Wound floor and wall exudate* is defined as fluid released from the wound floor and walls, including consistency (thin/watery, damp, or thick/dry) and distribution (none to more that 75% of the wound floor and/or walls).

   o *New edge* is defined as "presence or absence of new epithelial tissue at the rim of the open wound" (Cooper, 1990, p. 138), including amount (ranges from no new edge apparent to more than 75% of the wound), color (no edge apparent or pale pink), and extension over the wound (no new growth apparent, gnarled, undercut, or appropriate to wound and moving inward).

• *Suture material* is defined as presence or absence of suture material within the wound.

The *non-relational proposition* for the E *component* of the CTE structure is:

• Wound Status is measured by the Wound Characteristics Instrument (WCI).

Source: Cooper (1990).

A CTE STRUCTURE FOR DESCRIPTIVE QUALITATIVE RESEARCH

A journal article by Ballard, Robley, Barrett, Fraser, and Mendoza (2006) serves as an example of a report of descriptive qualitative research guided by Levine's Conservation Model. The purpose of their study was "to understand the remembered experiences of patients who were given NMBAs [neuromuscular blocking agents] and sedatives and/or analgesics to facilitate mechanical ventilation, improve hemodynamic status, and improve oxygenation while in the ICU [intensive care unit]" (p. 89).

The theory of remembered experiences was generated by means of a descriptive qualitative phenomenological approach (see Appendix A). The conceptual model concept is Conservation and its four dimensions—energy, structural integrity, personal integrity, and social integrity. The theory concept is Remembered Experiences. The four dimensions of Remembered Experiences are feeling of going back and forth, loss of control, almost dying, and feeling cared for.

Conservation and its four dimensions guided the conduct of the study and interpretation of the findings. Ballard et al. (2006) commented, "Levine's concept of conservation lends itself well to the experiences voiced by the patients in this study" (p. 92). Remembered Experiences and its four dimensions were discovered by means of constant comparative analysis (see Appendix B) of the study participants' oral answers to open-ended questions asked during unstructured in-depth interviews (Ballard et al., 2006).

The CTE structure constructed for Ballard et al.'s (2006) study is illustrated in Figure 4.7. The non-relational propositions for each component of the CTE structure are listed in Box 4.10.

BOX 4.10   An Example of a Conceptual–Theoretical–Empirical Structure for Levine's Conservation Model Descriptive Qualitative Research

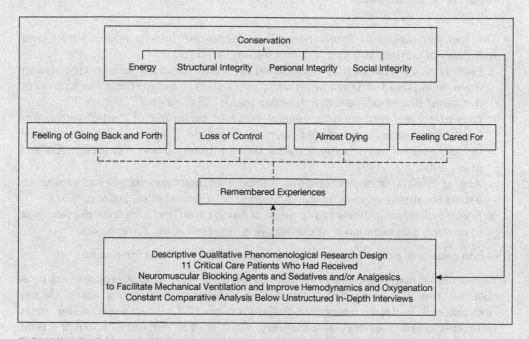

FIGURE 4.7 Conceptual–theoretical–empirical (CTE) structure for Levine's Conservation Model descriptive qualitative research—theory of remembered experiences.

The *non-relational propositions* for the *C component* of the conceptual–theoretical–empirical (CTE) structure are:

- *Conservation* is defined as "keeping together" (Levine, 1989, p. 331).
- The four dimensions of the concept are energy, structural integrity, personal integrity, and social integrity.
  - o *Energy* is defined as "balancing energy output and energy input to avoid excessive fatigue, that is, adequate rest, nutrition, and exercise" (Levine, 1988, p. 227).
  - o *Structural integrity* is defined as "maintaining or restoring the structure of the body, that is, preventing physical breakdown and promoting healing" (Levine, 1988, p. 227).
  - o *Personal integrity* is defined as "the maintenance or restoration of the patient's sense of identity, self-worth, and acknowledgment of uniqueness" (Levine, 1988, p. 227).
  - o *Social integrity* is defined as "acknowledgment of the patient as a social being" (Levine, 1988, p. 227).

The *non-relational propositions* for the *T component* of the CTE structure are:

- *Remembered experiences* is defined as negative and positive feelings of receiving "neuromuscular blocking agents and sedatives and/or analgesics to facilitate mechanical ventilation, improve hemodynamic stability, and improve oxygenation" (Ballard et al., 2006, p. 86).

(continued)

BOX 4.10   An Example of a Conceptual–Theoretical–Empirical Structure for Levine's Conservation Model Descriptive Qualitative Research   *(continued)*

- The four dimensions of Remembered Experiences are feeling of going back and forth, loss of control, almost dying, and feeling cared for.
  - o *Feeling of going back and forth* is defined as "a sense of being gone and then being there, being dead and then being alive; a vacillation…a weird dreamlike state with the unreal disembodiment that this state entails" (Ballard et al., 2006, p. 90).
  - o *Loss of control* is defined "a general sense of being out of control with every facet of existence…[including] time, money, and life…fighting [to regain control] or being tied down…being scared…being frightened and distressed" (Ballard et al., 2006, pp. 91–92).
  - o *Almost dying* is defined as "acknowledgment that death was close or had happened a number of times during the paralytic episode" (Ballard et al., 2006, p. 92).
  - o *Feeling cared for* is defined as "a sense of being cared [for]…despite the fear, loss of control, and experience of almost dying" (Ballard et al., 2006, p. 92).

The *non-relational proposition* for the *E component* of the CTE structure is:

- Remembered Experiences and its four dimensions were discovered in word data that are research participants' answers to open-ended questions asked during unstructured in-depth interviews. Ballard et al. (2006) explained, "The main questions asked of each participant were, What do you remember about the time when you were on the breathing machine and unable to move? and What events or conversations do you remember? Follow-up and clarifying probes (e.g., What was that like for you?) were used to elicit further meaning" (p. 89).

Source: Ballard, Robley, Barrett, Fraser, and Mendoza (2006).

A CTE STRUCTURE FOR CORRELATIONAL RESEARCH

Mefford and Alligood's (2011) journal article is an example of a report of Levine's Conservation Model–guided correlational research. The purpose of their study was to test a theory of health promotion of premature infants by means of a correlational path model research design (see Appendix A).

The sample for Mefford and Alligood's (2011) study included 235 preterm infants, born at less than 37 weeks gestation, who were hospitalized in a neonatal intensive care unit (NICU) and an associated intermediate care nursery (IMCN).

The conceptual model concepts are Conservation and its four dimensions (energy, structural integrity, personal integrity, and social integrity); Nursing Process as Conservation; and Health. The theory concepts are Physiological Immaturity, Structural Immaturity, Neurological Immaturity, Family System Characteristics, Intensity of Nursing Care, Consistency of Nursing Care, and Health Status at Discharge. The energy dimension of Conservation is represented by Physiological Immaturity; the structural integrity dimension of

Conservation is represented by Structural Immaturity; the personal integrity dimension of Conservation is represented by Neurological Immaturity; and the social integrity dimension of Conservation is represented by Family System Characteristics. Nursing Process as Conservation is represented by Intensity of Nursing Care and Consistency of Nursing Care. Health is represented by Health Status at Discharge.

Physiological Immaturity is measured by need for surfactant therapy and the Clinical Risk Index for Babies (CRIB; International Neonatal Network, 1993) scores for oxygenation and ventilation. Structural Immaturity is measured by two other components of the CRIB score—the infant's postconceptional age at birth and birth weight. Neurological Immaturity is measured by Apgar scores and degree of resuscitation at the time of the infant's birth. Family System Characteristics is measured by maternal demographics.

Intensity of Nursing Care is measured by direct nursing care hours during NICU and IMCN stay and numbers of other patients cared for by the nurse. Consistency of Nursing Care is measured by the shifts with care by the most frequent nurse caregiver and shifts with care by a first-time nurse caregiver. Health Status at Discharge is measured by the infant's postconceptional age and weight and morbidity score. Scores for all research instruments were analyzed using structural equation modeling to test the relations among the scores (see Appendix B).

The CTE structure constructed for Mefford and Alligood's (2011) study is illustrated in Figure 4.8. The non-relational and relational propositions for each component of the CTE structure are listed in Box 4.11.

A CTE STRUCTURE FOR EXPERIMENTAL RESEARCH

Mock, Krumm, et al.'s (2007) report of a randomized controlled clinical trial (RCCT; see Appendix A) is an example of Levine's Conservation Model–guided experimental research. Although the report is available only as an abstract, sufficient details are available for construction of the CTE structure, with supplemental content from a journal article by Mock, St. Ours, et al. (2007). The purpose of the Mock, Krumm, et al. (2007) study was "to determine the effects of a nurse-directed, home-based walking exercise program in maintaining physical functioning and managing symptoms during RT [radiation therapy] for prostate cancer" (p. 190).

The theory of the effects of walking exercise on general symptoms, fatigue, emotional distress, and physical function was tested using an experimental RCCT research design with random assignment of research participants to the experimental treatment group and the control treatment group. The research participants were 45 men who had stage I, II, or III prostate cancer and were receiving RT. The experimental treatment group received a walking exercise program, and the control treatment group received usual care. Data were collected before beginning RT and after 8 weeks of RT.

BOX 4.11   An Example of a Conceptual–Theoretical–Empirical Structure for Levine's Conservation Model Correlational Research

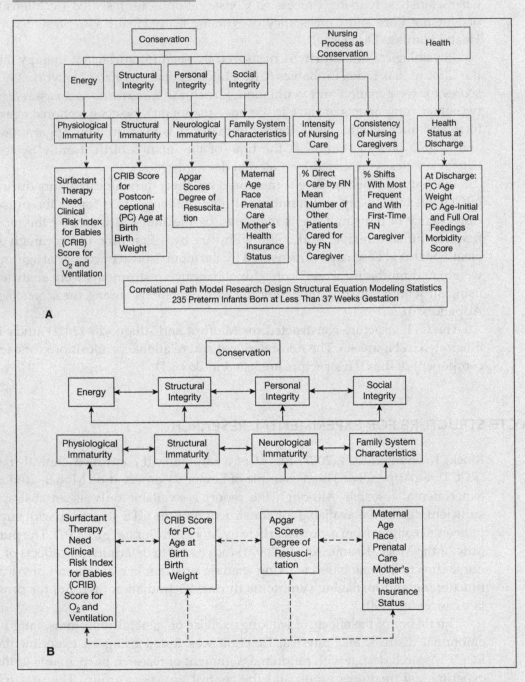

FIGURE 4.8 (A) Conceptual–theoretical–empirical (CTE) structure for Levine's Conservation Model correlational research—theory of health promotion of preterm infants: CTE linkages. (B) CTE structure for Levine's Conservation Model correlational research—theory of health promotion of preterm infants: C, T, and E interrelations. *(continued)*

(continued)

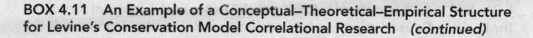

BOX 4.11 An Example of a Conceptual–Theoretical–Empirical Structure for Levine's Conservation Model Correlational Research *(continued)*

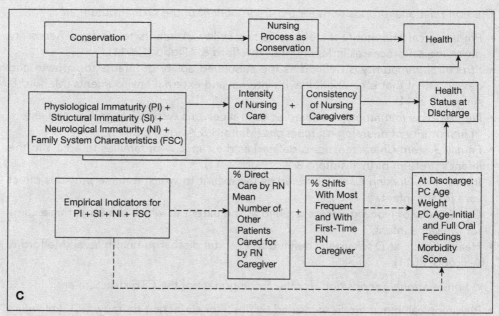

C

FIGURE 4.8 (C) CTE structure for Levine's Conservation Model correlational research—theory of health promotion of preterm infants: relational propositions.

The *non-relational propositions* for the *C component* of the conceptual–theoretical–empirical (CTE) structure are:

- *Conservation* is defined as "keeping together" (Levine, 1989, p. 331).
- The four dimensions of the concept are energy, structural integrity, personal integrity, and social integrity.
  - o *Energy* is defined as "balancing energy output and energy input to avoid excessive fatigue, that is, adequate rest, nutrition, and exercise" (Levine, 1988, p. 227).
  - o *Structural integrity* is defined as "maintaining or restoring the structure of the body, that is, preventing physical breakdown and promoting healing" (Levine, 1988, p. 227).
  - o *Personal integrity* is defined as "the maintenance or restoration of the patient's sense of identity, self-worth, and acknowledgment of uniqueness" (Levine, 1988, p. 227).
  - o *Social integrity* is defined as "acknowledgment of the patient as a social being" (Levine, 1988, p. 227).
- *Nursing Process as Conservation* is defined as a "scientific approach in the determination of nursing care" (Levine, 1966, p. 57).
- *Health* is defined as a pattern of adaptive change that is identified as such by each holistic being.

(continued)

BOX 4.11   An Example of a Conceptual–Theoretical–Empirical Structure for Levine's Conservation Model Correlational Research   *(continued)*

The *non-relational propositions* for the *T component* of the CTE structure are:

- *Physiological Immaturity* is defined as the ability of infants to perform necessary physiological processes independently (Mefford & Alligood, 2011).
- *Structural Immaturity* is defined as the continued ability of infants for growth and development that is compatible with internal and external environments (Mefford & Alligood, 2011).
- *Neurological Immaturity* is defined as central nervous system integration and extent of immaturity of neurological functions (Mefford & Alligood, 2011).
- *Family System Characteristics* is defined as the capacity of families to adjust to the infant's preterm birth (Mefford & Alligood, 2011).
- *Intensity of Nursing Care* is defined as the extent to which a nurse provides direct care for the infant.
- *Consistency of Nursing Care* is defined as the extent to which the same nurse cares for the same infant.
- *Health Status at Discharge* is defined as hospital discharge health level (Mefford & Alligood, 2011).

The *non-relational propositions* for the *E component* of the CTE structure are:

- Physiological Immaturity is measured by need for surfactant therapy, FiO_2 (minimum and maximum appropriate fraction of inspired oxygen), and base excess maximum, all during the first 12 hours of life (Mefford & Alligood, 2011). The FiO_2 scores are components of the Clinical Risk Index for Babies (CRIB; International Neonatal Network, 1993) scores for oxygenation (O_2) and ventilation.
- Structural Immaturity is measured by two components of the CRIB score-birth weight and postconceptual birth age (Mefford & Alligood, 2011).
- Neurological Immaturity is measured by 1- and 5-minute Apgar scores and extent of resuscitation required at time of delivery (Mefford & Alligood, 2011).
- Family System Characteristics is measured by the mother's age and race, as well as socioeconomic status, as measured by the proxies of extent of prenatal care and amount of health insurance (Mefford & Alligood, 2011).
- Intensity of Nursing Care is measured by percentage of registered nurse hours of the total of direct care while the infant was in a neonatal intensive care unit and while in an intermediate care nursery, and nurses' average amount of additional patient care while the infant was in a neonatal intensive care unit and in an intermediate care nursery (Mefford & Alligood, 2011).
- Consistency of Nursing Care is measured by percentage of shifts the infant was cared for by the same nurse and percentage of shifts the infant was cared for by a different nurse while in a neonatal intensive care unit and in an intermediate care nursery (Mefford & Alligood, 2011).
- Health Status at Discharge is measured by postconceptional age, weight, initial and full oral feeding age, and score for morbidity at the time of hospital discharge (Mefford & Alligood, 2011).

(continued)

BOX 4.11   An Example of a Conceptual–Theoretical–Empirical Structure for Levine's Conservation Model Correlational Research   *(continued)*

The *relational propositions* for the C and T components of the CTE structure are:

- The four dimensions of Conservation are interrelated.
- Therefore, Physiological, Structural, and Neurological Immaturity and Family System Characteristics are interrelated.
- Conservation is related to Nursing Process as Conservation.
- Therefore, Physiological Immaturity, Structural Immaturity, and Neurological Immaturity and Family System Characteristics are related to Intensity of Nursing Care and Consistency of Nursing Care.
- Nursing Process as Conservation has a positive effect on Health.
- Therefore, Intensity of Nursing Care and Consistency of Nursing Care are positively related to Health Status at Discharge.
- Conservation is related to Health.
- Therefore, Physiological Immaturity, Structural Immaturity, and Neurological Immaturity and Family System Characteristics are related to Health Status at Discharge.

The *relational propositions* for the E component of the CTE structure are:

- Surfactant therapy need and CRIB scores for O_2 and ventilation; CRIB scores for postconceptional age at birth and birth weight; Apgar scores and degree of resuscitation; and maternal age, race, prenatal care during pregnancy, and mother's health insurance status at the time of the infant's birth are interrelated.
- Surfactant therapy need, CRIB scores, Apgar scores, degree of resuscitation, maternal age, race, prenatal care during pregnancy, and mother's health insurance status at the time of the infant's birth are related to the percentage of direct care by the RN, mean number of other patients cared for by the RN caregiver, and percentage of shifts with most frequent and with first-time RN caregiver.
- Percentage of direct care by RN, mean number of other patients cared for by the RN caregiver, and percentage of shifts with most frequent and with first-time RN caregiver are related to postconceptional age at discharge, weight at discharge, postconceptional age at initial and full oral feedings, and morbidity scores.
- Surfactant therapy need, CRIB scores, Apgar scores, degree of resuscitation, maternal age, race, prenatal care during pregnancy, and mother's health insurance status at the time of the infant's birth are related to postconceptional age at discharge, weight at discharge, postconceptional age at initial and full oral feedings, and morbidity scores.

Source: Mefford and Alligood (2011).

The conceptual model concepts are the conservation of energy and conservation of structural integrity subdimensions of the intervention/action dimension of Nursing Process as Conservation and the energy and structural integrity dimensions of Conservation. One theory concept is Type of Nursing Intervention and its two dimensions—walking exercise program and usual care. The other theory concepts are General Symptoms, Fatigue, Emotional Distress, and Physical Function. Type of Nursing Intervention and its dimensions represent the conservation of energy and conservation of structural integrity subdimensions of the intervention/action dimension of Nursing Process as Conservation. General Symptoms, Fatigue, and Emotional Distress represent the energy dimension of Conservation, and Physical Function represents the structural integrity dimension of Conservation.

The walking exercise program dimension of Type of Nursing Intervention is operationalized by the experimental walking exercise program protocol. The usual care dimension of Type of Nursing Intervention is operationalized by the control usual care protocol. General Symptoms is measured by the Symptom Distress Scale (SDS; McCorkle & Young, 1978; Nuamah, Cooley, Fawcett, & McCorkle, 1999). Fatigue is measured by the Piper Fatigue Scale (Piper et al., 1998). Emotional Distress is measured by the Profile of Mood States (POMS; Shacham, 1983). Physical Function is measured by the Medical Outcomes Study—SF-36 physical functioning subscale (Ware & Sherbourne, 1992), the Physical Activity Questionnaire (Kohl et al., 1988), and treadmill tests of maximum rate of oxygen consumption (VO_2 max). Analyses of covariance (ANCOVA) statistics are used to analyze the data, with preradiation therapy scores as the covariates (see Appendix B).

The CTE structure constructed for Mock, Krumm, et al.'s (2007) study is illustrated in Figure 4.9. The non-relational and relational propositions for each component of the CTE structure are listed in Box 4.12.

A CTE STRUCTURE FOR MIXED-METHODS RESEARCH

No publications of mixed-methods research guided by Levine's Conservation Model could be located. Consequently, a hypothetical qualitative (qual) component was added to the quantitative experimental research (QUAN) conducted by Mock, Krumm, et al. (2007), based on content in Mock, St. Ours, et al. (2007).

The purpose of the QUAN portion of the study and the CTE structure for this portion of the study are the same as for the Mock, Krumm, et al. (2007) study discussed in the experimental research section of this chapter. The purpose of the hypothetical qual portion of the study is to describe the experimental research participants' thoughts about the walking exercise program. A simple descriptive research design is used (see Appendix A). The research participants are men with prostate cancer who are receiving RT and had been randomly assigned to the walking exercise program.

The conceptual model concept for the hypothetical qual portion of the study is Nursing Process as Conservation, with the relevant dimension of interaction/ action and the relevant subdimensions of conservation of energy and conservation of structural integrity. These subdimensions guided the selection of the empirical indicator and the analysis of the data for the QUAL portion of the study. The theory concept for the hypothetical QUAL portion of the study is

BOX 4.12 An Example of a Conceptual–Theoretical–Empirical Structure for Levine's Conservation Model Experimental Research

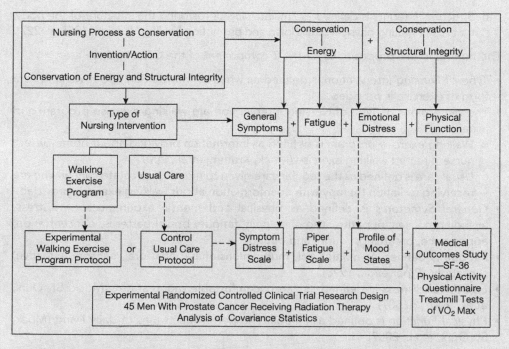

FIGURE 4.9 Conceptual–theoretical–empirical (CTE) structure for Levine's Conservation Model Experimental Research—theory of the effects of walking exercise on general symptoms: fatigue, emotional distress, and physical function.

VO₂ Max, maximum rate of oxygen consumption.

The *non-relational propositions* for the *C component* of the conceptual–theoretical–empirical (CTE) structure are:

- *Nursing Process as Conservation* is defined as a "scientific approach in the determination of nursing care" (Levine, 1966, p. 57).
- The relevant dimension of Nursing Process as Conservation is intervention/action.
  - *Intervention/action* is defined as a test of the hypothesis formulated by trophicognosis.
  - The two relevant subdimensions of intervention/action are conservation of energy and conservation of structural integrity.
    - *Conservation of energy* is defined as therapeutic nursing intervention that is targeted to the patient's energy through an adequate deposit of energy resources and regulation of the expenditure of energy.
    - *Conservation of structural integrity* is defined as therapeutic nursing intervention that is targeted to the patient's structural integrity through maintenance or restoration of the structure of the body cells, tissues, and organs.
- *Conservation* is defined as "keeping together" (Levine, 1989, p. 331).
- The two relevant dimensions of Conservation are energy and structural integrity.
  - *Energy* is defined as "balancing energy output and energy input to avoid excessive fatigue, that is, adequate rest, nutrition, and exercise" (Levine, 1988, p. 227).

(continued)

BOX 4.12 An Example of a Conceptual–Theoretical–Empirical Structure for Levine's Conservation Model Experimental Research *(continued)*

> o *Structural integrity* is defined as "maintaining or restoring the structure of the body, that is, preventing physical breakdown and promoting healing" (Levine, 1988, p. 227).

The *non-relational propositions* for the *T component* of the CTE structure are:

- *Type of Nursing Intervention* is defined as whether information about walking as a form of exercise is provided.
- The dimensions of Type of Nursing Intervention are walking exercise program and usual care.
  - o *Walking exercise program* is defined as information provided about home-based, nurse-directed walking exercise (Mock, Krumm, et al., 2007)
  - o *Usual care* is defined as the regular care given to men with prostate cancer who are receiving radiation therapy with no information about walking exercise provided.
- *General Symptoms* is defined as physical and mental experiences of distress, including nausea, appetite, insomnia, pain, fatigue, bowel patterns, concentration, appearance, breathing, cough, and outlook.
- *Fatigue* is defined as multicausal, multidimensional (behavioral, sensory, affective) sensations (Piper et al., 1998).
- *Emotional distress* is defined as "an uncomfortable mood state" (Mock, St. Ours, et al., 2007, p. 507).
- *Physical Function* is defined as an ability to perform activities of daily living (Mock, St. Ours, et al., 2007).

The *non-relational propositions* for the *E component* of the CTE structure are:

- Walking Exercise Program is operationalized by the experimental walking exercise program protocol, which stipulates brisk walking five to six times each week, increasing incrementally from 20 to 30 minutes (Mock, Krumm, et al., 2007).
- Usual Care is operationalized by the control usual care protocol, which includes no explicit information about exercise.
- General Symptoms is measured by the Symptom Distress Scale (SDS; McCorkle & Young, 1978; Nuamah, Cooley, Fawcett, & McCorkle, 1999). The SDS includes 13 items (presence of nausea, intensity of nausea, appetite, insomnia, presence of pain, intensity of pain, fatigue, bowel patterns, concentration, appearance, breathing, cough, and outlook that are rated on 5-point scale of 1 = no distress to 5 = extensive distress.
- Fatigue is measured by the Piper Fatigue Scale (PFS; Piper et al., 1998). Piper et al. (1998) explained that the PFS is made up of 22 items that measure overall fatigue and the behavioral/severity (six items), affective meaning (five items), sensory (five items), and cognitive/mood (six items) dimensions of subjective fatigue. Items are rated on a scale of 1 to 10 "that vary from the generic [none to a great deal] to the specific [e.g., able to concentrate to unable to concentrate]" (Piper et al., 1998, p. 680).
- Emotional Distress is measured by the Profile of Mood States (POMS; Shacham, 1983). The POMS subscales and their items are: depression (unhappy, sad, blue, hopeless, discouraged, miserable, helpless, worthless), vigor (lively, active, energetic, cheerful, full of pep, vigorous), confusion (confused, unable to concentrate, bewildered,

(continued)

BOX 4.12   An Example of a Conceptual–Theoretical–Empirical Structure for Levine's Conservation Model Experimental Research   (continued)

forgetful, uncertain about things), tension (tense, on edge, uneasy, restless, nervous, anxious), anger (angry, peeved, grovely, annoyed, resentful, bitter, furious), and fatigue (worn out, fatigued, exhausted, weary, bushed) (Shacham, 1983, p. 306). Each item is rated on the 5-point scale of "not at all" to "extremely."

- Physical Function is measured by the Medical Outcomes Study—SF-36 physical functioning subscale (MOS SF-36; Ware & Sherbourne, 1992), the Physical Activity Questionnaire (PAQ; Kohl et al., 1988), and treadmill tests of VO_2 Max.
  o The MOS SF-36 physical functioning subscale includes 10 items that are rated as "Yes, limited a lot," "Yes, limited a little," or "No, not limited at all" (Ware & Sherbourne, 1992, p. 483) The stem for the subscale is: "The following items are about activities you might do during a typical day. Does your health now limit you in these activities? If so, how much?" (Ware & Sherbourne, 1992, p. 482).
  o The PAQ included five items addressing recall of exercise and general physical activities during the past 3 months, including "strenuous racket sports; running; walking and jogging; bicycling; [and] swimming" (Kohl et al., 1988, p. 1231) that are answered "Yes" or "No."
  o Maximum rate of oxygen consumption (VO_2 max) is measured during treadmill walking.

The *relational propositions* for the C and T components of the CTE structure are:

- Nursing Process as Conservation is related to Conservation.
- Therefore, Type of Nursing Intervention is related to General Symptoms, Fatigue, Emotional Distress, and Physical Function.

The *relational proposition* for the E component of the CTE structure is:

- Participants who follow the walking exercise program protocol will have better scores on the Symptom Distress Scale, the PFS, POMS, MOS—SF-36, the PAQ, and the treadmill tests of VO_2 max than participants who receive usual care.

Source: Mock, Krumm, et al. (2007).

Intervention Thoughts and its four dimensions—personal reflections, progress, difficulties, and frustrations. The theory concept and its dimensions were generated from the participants' expressive narratives discovered by content analysis (see Appendix B) of their daily logs.

The CTE structure constructed for the hypothetical mixed-methods version of Mock, Krumm, et al.'s (2007) study is illustrated in Figure 4.10. The nonrelational and relational propositions for each component of the CTE structure are listed in Box 4.13.

BOX 4.13   An Example of a Conceptual–Theoretical–Empirical Structure for Levine's Conservation Model Mixed-Methods Research

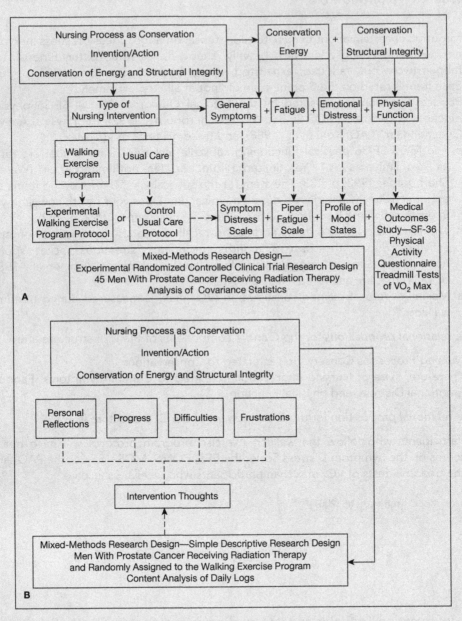

FIGURE 4.10 (A) Conceptual–theoretical–empirical (CTE) structure for Levine's Conservation Model mixed-methods research—theory of the effects of walking exercise on general symptoms, fatigue, emotional distress, and physical function— quantitative portion. (B) Conceptual–theoretical–empirical (CTE) structure for Levine's Conservation Model mixed-method research—theory of effects of walking exercise on symptoms and physical function—qualitative portion.

VO₂ Max, maximum rate of oxygen consumption.

(continued)

BOX 4.13   An Example of a Conceptual–Theoretical–Empirical Structure for Levine's Conservation Model Mixed-Methods Research   *(continued)*

The *non-relational propositions* for the *C component* of the conceptual–theoretical–empirical (CTE) structure for the hypothetical qualitative portion of the study are:

- *Nursing Process as Conservation* is defined as a "scientific approach in the determination of nursing care" (Levine, 1966, p. 57).
- The relevant dimension of Nursing Process as Conservation is intervention/action.
  - o *Intervention/action* is defined as a test of the hypothesis formulated by trophicognosis.
  - o The two relevant subdimensions of intervention/action are conservation of energy and conservation of structural integrity.
    - ▪ *Conservation of energy* is defined as therapeutic nursing intervention that is targeted to the patient's energy through an adequate deposit of energy resources and regulation of the expenditure of energy.
    - ▪ *Conservation of structural integrity* is defined as therapeutic nursing intervention that is targeted to the patient's structural integrity through maintenance or restoration of the structure of the body cells, tissues, and organs.

The *non-relational propositions* for the *T component* of the CTE structure for the hypothetical qualitative portion of the study are:

- *Intervention Thoughts* is defined as ideas about participating in the experimental walking exercise program.
- The four dimensions of Intervention Thoughts are personal reflections, progress, difficulties, and frustrations.
  - o *Personal reflections* is defined as thoughts about participating in the experimental walking exercise program.
  - o *Progress* is defined as thoughts about following the experimental walking exercise program protocol.
  - o *Difficulties* is defined as thoughts about problems with following the experimental walking exercise program protocol.
  - o *Frustrations* is defined as thoughts about disappointments about problems with following the experimental walking exercise program protocol.

The *non-relational proposition* for the *E component* of the CTE structure for the hypothetical qualitative portion of the study is:

- Intervention Thoughts and its dimensions were generated from content analysis of men's expressive narratives recorded in daily logs.

Source: Constructed for this chapter from Mock, Krumm, et al. (2007) and Mock, St. Ours, et al. (2007). See Box 4.12 for the concepts and propositions for the quantitative portion of the study.

CONCLUSION

Levine's Conservation Model represents a substantial contribution to the discipline of nursing by focusing attention on human wholeness, which is the central feature of the model. Levine (1995) stated, "I introduced . . . [wholeness] with the

Conservation Principles in 1964, and it has remained a hallmark of my work ever since" (p. 262).

Grindley and Paradowski (1991) maintained that "the adaptability of the model is one of its greatest strengths. The conservation principles have easily stood the test of time and the impact of technology" (p. 207). They went on to say:

> Individuals continue to be unique; they cope with ever-increasing assaults on their energies. The constant barrage on their integrities by the world around them reinforces the fact that the nurse must be ever alert to the potential and actual impact of these assaults. Holistic care touches the individual, the family, and the community. Levine's [propositions about conservation] are applicable not only to individuals but also to a larger group, the others who are significant to them. (pp. 207–208)

The comprehensive utility of Levine's Conservation Model is evident in the examples of its use as a guide for practice, quality improvement projects, and research given in this chapter. Schaefer (2002) commented, Levine's Conservation Model "has continued to have utility for nursing practice and research [and quality improvement projects] and is receiving increased recognition in this twenty-first century" (p. 219).

NOTE

1. Portions of this chapter are adapted from Fawcett and DeSanto-Madeya (2013, chapter 6), with permission.

REFERENCES

Ballard, N., Robley, L., Barrett, D., Fraser, D., & Mendoza, I. (2006). Patients' recollections of therapeutic paralysis in the intensive care unit. *American Journal of Critical Care, 15*, 86–94.

Burd, C., Langemo, D. K., Olson, B., Hanson, D., Hunter, S., & Sauvage, T. (1992). Skin problems: Epidemiology of pressure ulcers in a skilled care facility. *Journal of Gerontological Nursing, 18*(9), 29–39.

Burd, C., Olson, B., Langemo, D., Hunter, S., Hanson, D., Osowski, K. F., & Sauvage, T. (1994). Skin care strategies in a skilled nursing home. *Journal of Gerontological Nursing, 20*(11), 28–34.

Cooper, D. M. (1990). *Development and testing of an instrument to assess the visual characteristics of open, soft tissue wounds*. (Doctoral dissertation). Retrieved from ProQuest Dissertations and Theses Full Text (Dissertation Number 9026541; ProQuest Document ID 303887787).

Fawcett, J. (2014, September). Levine's conservation model: Bibliography update July 2012–September 2014. Unpublished.

Fawcett, J., & DeSanto-Madeya, S. (2013). *Contemporary nursing knowledge: Analysis and evaluation of nursing conceptual models and theories* (3rd ed.). Philadelphia, PA: F. A. Davis.

Grindley, J., & Paradowski, M. (1991). Developing an undergraduate program using Levine's model. In K. M. Schaefer & J. B. Pond (Eds.), *Levine's conservation model: A framework for nursing practice* (pp. 199–208). Philadelphia, PA: F. A. Davis.

Hanson, D. S., Langemo, D., Olson, B., Hunter, S., & Burd, C. (1994). Evaluation of pressure ulcer prevalence rates for hospice patients post-implementation of pressure ulcer protocols. *The American Journal of Hospice & Palliative Care, 11*(6), 14–19.

Hanson, D., Langemo, D. K., Olson, B., Hunter, S., Sauvage, T. R., Burd, C., & Cathcart-Silberberg, T. (1991). The prevalence and incidence of pressure ulcers in the hospice setting: Analysis of two methodologies. *American Journal of Hospice & Palliative Care, 8*(5), 18–22.

Hunter, S. M., Cathcart-Silberberg, T., Langemo, D. K., Olson, B., Hanson, D., Burd, C., & Sauvage, T. R. (1992). Pressure ulcer prevalence and incidence in a rehabilitation hospital. *Rehabilitation Nursing, 17*, 239–242.

Hunter, S. M., Langemo, D. K., Olson, B., Hanson, D., Cathcart-Silberberg, T., Burd, C., & Sauvage, T. R. (1995). The effectiveness of skin care protocols for pressure ulcers. *Rehabilitation Nursing, 20*, 250–255.

International Neonatal Network. (1993). The CRIB (clinical risk index for babies) score: A tool for assessing initial neonatal risk and comparing performance of neonatal intensive care units. *Lancet, 342*, 193–198.

Kohl, H. W., Blair, S. N., Paffenbarger, R. S., Macera, C. A., & Kronenfeld, J. J. (1988). A mail survey of physical activity habits as related to measured physical fitness. *American Journal of Epidemiology, 127*, 1228–1239.

Langemo, D. K., Olson, B., Hanson, D., Burd, C., Cathcart-Silberberg, T., & Hunter, S. (1990). Prevalence of pressure ulcers in five patient care settings. *Journal of Enterostomal Therapy, 17*, 187–192.

Langemo, D., Olson, B., Hanson, D., Hunter, S., Cathcart-Silberberg, T., & Sauvage, T. (1993). Pressure ulcer research: Prevalence, incidence, and evaluation of effectiveness of protocols. *The Prairie Rose, 62*(2), 13–16.

Langemo, D. K., Olson, B., Hunter, S., Burd, C., Hansen, D., & Cathcart-Silberberg, T. (1989). Incidence of pressure sores in acute care, rehabilitation, extended care, home health, and hospice in one locale. *Decubitus, 2*(2), 42.

Langemo, D. K., Olson, B., Hunter, S., Hanson, D., Burd, C., & Cathcart-Silberberg, T. (1991). Incidence and prediction of pressure ulcers in five patient care settings. *Decubitus, 4*(3), 25–26, 28, 30, 32, 36.

Levine, M. E. (1966). Trophicognosis: An alternative to nursing diagnosis. In *American Nurses' Association Regional Clinical Conference* (Vol. 2, pp. 55–70). New York, NY: American Nurses Association.

Levine, M. E. (1969). The pursuit of wholeness. *The American Journal of Nursing, 69*(1), 93–98.

Levine, M. E. (1973). *Introduction to clinical nursing* (2nd ed.). Philadelphia, PA: F. A. Davis.

Levine, M. E. (1988). Myra Levine. In T. M. Schorr & A. Zimmerman, *Making choices. Taking chances. Nurse leaders tell their stories* (pp. 215–228). St. Louis, MO: Mosby.

Levine, M. E. (1989). The conservation principles of nursing: Twenty years later. In J. P. Riehl (Ed.), *Conceptual models for nursing practice* (3rd ed., pp. 325–337). Norwalk, CT: Appleton & Lange.

Levine, M. E. (1990). Conservation and integrity. In M. E. Parker (Ed.), *Nursing theories in practice* (pp. 189–201). New York, NY: National League for Nursing.

Levine, M. E. (1991). The conservation principles: A model for health. In K. M. Schaefer and J. B. Pond (Eds.), *Levine's conservation model: A framework for nursing practice* (pp. 1–11). Philadelphia, PA: F. A. Davis.

Levine, M. E. (1995). Myra Levine responds [Letter to the editor]. *Image: Journal of Nursing Scholarship, 27*, 262.

Levine, M. E. (1996). The conservation principles: A retrospective. *Nursing Science Quarterly, 9*, 38–41.

McCall, B. H. (1991). Neurological intensive monitoring system: Unit assessment tool. In K. M. Schaefer & J. B. Pond (Eds.), *Levine's conservation model: A framework for nursing practice* (pp. 83–90). Philadelphia, PA: F. A. Davis.

McCorkle, R., & Young, K. (1978). Development of a symptom distress scale. *Cancer Nursing, 1,* 373–378.

Mefford, L. C., & Alligood M. R. (2011). Testing a theory of health promotion for preterm infants based on Levine's conservation model of nursing. *Journal of Theory Construction and Testing, 15*(2), 41–47.

Melnyk, B. M., & Fineout-Overholt, E. (2005). *Evidence-based practice in nursing and healthcare: A guide to best practice.* Philadelphia, PA: Lippincott Williams and Wilkins.

Mock, V., Krumm, S., Belcher, A., Stewart, K., DeWeese, T., Shang, J., & Hall, S. (2007). Exercise during prostate cancer treatment: Effects on functional status and symptoms. *Oncology Nursing Forum, 34,* 189–190 [Abstract].

Mock, V., St. Ours, C., Hall, S., Bositis, A., Tillery, M., Belcher, A., . . . McCorkle, R. (2007). Using a conceptual model in nursing research—mitigating fatigue in cancer patients. *Journal of Advanced Nursing, 58,* 503–512.

Nuamah, I. F., Cooley, M. E., Fawcett, J., & McCorkle, R. (1999). Testing a theory for health-related quality of life in cancer patients: A structural equation approach. *Research in Nursing & Health, 22,* 231–242.

Odesina, V., Bellini, S., Leger, R., Bona, R., Delaney, C., Andemariam, B., . . . Goodrich, S. E. (2010). Evidence-based sickle cell pain management in the emergency department. *Advanced Emergency Nursing Journal, 32,* 102–111.

Olson, B., Langemo, D., Burd, C., Hanson, D., Hunter, S., & Cathcart-Silberberg, T. (1996). Pressure ulcer incidence in an acute care setting. *Journal of Wound, Ostomy, and Continence Nursing, 23,* 15–22.

Piper, B. F., Dibble, S. L., Dodd, M. J., Weiss, M. C., Slaughter, R. E., & Paul, S. M. (1998). The revised Piper Fatigue Scale: Psychometric evaluation in women with breast cancer. *Oncology Nursing Forum, 25,* 677–684.

Popham, W. J. (1978). *Criterion-referenced measurement.* Englewood Cliffs, NJ: Prentice-Hall.

Schaefer, K. M. (1991). Levine's conservation principles and research. In K. M. Schaefer & J. B. Pond (Eds.), *Levine's conservation model: A framework for nursing practice* (pp. 45–59). Philadelphia, PA: F. A. Davis.

Schaefer, K. M. (2002). Myra Estrin Levine: The conservation model. In A. Marriner Tomey & M. R. Alligood (Eds.), *Nursing theorists and their work* (5th ed., pp. 212–225). St. Louis, MO: Mosby.

Schaefer, K. M. (2010). Myra Levine's conservation model. In M. E. Parker & M. C. Smith (Eds.), *Nursing theories and nursing practice* (3rd ed., pp. 83–103). Philadelphia, PA: F. A. Davis.

Shacham, S. (1983). A shortened version of the Profile of Mood States. *Journal of Personality Assessment, 47,* 305–306.

Tanabe, P., Myers, R., Zosel, A., Brice, J., Ansari, A. H., Evans, J., . . . Paice, J. A. (2007). Emergency department management of acute pain episodes in sickle cell disease. *Academic Emergency Medicine, 14,* 419–425.

Venes, D. (Ed.). (2013). *Taber's cylcopedic medical dictionary* (22nd ed.). Philadelphia, PA: F. A. Davis.

Ware, J. E., & Sherbourne, C. D. (1992). The MOS 36-item short-form health survey (SF-36). I. Conceptual framework and item selection. *Medical Care, 30,* 473–483.

CHAPTER 5

NEUMAN'S SYSTEMS MODEL[1]

Betty Neuman's Systems Model focuses on client system wellness and the environmental stressors that threaten optimal client system stability (Neuman, 2011). The goal of nursing guided by Neuman's Systems Model is facilitation of optimal wellness of client systems through retention, attainment, or maintenance of client system stability.

NEUMAN'S SYSTEMS MODEL: CONCEPTS AND NON-RELATIONAL PROPOSITIONS

This section of the chapter includes the concepts of Neuman's Systems Model and the definitions (non-relational propositions) of the concepts and dimensions of the multidimensional concepts (Neuman, 2011).

Client/Client System is defined as an open system that interacts with the internal and external environments. The four dimensions of the concept are individual, family, community, and social issue.

Individual is defined as an individual person.

Family is defined as a type of group.

Community is defined as a type of group.

Social issue is defined as a policy or major concern of society.

Interacting Variables is defined as the five components of the client system that function more or less harmoniously in interactions with internal and external environmental stressors. The extent of the interactions between and among the five variables determines how much resistance a client system has to environmental stressors. The five dimensions of the concept are physiological variables, psychological variables, sociocultural variables, developmental variables, and spiritual variables.

Physiological variable is defined as the structures and functions of the physical body.

Psychological variable is defined as internal and external psychological processes and interactions with others.

Sociocultural variable is defined as the influences of social and cultural aspects of life.

Developmental variable is defined as processes of growth and development across the life span.

Spiritual variable is defined as beliefs and values about the meaning of life and the world, of which the client system may be fully aware to not at all aware.

Central Core is defined as the basic structure of the client system, which is made up of basic survival factors that are common to all human beings.

Normal Line of Defense is defined as the client system's normal or usual wellness level, which reflects a typical yet evolving range of responses to environmental stressors; expansion of the normal line of defense reflects an enhanced wellness state, whereas contraction reflects a diminished state of wellness.

Flexible Line of Defense is defined as the outer boundary of the client system, which is a buffer that protects the client system's normal line of defense from stressor invasion; the flexible line of defense is highly dynamic in that it can rapidly expand away from the normal line of defense, offering greater protection, or rapidly draw closer to the normal line of defense, offering less protection.

Lines of Resistance is defined as internal factors that protect the central core and support return of the client system to wellness at the same or a higher state of wellness.

Internal Environment is defined as all forces or interacting factors that are internal to the client system, including intrapersonal stressors.

External Environment is defined as all forces or interacting factors that are external to the client system, including interpersonal and extrapersonal stressors.

Created Environment is defined as the client system's perception of his or her life and surroundings, his or her construction of reality (Neuman, 2001).

Stressors is defined as internal and external forces that produce tensions that may be beneficial or noxious. The three dimensions of the concept are intrapersonal stressors, interpersonal stressors, and extrapersonal stresssors.

Intrapersonal stressors is defined as internal environmental forces.

Interpersonal stressors is defined as proximal external environmental forces.

Extrapersonal stressors is defined as distal external environmental forces.

Health/Wellness/Optimal Client System Stability is defined as "the best possible wellness state at any given time" (Neuman, 2011, p. 23).

Variances From Wellness is defined as "varying degrees of system instability [that] are caused by stressor invasion of the normal line of defense" (Neuman, 2011, p. 24).

Illness is defined as "a state of insufficiency with disrupting needs unsatisfied" (Neuman, 2011, p. 24).

Reconstitution is defined as "the successful mobilization of client resources to prevent further stressor reaction or regression; it represents a dynamic state of adjustment to stressors and integration of all necessary factors towards optimal use of existing resources for client system stability or wellness maintenance.... Complete reconstitution may progress well beyond the previously determined normal line of defense or usual wellness state, it may stabilize the system at a lower level, or it may return to the level prior to illness.... [If reconstitution does not occur,] death occurs as a result of failure of the basic structure" (Neuman, 2011, pp. 28–29).

Prevention as Intervention is defined as the goals and outcomes components of Neuman's System Model Nursing Process Format. The three dimensions of the concept of Prevention as Intervention are primary prevention as intervention, secondary prevention as intervention, and tertiary prevention as intervention.

> *Primary prevention as intervention* is defined as retention of wellness by increasing the strength of the flexible line of defense by means of prevention of stress and reducing risk factors (Neuman, 2011).

> *Secondary prevention as intervention* is defined as attainment of wellness by increasing the strength of the lines of resistance by means of symptom management and treatment (Neuman, 2011).

> *Tertiary prevention as intervention* is defined as maintenance of wellness by protecting the attainment of wellness from secondary prevention as intervention by means of support of the client system's strengths and energy reserves (Neuman, 2011).

NEUMAN'S SYSTEMS MODEL: RELATIONAL PROPOSITIONS

The statements of associations (relational propositions) among the concepts of Neuman's Systems Model are listed here.

- The physiological, psychological, sociocultural, developmental, and spiritual variables are interrelated.
- The relation between Stressors and the Normal Line of Defense is moderated by the Flexible Line of Defense.

- The relation between Stressors and the Lines of Resistance is mediated by the Normal Line of Defense.
- The Lines of Resistance are positively related to the Central Core.
- Prevention as Intervention and its dimensions have a positive effect on the Flexible Line of Defense, the Normal Line of Defense, and the Lines of Resistance.
- Prevention as Intervention and its dimensions have a positive effect on Optimal Client System Stability.

NEUMAN'S SYSTEMS MODEL: APPLICATION TO NURSING PRACTICE

The guidelines for Neuman's Systems Model nursing practice are listed in Box 5.1. A diagram of the practice methodology for Neuman's Systems Model, which is called the Nursing Process Format, is illustrated in Figure 5.1.

A practice tool that includes all parts of the practice methodology is given in Box 5.2.

A Conceptual–Theoretical–Empirical Structure for Assessment

A portion of Fashinpaur's (2002) book chapter provides an example of Neuman's Systems Model nursing practice focused on assessment. She developed the Neuman Postpartum Mood Questionnaire (NPMQ) to screen for postpartum mood disorders (PPMD). Fashinpaur (2002) explained that the NPMQ "is a [postpartum mood disorders] assessment tool intended for use in initiating dialogue between the nurse and new mother about her postpartum emotional status that will provide data for the development of a nursing diagnosis" (p. 77).

The theory is assessment of the occurrence of PPMD. The conceptual model concept is Interacting Variables with its five dimensions—physiological variable, psychological variable, sociocultural variable, developmental variable, and spiritual variable. The theory concept is PPMD and its five dimensions—physiology; cognition; feelings about partner, baby, and motherhood; history of depression; and spirituality.

Interacting Variables is represented by PPMD. The physiological variable dimension of Interacting Variables is represented by the physiology dimension of PPMD; the psychological variable dimension of Interacting Variables is represented by the cognition dimension of PPMD; the sociocultural variable dimension of Interacting Variables is represented by the feelings about partner, baby, and motherhood dimension of PPMD; the developmental variable dimension of Interacting Variables is represented by the history of depression dimension of PPMD; and the spiritual variable dimension of Interacting Variables is represented by the spirituality dimension of PPMD. All five dimensions of PPMD are measured by the NPMQ.

BOX 5.1   Guidelines for Neuman's Systems Model Nursing Practice

The purpose of nursing practice is to assist client systems in retaining, attaining, or maintaining the optimal system stability achievable at a given point in time.

Practice problems of interest are the client system's actual or potential reactions to stressors.

Settings for practice include any health care or community-based setting, as well as situations that involve virtual contact between client systems and caregivers using distance technology and the Internet.

Participants in practice include client systems who are faced with actual or potential stressors, along with their health professional or layperson caregivers, who come together in physical or virtual spaces. Individuals, families, groups, communities, and entire health care teams are regarded as human client systems. The client system and the caregiver are engaged in a reciprocal partnership, the goal of which is to assist the client system to achieve the highest possible level of system stability.

The practice process is the Neuman Systems Model Nursing Process Format, which encompasses three components—diagnosis, goals, and outcomes.

Diagnoses may be classified in a taxonomy, using five organizing principles derived from the Neuman's Systems Model—(a) human client system (individual, family, group, community); (b) level of response (primary, secondary, tertiary); (c) interacting variable(s) responding to the stressor (physiological, psychological, sociocultural, developmental, spiritual); and (d) type of stressor (intrapersonal, interpersonal, extrapersonal).

Goals for practice are determined through a process of negotiation between the client system and caregiver that involves the client system as a full participant in determining the desired result(s), to the extent possible.

Caregiver actions used to assist the client system to achieve optimum system stability occur as primary, secondary, or tertiary prevention as interventions, depending on the degree to which stressors have penetrated the client system's lines of defense and resistance.

Outcomes may be general or specific to the particular client system. General outcomes are statements about the concepts of Neuman's Systems Model that are derived from the content of the model. Client system–specific outcomes involve application of the general statements to particular situations.

Practice effectiveness depends on the application of research findings—that is, evidence—to direct practice. In turn, problems encountered in practice give rise to new research questions.

Adapted from Fawcett and DeSanto-Madeya (2013), with permission.

The conceptual–theoretical–empirical (CTE) structure constructed from the content of this portion of Fashinpaur's (2002) book chapter is illustrated in Figure 5.2. The non-relational propositions for each component of the CTE structure are listed in Box 5.3.

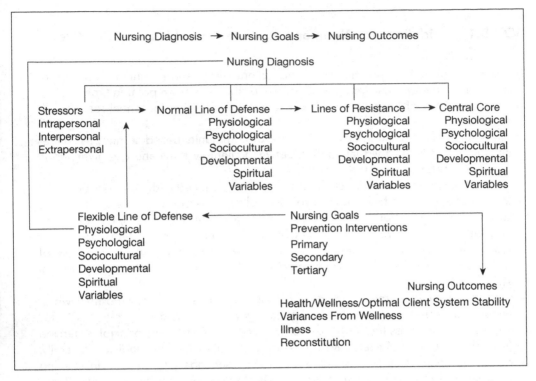

FIGURE 5.1 Neuman's Systems Model practice methodology: The nursing process format.

A CTE Structure for Intervention

Another portion of Fashinpaur's (2002) book chapter provides an example of Neuman's Systems Model nursing practice focused on intervention. Fashinpaur (2002) pointed out that "By implementing these [primary] prevention interventions…nurses will strengthen the flexible defense lines of the systems of the women and families with whom they work, thus preventing PPMD experiences. Primary prevention intervention will reduce or eliminate the impact of PPMD stressors on the normal defense lines and lines of resistance of childbearing client systems" (p. 84).

The theory is effect of PPMD information on reduction of occurrence of PPMD. One conceptual model concept is Prevention as Intervention, and the relevant dimension is primary prevention as intervention. The other conceptual model concept is Flexible Line of Defense.

The theory concepts are Postpartum Mood Disorders Information and Postpartum Mood Disorders (PPMD). PPMD Information represents the primary prevention as intervention dimension of Prevention as Intervention, and is operationalized by the PPMD Information protocol. PPMD represents the Flexible Line of Defense, and is measured by the NPMQ (Fashinpaur, 2002).

BOX 5.2   The Neuman's Systems Model Practice Methodology Tool

NURSING DIAGNOSIS

Physiological Variable

How do you usually feel physically? (Normal line of defense)
How do you feel physically today? (Flexible line of defense)
What happened to make you feel this way? (Stressors)

Psychological Variable

How do you usually feel emotionally? (Normal line of defense)
How do you feel emotionally today? (Flexible line of defense)
What happened to make you feel this way? (Stressors)

Sociocultural Variable

Please tell me about your lifestyle and culture. (Normal line of defense)
What changes have you experienced in your lifestyle and culture recently? (Flexible line of defense)
What has happened to result in these changes? (Stressors)

Developmental Variable

What are your current goals for yourself? (Normal line of defense)
In what ways have your personal goals changed recently? (Flexible line of defense)
What has happened to result in these changes? (Stressors)

Spiritual Variable

What are your spiritual beliefs? What gives your life meaning? What gives you hope? (Normal line of defense)
Have your spiritual beliefs, ideas about meaning in life, and/or sources of hope changed recently? (Flexible line of defense)
What has happened to result in this change? (Stressors)

NURSING GOALS

The nurse and the client system identify goals for primary, secondary, and/or tertiary prevention as intervention.

NURSING OUTCOMES

The nurse and the client system implement primary, secondary, and/or tertiary prevention as interventions and evaluate outcomes.

Adapted from Fawcett and DeSanto-Madeya (2013).

The CTE structure constructed from the content of this portion of Fashinpaur's (2002) book chapter is illustrated in Figure 5.3. The non-relational and relational propositions for each component of the CTE structure are listed in Box 5.4.

BOX 5.3   An Example of a Conceptual–Theoretical–Empirical Structure for Neuman's Systems Nursing Practice: Assessment

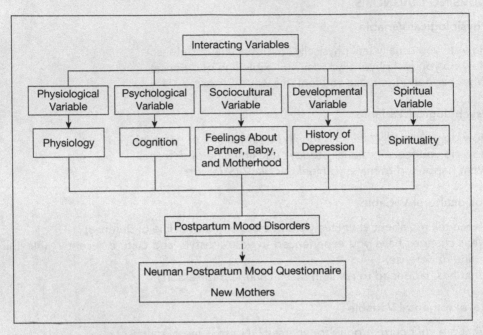

FIGURE 5.2 Conceptual–theoretical–empirical (CTE) structure for Neuman's System Model nursing practice: Assessment—theory of assessment of the occurrence of postpartum mood disorders.

The *non-relational propositions* for the *C component* of the conceptual–theoretical–empirical (CTE) structure are:

- *Interacting Variables* is defined as the five components of the client system, which function more or less harmoniously in interactions with internal and external environmental stressors. The extent of the interactions between and among the five variables determines how much resistance a client system has to environmental stressors.
- The five dimensions of Interacting Variables are physiological variable, psychological variable, sociocultural variable, developmental variable, and spiritual variable.
  - o *Physiological variable* is defined as the structures and functions of the physical body (Neuman, 2011).
  - o *Psychological variable* is defined as "mental processes and interactive environmental effects, both internally and externally" (Neuman, 2011, p. 16).
  - o *Sociocultural variable* is defined as "combined effects of social cultural conditions and influences" (Neuman, 2011, p. 16).
  - o *Developmental variable* is defined as "age-related development[al] processes and activities" (Neuman, 2011, p. 16).

(continued)

BOX 5.3 An Example of a Conceptual–Theoretical–Empirical Structure for Neuman's Systems Nursing Practice: Assessment *(continued)*

---

    o *Spiritual variable* is defined as "spiritual beliefs and influences...[which are] on a continuum of dormant, unacceptable, or undeveloped to recognition, development, and positive system influence" (Neuman, 2011, pp. 16–17).

The *non-relational propositions* for the *T component* of the CTE structure are:

- *Postpartum Mood Disorder* (PPMD) is defined as "an unexpected illness that robs the new mother, and consequently other family members, of happiness" (Fashinpaur, 2002, p. 74). PPDMs include postpartum major depression, new-onset obsessive-compulsive disorder, and postpartum psychosis. Baby blues are not considered a PPMD (Fashinpaur, 2002).
- The five dimensions of PPMDs are physiology; cognition; feelings about partner, baby, and motherhood; history of depression; and spirituality.
  - o *Physiology* is defined as sleep and/or appetite disturbances (Fashinpaur, 2002).
  - o *Cognition* is defined as feelings of sadness, anxiety, or fear (Fashinpaur, 2002).
  - o *Feelings about partner, baby, and motherhood* is defined as feelings of distance from partner and/or baby and feelings about self as mother (Fashinpaur, 2002).
  - o *History of depression* is defined as past experiences of depression of new mother and/or family members (Fashinpaur, 2002).
  - o *Spirituality* is defined as feelings of hopelessness and feelings about who the new mother is as a person (Fashinpaur, 2002).

The *non-relational propositions* for the *E component* of the CTE structure are:

- The five dimensions of PPMDs are assessed by the Neuman Postpartum Mood Questionnaire (NPMQ). The NPMQ includes 21 questions that ask the new mother about "potential reactions to PPMD stressors" (Fashinpaur, 2002, p. 77). The possible answers to the questions are "Yes" or "No." Scores are not computed for answers but rather the answers are used to "facilitate mutually collaborative exploration of each item" by the nurse and new mother (Fashinpaur, 2002, p. 78). The NPMQ may be used for self-report by new mothers or as an interview guide used by the nurse.

Source: Fashinpaur (2002).

NEUMAN'S SYSTEMS MODEL: APPLICATION TO QUALITY IMPROVEMENT PROJECTS

The guidelines for Neuman's Systems Model quality improvement (QI) projects are listed in Box 5.5.

A CTE Structure for a QI Project

Hammonds's (2012) journal article is an example of a report of a Neuman's Systems Model–guided QI project. Hammonds stated that the purpose of her

BOX 5.4 An Example of a Conceptual–Theoretical–Empirical Structure for Neuman's Systems Nursing Practice: Intervention

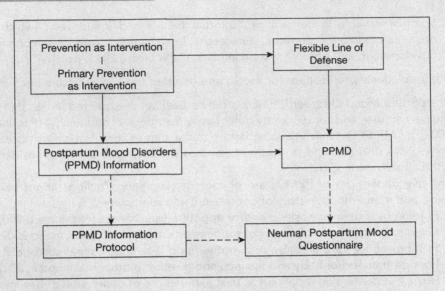

FIGURE 5.3 Conceptual–theoretical–empirical (CTE) structure for Neuman's Systems Model nursing practice: Intervention—theory of the effect of PPMD Information on reduction of occurrence of PPMD.

The *non-relational propositions* for the *C component* of the conceptual–theoretical–empirical (CTE) structure are:

- *Prevention as Intervention* is defined as the goals and outcomes components of Neuman's System Model Nursing Process Format.
- The relevant dimension of Prevention as Intervention is primary prevention as intervention.
  - o *Primary prevention as intervention* is defined as retention of wellness by increasing the strength of the flexible line of defense by means of prevention of stress and reducing risk factors (Neuman, 2011).
- *Flexible Line of Defense* is defined as the outer boundary of the client system, which is a buffer that protects the client system's normal line of defense from stressor invasion; the flexible line of defense is highly dynamic in that it can rapidly expand away from the normal line of defense, offering greater protection, or rapidly draw closer to the normal line of defense, offering less protection.

The *non-relational propositions* for the *T component* of the CTE structure are:

- *Postpartum Mood Disorders (PPMD) Information* is defined as educational materials about PPMD.

(continued)

BOX 5.4   An Example of a Conceptual–Theoretical–Empirical Structure for Neuman's Systems Nursing Practice: Intervention   *(continued)*

- *PPMD* is defined as "an unexpected illness that robs the new mother, and consequently other family members, of happiness" (Fashinpaur, 2002, p. 74). PPMDs include postpartum major depression, new-onset obsessive-compulsive disorder, and postpartum psychosis. Baby blues are not considered a PPMD (Fashinpaur, 2002).
- The five dimensions of PPMD are physiology; cognition; feelings about partner, baby, and motherhood; history of depression; and spirituality.
  - o *Physiology* is defined as sleep and/or appetite disturbances (Fashinpaur, 2002).
  - o *Cognition* is defined as feelings of sadness, anxiety, or fear (Fashinpaur, 2002).
  - o *Feelings about partner, baby, and motherhood* is defined as feelings of distance from partner and/or baby and feelings about self as mother (Fashinpaur, 2002).
  - o *History of depression* is defined as past experiences of depression of new mother and/or family members (Fashinpaur, 2002).
  - o *Spirituality* is defined as feelings of hopelessness and feelings about who the new mother is as a person (Fashinpaur, 2002).

The *non-relational propositions* for the *E* component of the CTE structure are:

- PPMD Information is operationalized by the PPMD Information protocol. Fashinpaur (2002) recommended that information about types, time of occurrence, and signs and symptoms of PPMD should be provided to nurses, nurse midwives, nurse practitioners, nurse counselors, visiting nurses, lactation consultants, obstetricians, pediatricians, and new mothers and should be included in the curriculum of childbirth education classes and nursing education programs. She also indicated that PPMD Information should be more widely disseminated via publications and presentations at conferences and group meetings of new mothers and parents, and should be made available in public libraries and community resource centers for women.
- The five dimensions of PPMD are measured by the Neuman Postpartum Mood Questionnaire (NPMQ). The NPMQ includes 21 questions that ask the new mother about "potential reactions to PPMD stressors" (Fashinpaur, 2002, p. 77). The possible answers to the questions are "Yes" or "No." Scores are not computed for answers but rather the answers are used to "facilitate mutually collaborative exploration of each item" by the nurse and new mother (Fashinpaur, 2002, p. 78). The NPMQ may be used for self-report by new mothers or as an interview guide used by the nurse.

The *relational propositions* for the *C* and *T* components of the CTE structure are:

- The primary prevention as intervention dimension of Prevention as Intervention has a positive effect on the Flexible Line of Defense, such that use of primary prevention as intervention strengthens the Flexible Line of Defense.
- Therefore, PPMD Information has a negative effect on occurrence of PPMD, that is, reduces the occurrence of PPMD.

(continued)

BOX 5.4 An Example of a Conceptual–Theoretical–Empirical Structure for Neuman's Systems Nursing Practice: Intervention *(continued)*

The *relational proposition* for the *E component* of the CTE structure is:

- Provision of the PPMD Information protocol will reduce the number of "Yes" responses to the NPMQ items, which indicates a reduction in the occurrence of PPMDs.

Source: Fashinpaur (2002).

BOX 5.5 Guidelines for Neuman's Systems Model Quality Improvement Projects

The purpose of quality improvement (QI) projects is to test the effectiveness of nurses' use of Neuman's Prevention as Intervention modalities (primary, secondary, and/or tertiary prevention as intervention) on nurses' and/or client systems' optimal system stability.

The phenomenon of interest for a QI project is the extent of nurses' use of Prevention as Intervention Nursing modalities (primary prevention as intervention, secondary prevention as intervention, tertiary prevention as intervention) on nurses' and/or clients' optimal system stability.

Data for QI projects are to be collected from client systems (including nurses) in various settings, such as clients' homes, nurses' private offices, ambulatory clinics, hospitals, and communities.

Any methodological theory of change or QI may be used to guide the design of the QI project and the times for data collection. Checklists, rating scales, and responses to open-ended questions may be used to determine the extent to which nurses actually implement Prevention as Intervention modalities. Descriptive statistics may be used to analyze data obtained from checklists or rating scales, and content analysis may be used to identify categories or themes found in responses to open-ended questions.

The results of Neuman's Systems Model–based QI projects enhance understanding of how using Prevention as Intervention modalities influences optimal client system stability.

QI project was to determine whether outpatient clinic oncology nurses' use of the Distress Thermometer facilitates identification of distress and referral for support for clients diagnosed with breast cancer attending an outpatient clinic.

The theory is the theory of outcomes of use of the Distress Thermometer. One conceptual model concept is Prevention as Intervention and its three dimensions—primary prevention as intervention, secondary prevention as intervention, and tertiary prevention as intervention. The other conceptual model concept is Flexible Line of Defense. One theory concept is Distress Nursing Interventions; its dimensions are education, implementation, and referral. The other theory concept is Distress.

The primary prevention as intervention dimension of Prevention as Intervention is represented by the education dimension of Distress Nursing Interventions; the secondary prevention as intervention dimension is represented by the implementation dimension of Distress Nursing Interventions; and the tertiary prevention as intervention dimension is represented by the referral dimension of Distress Nursing Interventions. The Flexible Line of Defense is represented by Distress.

Distress Nursing Interventions is operationalized by the Distress Nursing Interventions protocol. Hammonds (2012) explained that the protocol is guided by the Johns Hopkins Nursing evidence-based practice model and guidelines and the practice question, evidence, and translation (PET) model (Newhouse, Dearholt, Poe, Pugh, & White, 2007), which is a QI methodological theory (see Appendix A). Distress is measured by the Distress Thermometer (National Comprehensive Cancer Network, 2012, 2013) and a chart audit to determine the number of clients who experienced distress and the number of clients who were referred for support. Hammonds (2012) used descriptive statistics (frequencies, calculated as absolute risk; see Appendix B) to analyze the data.

The CTE structure constructed from an interpretation of Hammonds' (2012) journal article is illustrated in Figure 5.4. The non-relational and relational propositions for each component of the CTE structure are listed in Box 5.6.

NEUMAN'S SYSTEMS MODEL: APPLICATION TO NURSING RESEARCH

The guidelines for Neuman's Systems Model nursing research are listed in Box 5.7.

A CTE Structure for a Systematic Literature Review

Skalski, DiGerolamo, and Gigliotti's (2006) journal article is an example of a literature review guided by Neuman's Systems Model. The purpose of their integrative literature review was "to identify and categorize client systems stressors in NSM [Neuman's Systems Model]-based studies" (p. 71).

Skalski et al. (2006) explained, "The NSM research literature from 1983 to February 2005 was searched using Fawcett's (2005) NSM bibliography and a follow-up review of the [Cumulative Index to Nursing and Allied Health Literature] CINAHL database using the keywords 'Neuman's systems model' and 'stressors'" (p. 71). They applied Cooper's (1989) five-stage integrative review method (see Appendix A) to 13 studies of stressors from a total of 87 research reports they had identified and reviewed.

BOX 5.6 An Example of a Neuman's Systems Model Quality Improvement Project

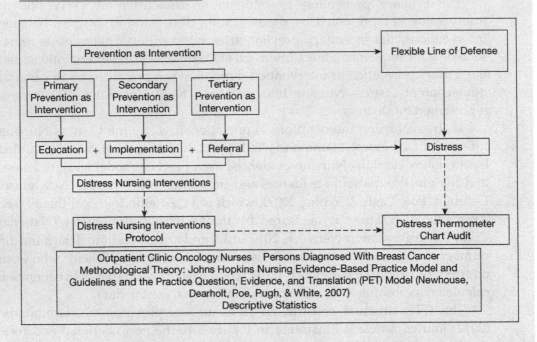

FIGURE 5.4 Conceptual–theoretical–empirical (CTE) structure for a Neuman's Systems Model quality improvement project—theory of outcomes of use of the distress thermometer.

The *non-relational propositions* for the C *component* of the conceptual–theoretical–empirical (CTE) structure are:

- *Prevention as Intervention* is defined as the goals and outcomes components of Neuman's System Model Nursing Process Format.
- The relevant dimensions of Prevention as Intervention are primary prevention as intervention, secondary prevention as intervention, and tertiary prevention as intervention.
  - *Primary prevention as intervention* is defined as retention of wellness by increasing the strength of the flexible line of defense by means of prevention of stress and reducing risk factors (Neuman, 2011).
  - *Secondary prevention as intervention* is defined as attainment of wellness by increasing the strength of the lines of resistance by means of symptom management and treatment (Neuman, 2011).
  - *Tertiary prevention as intervention* is defined as maintenance of wellness by protecting the attainment of wellness from secondary prevention as intervention by means of support of the client system's strengths and energy reserves (Neuman, 2011).

(continued)

BOX 5.6   An Example of a Neuman's Systems Model Quality Improvement Project   (continued)

- *Flexible Line of Defense* is defined as the outer boundary of the client system, which is a buffer that protects the client system's normal line of defense from stressor invasion; the flexible line of defense is highly dynamic in that it can rapidly expand away from the normal line of defense, offering greater protection, or rapidly draw closer to the normal line of defense, offering less protection.

The *non-relational propositions* for the *T component* of the CTE structure are:

- *Distress Nursing Interventions* is defined as actions taken by nurses on behalf of clients who may experience distress.
- The dimensions of Distress Nursing Interventions are education, implementation, and referral.
  - o *Education* is defined as "educating [clients] about distress and cancer" (Hammonds, 2012, p. 493).
  - o *Implementation* is defined as "administering the Distress Thermometer" (Hammonds, 2012, p. 493).
  - o *Referral* is defined as "referring [clients] for additional evaluation and support" (Hammonds, 2012, p. 493).
- *Distress* is defined as "disturbing psychological, social, and spiritual discomfort of varying intensity experienced by [clients] with cancer" (National Comprehensive Cancer Network, as cited in Hammonds, 2012, p. 491).

The *non-relational propositions* for the *E component* of the CTE structure are:

- Distress Nursing Interventions is operationalized by the Distress Nursing Intervention protocol. The protocol content and processes are guided by the Johns Hopkins Nursing evidence-based practice model and guidelines and the practice question, evidence, and translation (PET) model (Newhouse, Dearholt, Poe, Pugh, & White, 2007), which is a methodological theory for quality improvement. Hammonds (2012) explained, "In the Johns Hopkins Nursing model, nurses evaluate evidence for implementing a quality improvement project, whereas the PET model is used for successfully implementing that project.... A clinic nurse discussed the commonness of distress with cancer, and the Distress Thermometer was administered. A clinic nurse discussed the individual responses with each [client], collected the [Distress Thermometer], offered a referral for support to [clients] with [Distress Thermometer] scores of 4 or higher, and arranged referrals for [clients] who agreed to them. Options for referral included psychiatric mental health nurse practitioner, social worker, chaplain, dietitian, primary care provider, and oncology provider" (p. 493).
- Distress is measured by the Distress Thermometer (National Comprehensive Cancer Network, 2012, 2013) and a chart audit to determine the number of clients who experienced distress and the number of clients who were referred for support. The Distress Thermometer includes a vertical illustration of a thermometer, on which the amount of distress is rated on a scale of 0 = no distress to 10 = extreme distress. The Distress Thermometer also includes a checklist of practical, family, emotional, and physical problems, which are answered as "Yes" or "No," as well as spiritual/religious concerns. A space to add other problems is also provided.

(continued)

BOX 5.6 An Example of a Neuman's Systems Model Quality Improvement Project *(continued)*

The *relational propositions* for the C and T components of the CTE structure are:

- Prevention as Intervention and its dimensions have a positive effect on the Flexible Line of Defense, such that use of primary, secondary, and tertiary preventions as interventions strengthens the Flexible Line of Defense.
- Therefore, Distress Nursing Interventions have a positive effect on Distress, such that use of the Distress Nursing Interventions increases identification of clients experiencing distress and referral of those clients for support.

The *relational proposition* for the E component of the CTE structure is:

- Implementation of the Distress Nursing Interventions protocol increases outpatient clinical oncology nurses' identification of distress experienced by clients with breast cancer and increases referral for support for the clients whose Distress Thermometer score is 4 or higher.

Source: Hammonds (2012).

Skalski et al. (2006) explicitly labeled the results of their literature review as the theory of caregiver role strain. The conceptual model concept Stressors and its three dimensions—intrapersonal stressors, interpersonal stressors, and extrapersonal stressors—guided the literature review. The theory concept that emerged from the literature review is Stress and its three dimensions—caregiver responsibility, role conflict/role fatigue/role stress, and caregiver role strain.

The CTE structure constructed for Skalski et al.'s (2006) literature review is illustrated in Figure 5.5. The non-relational propositions for each component of the CTE structure are listed in Box 5.8. Two relational propositions for the T component that were generated from the results of the literature review also are included in Box 5.8.

A CTE Structure for Instrument Development

Carrigg and Weber's (1997) report of the development and psychometric testing of the Spiritual Care Scale (SCS) is a source for construction of a Neuman's Systems Model CTE structure for instrument development.

The theory is spiritual care. The conceptual model concept is Interacting Variables and its relevant dimension is spiritual variable. The theory concept is Spiritual Care, which has four dimensions—faith, empowerment, meaningfulness, and psychosocial care. The spiritual variable dimension of Interacting Variables is represented by Spiritual Care and its dimensions.

Spiritual Care and its dimensions are measured by the SCS. Items for the SCS were generated by content analysis (see Appendix B) of expert nurses'

BOX 5.7 Guidelines for Neuman's Systems Model Research

One purpose of Neuman's Systems Model–based research is to predict the effects of primary, secondary, and tertiary prevention interventions on retention, attainment, and maintenance of client system stability. Another purpose is to determine the cost, benefit, and utility of prevention interventions.

The phenomena of interest encompass the physiological, psychological, sociocultural, developmental, and spiritual variables; the properties of the central core of the client/ client system; the properties of the flexible and normal lines of defense and the lines of resistance; the characteristics of the internal, external, and created environments; the characteristics of intrapersonal, interpersonal, and extrapersonal stressors; and the elements of primary, secondary, and tertiary prevention interventions.

The precise problems to be studied are those dealing with the impact of stressors on client system stability with regard to physiological, psychological, sociocultural, developmental, and spiritual variables, as well as the lines of defense and resistance.

Research designs encompass both inductive and deductive research using qualitative, quantitative, and/or mixed-methods designs and appropriate instruments. Data encompass both the client system's and the researcher's perceptions, and may be collected in inpatient, ambulatory, home, and community settings.

Research participants can be a client system of individuals, families, groups, communities, organizations, or collaborative relationships between two or more individuals. The researcher also is a participant in the research and contributes his or her perceptions of the client system's perceptions and responses.

Data analysis techniques associated with both qualitative and quantitative methods are appropriate. Quantitative methods of data analysis should consider the flexible line of defense as a moderator variable and the lines of resistance as a mediator variable. Secondary data analysis techniques may be used to recast existing research findings within the context of Neuman's Systems Model.

Neuman's Systems Model–based research findings advance understanding of the influence of prevention interventions on the relation between stressors and client system stability. Research is linked to practice through the use of research findings as the evidence to direct practice. In turn, problems encountered in practice give rise to new research questions.

Adapted from Fawcett and DeSanto-Madeya (2013), with permission.

written responses to questions about spiritual care and psychosocial care. The SCS items are arranged in two subscales: spiritual component, which includes items for the faith, empowerment, and meaningfulness dimensions of Spiritual Care; and psychosocial component, which includes items for the psychosocial care dimension. The two subscales allow users of the SCS to distinguish the spiritual component from the psychosocial component of spiritual care. Carrigg and Weber (1997) estimated the psychometric properties for the SCS, including adequate internal consistency reliability with Cronbach's alpha, and construct validity with factor analysis (see Appendix B), using a sample of 144 nurses.

The CTE structure constructed for Carrigg and Weber's (1990) instrument development research, with supplemental information from a journal article by

BOX 5.8   An Example of a Conceptual–Theoretical–Empirical Structure for a Neuman's Systems Model Literature Review

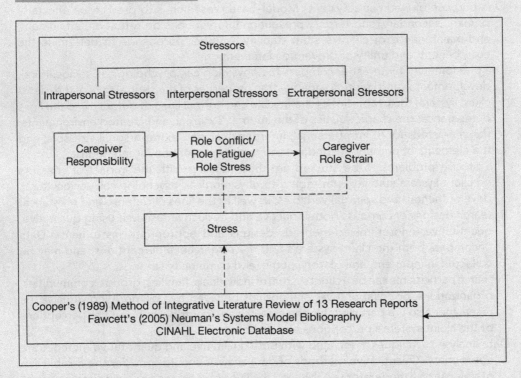

FIGURE 5.5 Conceptual–theoretical–empirical (CTE) structure for Neuman's Systems Model literature review—theory of caregiver role strain.

CINAHL, Cumulative Index of Nursing and Allied Health Literature.

The *non-relational propositions* for the *C component* of the conceptual–theoretical–empirical (CTE) structure are:

- *Stressors* is defined as "tension producing stimuli or forces occurring within the internal and external environmental boundaries of the client system" (Neuman, 2011, p. 22).
- The three dimensions of Stressors are intrapersonal stressors, interpersonal stressors, and extrapersonal stresssors.
  - o *Intrapersonal stressors* is defined as internal environmental forces (Neuman, 2011).
  - o *Interpersonal stressors* is defined as proximal external environmental forces (Neuman, 2011).
  - o *Extrapersonal stressors* is defined as distal external environmental forces (Neuman, 2011).

(continued)

BOX 5.8   An Example of a Conceptual–Theoretical–Empirical Structure for a Neuman's Systems Model Literature Review   *(continued)*

The *non-relational propositions* for the *T component* of the CTE structure are:

- *Stress* is defined as needs, concerns, and problems excountered by caregivers.
- The three dimensions of Stress are caregiver responsibility, role conflict/role fatigue/role stress, and caregiver role strain.
  - o *Caregiver responsibilty* is defined as stress arising from expectations of people who are obligated to care for others.
  - o *Role conflict/role fatigue/role stress* is defined as conflicts, fatigue, and stress arising from expected performance of caregivers' activities.
  - o *Caregiver role strain* is defined as "profound depression unless mediated by emotional and tangible support from family and friends, tangible and informational support from social services, and informational support from health care professionals" (Skalski et al., 2006, p. 76).

The *non-relational propositions* for the *E component* of the CTE structure are:

- Stress and its three dimensions were extracted from an integrative literature review of 13 Neuman's Systems Model studies of stressors.

The *relational propositions* for the *T component* of the CTE structure are:

- Caregiver responsibilty is related to role conflict/role fatigue/role stress.
- Role conflict/role fatigue/role stress is related to caregiver role strain.

Source: Skalski, DiGerolamo, and Gigliotti (2006).

Weber and Carrigg (1997), is illustrated in Figure 5.6. The non-relational propositions for each component of the CTE structure are listed in Box 5.9.

A CTE Structure for Descriptive Qualitative Research

Lowry's (2012) journal article is an example of a report of descriptive qualitative research (see Appendix A) guided by Neuman's Systems Model. Lowry explained:

> The purposes of this study were to a) explore the meaning of spirituality as described by aging adults in various states of health, b) describe the relationship between spirituality and health, c) describe client expectations of healthcare providers related to spirituality, d) compare the identified meanings with the definition of spirituality proposed by Dr. Betty Neuman, and e) validate the Neuman systems model (NSM) as a credible framework for guiding the practice of holistic nursing. (p. 356)

The study participants were older adults who represented one of three levels of health: "those who are well and living independently, those who have health

BOX 5.9   An Example of a Conceptual–Theoretical–Empirical Structure for Neuman's Systems Model Instrument Development

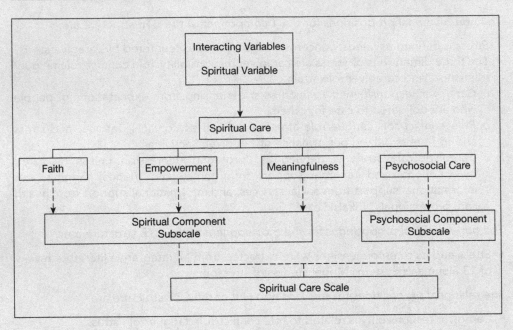

FIGURE 5.6 Conceptual–theoretical–empirical (CTE) structure for Neuman's Systems Model instrument development research—theory of spiritual care.

The *non-relational propositions* for the *C component* of the conceptual–theoretical–empirical (CTE) structure are:

- *Interacting Variables* is defined as the five components of the client system, which function more or less harmoniously in interactions with internal and external environmental stressors. The extent of the interactions between and among the five variables determines how much resistance a client system has to environmental stressors.
- The relevant dimension of Interacting Variables is spiritual variable.
  - *Spiritual variable* is defined as "spiritual beliefs and influences...[which are] on a continuum of dormant, unacceptable, or undeveloped to recognition, development, and positive system influence" (Neuman, 2011, pp. 16–17).

The *non-relational propositions* for the *T component* of the CTE structure are:

- *Spiritual Care* is defined as nursing practice directed toward religious and other spiritual problems experienced by client systems. Spritual care involves "listening,

(continued)

BOX 5.9 An Example of a Conceptual–Theoretical–Empirical Structure for Neuman's Systems Model Instrument Development *(continued)*

talking and praying with...[clients] at their request...affirming an individual's inner resources for renewal and self-fulfillment that connect one to a higher power...paying attention to the [client's] need for practicing/observing values and beliefs that guide [his or her] life...meeting the [clients] where they are in their life experience and relationship with God (if any) to aid them further on their journey" (Weber & Carrigg, 1997, p. 32).

- The dimensions of Spiritual Care are faith, empowerment, meaningfulness, and psychosocial care.
  o *Faith* is defined as belief in and acceptance of the doctrines of a religion or personal spirituality.
  o *Empowerment* is defined as a feeling of control over one's own life and life circumstances.
  o *Meaningfulness* is defined as identification of the significance of one's own life and life circumstances.
  o *Psychosocial care* is defined as "listening, touching, and being respectful," directed toward psychological and social problems experienced by client systems (Weber & Carrigg, 1997, p. 32).

The *non-relational proposition* for the *E component* of the CTE structure is:

- Spiritual Care is measured by the Spiritual Care Scale (SCS; Carrigg & Weber, 1997). The SCS contains 27 items arranged in two subscales: spiritual component, which includes items for faith, empowerment, and meaningfulness; and psychosocial component, which includes psychosocial care items. The items are rated on a 4-point scale of "strongly disagree" to "strongly agree."

Source: Carrigg and Weber (1997).

deficits requiring assisted living, and those requiring skilled care" (Lowry, 2012, p. 358). Study participants were interviewed in focus groups using a structured interview guide containing seven questions, some of which were adapted from Neuman's Systems Model Assessment Format (Neuman, 2002).

The theory is the meaning of spirituality. The conceptual model concept is Interacting Variables; the relevant dimension is spiritual variable. The spiritual variable dimension of Interacting Variables is represented by the theory concept of Meaning of Spirituality. The three dimensions of Meaning of Spirituality are spirituality is connection to God, positive spirituality contributes to personal wholeness and health, and integrate spirituality into client system care. Meaning of Spirituality and its dimensions were discovered in the transcriptions of the tape-recorded focus group interviews, using van Manen's (2001) data analysis method of descriptive interpretation (see Appendix B).

The CTE structure constructed from the content of Lowry's (2012) journal article is illustrated in Figure 5.7. The non-relational propositions for each component of the CTE structure are listed in Box 5.10.

BOX 5.10   An Example of Neuman's Systems Model Descriptive Qualitative Research

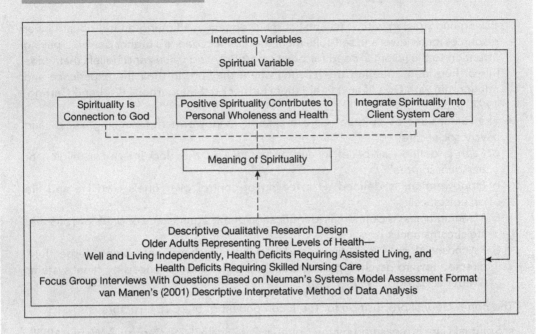

FIGURE 5.7 Conceptual–theoretical–empirical (CTE) structure for Neuman's Systems Model descriptive qualitative research—theory of the meaning of spirituality.

The *non-relational propositions* for the *C component* of the conceptual–theoretical–empirical (CTE) structure are:

- *Interacting Variables* is defined as the five components of the client system, which function more or less harmoniously in interactions with internal and external environmental stressors. The extent of the interactions between and among the five variables determines how much resistance a client system has to environmental stressors.
- The relevant dimension of Interacting Variables is spiritual variable.
  o *Spiritual variable* is defined as "spiritual beliefs and influences...[which are] on a continuum of dormant, unacceptable, or undeveloped to recognition, development, and positive system influence" (Neuman, 2011, pp. 16–17).

The *non-relational propositions* for the *T component* of the CTE structure are:

- *Meaning of Spirituality* is defined as participants' perceptions of the meaning of spirituality and their personal expressions of spirituality (Lowry, 2012).

(continued)

BOX 5.10   An Example of Neuman's Systems Model Descriptive Qualitative Research   (continued)

- The dimensions of Meaning of Spirituality are spirituality is connection to God, positive spirituality contributes to personal wholeness and health, and integrate spirituality into client system care.
    - *Spirituality is connection to God* is defined as "an individual, conscious, committed connection to God [or Christ], who gives unfailing love, comfort, and support that prompts a human response" (Lowry, 2012, p. 358).
    - *Positive spirituality contributes to personal wholeness and health* is defined as "spirituality [having] a positive influence on [participants'] state of health and feelings of wellbeing" (Lowry, 2012, p. 359).
    - *Integrate spirituality into client system care* is defined as participants' desire to have "healthcare professionals to consider their spiritual needs" (Lowry, 2012, p. 359).

The *non-relational proposition* for the *E component* of the CTE structure is:

- Meaning of Spirituality and its dimensions were discovered in participants' responses to seven focus group interview questions based on Neuman's Systems Model Assessment Format (Neuman, 2002). The questions are listed here; the statements in parentheses are items from Neuman's Systems Model Assessment Format.
    1. What does spirituality mean to you? (Identify your major health concerns.)
    2. How do you express your spirituality? (Describe your lifestyle patterns.)
    3. What other words do you associate with spirituality?
    4. In what situations does your spirituality help you to cope? (How have you coped with this problem in the past?)
    5. How does your spirituality affect your health or feelings of well-being? (How will you cope with this problem in the future? How can you help yourself?)
    6. What do you expect health care professionals to do for you related to your spiritual needs? (What do you expect from caregivers and others?)
    7. Do you think that health care professionals should be taught how to meet spiritual needs of persons?

Source: Lowry (2012).

A CTE Structure for Correlational Research

Pines et al.'s (2012) journal article is an example of a report of correlational research. The purpose of their study was:

> To examine relations of stress resiliency, psychological empowerment, selected demographic characteristics (age, ethnicity, semester in school) and [interpersonal conflict to] conflict management styles of [166] baccalaureate nursing students [and freshmen pre-nursing students] enrolled in [one of six courses in] a private Hispanic-serving university. (p. 1485)

The theory of the relations of stress resiliency, psychological empowerment, age, ethnicity, semester in school, and interpersonal conflict to conflict management style was tested using a correlational regression model research design (see Appendix A) with multiple regression statistics used to analyze the data (see Appendix B). The conceptual model concepts are Interacting Variables and Stressors. The relevant dimensions of Interacting Variables are psychological variable, sociocultural variable, and developmental variable. The relevant dimension of Stressors is interpersonal stressors. The theory concepts are Stress Resiliency, Psychological Empowerment, Conflict Management Style, Ethnicity, Age, Semester in School, and Interpersonal Conflict.

The psychological variable dimension of Interacting Variables is represented by Stress Resiliency, Psychological Empowerment, and Conflict Management Style. The sociocultural variable dimension is represented by Ethnicity, and the developmental variable dimension is represented by Age and Semester in School. The interpersonal stressors dimension of Stressors is represented by Interpersonal Conflict.

Stress Resiliency is measured by the Stress Resiliency Profile (Thomas & Tymon, 1992), Psychological Empowerment is measured by the Psychological Empowerment Instrument (Spreitzer, 1995), and Conflict Management Style is measured by the Conflict Mode Instrument (Kilmann & Thomas, 1977; Thomas & Kilman, 1974). Ethnicity, Age, and Interpersonal Conflict are measured by items on a Demographic Inventory developed by Pines et al. (2012). Pines et al. (2012) did not indicate how Semester in School was measured.

The CTE structure constructed from the content of Pines et al.'s (2012) journal article is illustrated in Figure 5.8. The non-relational and relational propositions for each component of the CTE structure are listed in Box 5.11.

A CTE Structure for Experimental Research

Pines et al.'s (2014) journal article is an example of a report of experimental research. The purpose of their study "was to determine whether nursing students who participate in simulated training exercises that manage intimidating and disruptive behaviors of others have increased perceptions of [stress] resiliency, psychological empowerment, and conflict management styles after training" (p. 85).

The study participants were 60 upper division baccalaureate nursing students who were enrolled in a psychiatric-mental health nursing course during one semester and a leadership/management nursing course during the subsequent semester. The students received the simulated training exercises for both semesters. The study was conducted as a quasi-experimental one group pretest (prior to starting the training exercises)–posttest (after completing the training exercises) research design (see Appendix A). Pretest–posttest differences were tested with paired t-test statistics (see Appendix B).

The theory is the effects of simulated conflict management training exercises on stress resiliency, psychological empowerment, and conflict management

BOX 5.11   An Example of Neuman's Systems Model Correlational Research

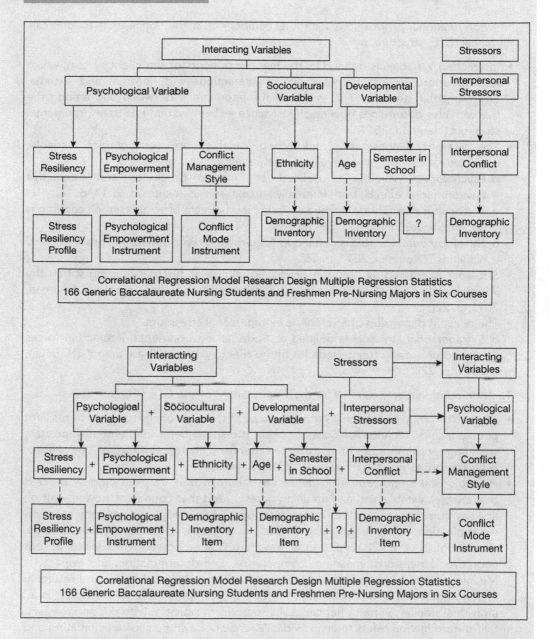

FIGURE 5.8 Conceptual–theoretical–empirical (CTE) structure for Neuman's Systems Model correlational research—theory of the relations of stress resiliency, psychological empowerment, ethnicity, age, semester in school, and interpersonal conflict to conflict management style.

(continued)

BOX 5.11   An Example of Neuman's Systems Model Correlational Research   *(continued)*

The *non-relational propositions* for the *C component* of the conceptual–theoretical–empirical (CTE) structure are:

- *Interacting Variables* is defined as the five components of the client system, which function more or less harmoniously in interactions with internal and external environmental stressors. The extent of the interactions between and among the five variables determines how much resistance a client system has to environmental stressors (Neuman, 2011).
- The relevant dimensions of Interacting Variables are psychological variable, sociocultural variable, and developmental variable.
  o *Psychological variable* is defined as "mental processes and interactive environmental effects, both internally and externally" (Neuman, 2011, p. 16).
  o *Sociocultural variable* is defined as "combined effects of social cultural conditions and influences" (Neuman, 2011, p. 16).
  o *Developmental variable* is defined as "age-related development[al] processes and activities" (Neuman, 2011, p. 16).
- *Stressors* is defined as "tension producing stimuli or forces occurring within the internal and external environmental boundaries of the client system" (Neuman, 2011, p. 22).
- The relevant dimension of Stressors is extrapersonal stresssors.
  o *Extrapersonal stressors* is defined as "external environmental interaction forces that occur outside the boundaries of the client system at distal range" (Neuman, 2011, p. 22).

The *non-relational propositions* for the *T component* of the CTE structure are:

- *Stress Resiliency* is defined as a human trait; "[t]he personal attributes of resilient people include an 'internal locus of control pro-social behaviour, empathy, positive self-image, optimism, and the ability to organize daily responsibilities'" (McAllister & McKinnon, as cited in Pines et al., 2012, p. 1483).
- *Psychological Empowerment* is defined as a human trait; "a psychological process that enables establishing and attaining goals...[and that connotes] 'power, control, ability, competence, self-efficacy, autonomy, knowledge, development, self-determination, and strengthening of one's own group in society'" (Uner & Turan, cited in Pines et al., 2012, p. 1483). "Psychological empowerment consists of four cognitive dimensions: meaning, competence, self-determination and impact.... Meaning is the value an individual attributes to personal work goals and results in high commitment and concentration of energy; competence or self-efficacy, is an individual's beliefs in his or her capability to perform activities with skill and mastery. Self-determination refers to an individual's sense of having a choice in initiating and regulating actions and work behaviours; and impact reflects the degree to which an individual can influence strategic or operating outcomes at work" (Pines et al., 2012, pp. 1483–1484).
- *Conflict Management Style* is defined as "an individual's behaviour in conflict situations in which the concerns of two people appear to be incompatible. In

(continued)

BOX 5.11   An Example of Neuman's Systems Model Correlational Research   *(continued)*

conflict situations, a person's behaviour can be described along two dimensions: (1) assertiveness, defined as the extent to which the individual attempts to satisfy his or her own concerns; (2) cooperativeness, defined as the extent to which the individual attempts to satisfy other people's concerns. Assertiveness and cooperativeness can be used to define five methods of dealing with conflict: competing, collaborating, compromising, avoiding and accommodating" (Pines et al., 2012, p. 1486).

- *Ethnicity* is defined as self-identification as African American, Asian/Pacific Islander, Caucasian, Hispanic, or other (Pines et al., 2012).
- *Age* is defined as number of years since birth.
- *Semester in School* is not defined but can be inferred to be the first through the eighth term at a university.
- *Interpersonal Conflict* is defined "as any act of aggression or hostility perpetrated by a colleague on another colleague ... including emotional, physical and verbal threats and intimidating covert or overt aggressive behaviours, and innuendoes or criticism" (Pines et al., 2012, p. 1483).

The *non-relational propositions* for the *E component* of the CTE structure are as follows:

- Stress Resiliency is measured by the Stress Resiliency Profile (Thomas & Tymon, 1992). This instrument contains 18 items that describe how an individual thinks he or she is performing, which are rated on a scale of 1 = strongly disagree to 7 = strongly agree.
- Psychological Empowerment is measured by the Psychological Empowerment Instrument (PEI; Spreitzer, 1995). The PEI is made up of 12 items arranged in four subscales (meaning, competence, self-determination, and impact). Items are rated on a 7-point scale of "very strongly disagree" to "very strongly agree."
- Conflict Management Style is measured by the Conflict Mode Instrument (Thomas & Kilmann, 1974; Kilmann & Thomas, 1977). This instrument includes "30 pairs of statements describing possible behavioural responses. Participants were asked to choose one statement from each pair to indicate how they would behave if they found their own wishes differing from those of another person. In each of the five methods of dealing with conflict [competing, collaborating, compromising, avoiding and accommodating], possible scores range from 0 for very low use to 12 for very high use" (Pines et al., 2012, p. 1486).
- Ethnicity is measured by an item on the investigator-developed Demographic Inventory (Pines et al., 2012).
- Age is measured by an item on the investigator-developed Demographic Inventory (Pines et al., 2012).
- Semester in School—The way in which this concept is measured is not mentioned by Pines et al. (2012) but can be inferred to be an item on the Demographic Inventory.
- Interpersonal Conflict is measured by two items on the investigator-developed Demographic Inventory. One item is a forced choice question that asks the person whether he or she had experienced interpersonal conflict in the workplace. The other item is an open-ended question asking the person to describe the interpersonal conflict (Pines et al., 2012).

(continued)

> **BOX 5.11 An Example of Neuman's Systems Model Correlational Research** *(continued)*
>
> The *relational propositions* for the C and T components of the CTE structure are:
>
> - The psychological, sociocultural, and developmental variables are interrelated.
> - Therefore Stress Resiliency, Psychological Empowerment, Ethnicity, Age, Semester in School, and Interpersonal Conflict are related to Conflict Management Style.
>
> The *relational proposition* for the E component of the CTE structure is as follows:
>
> - Scores on the Stress Resiliency Profile, Psychological Empowerment Instrument, and Demographic Inventory items are related to scores on the Conflict Mode Instrument.
>
> *Source:* Pines et al. (2012).

style. One conceptual model concept is Prevention as Intervention; the relevant dimension is primary prevention as intervention. The other conceptual model concept is Flexible Line of Defense. The theory concepts are Simulated Conflict Management Training Exercises, Stress Resiliency, Psychological Empowerment, and Conflict Management Style. The primary prevention as intervention dimension of Prevention as Intervention is represented by Simulate Conflict Management Training Exercises. The Flexible Line of Defense is represented by Stress Resiliency, Psychological Empowerment, and Conflict Management Style. Simulated Conflict Management Training Exercises is operationalized by the Simulated Conflict Management Training Exercises protocol. Stress Resiliency is measured by the Stress Resiliency Profile (Thomas & Tymon, 1992), Psychological Empowerment is measured by the Psychological Empowerment Instrument (Spreitzer, 1995), and Conflict Management Style is measured by the Conflict Mode Instrument (Kilmann & Thomas, 1977; Thomas & Kilmann, 1974) and the DESC Self-Assessment Tool from the Agency for Health Care Research and Quality TeamSTEPPS program (Agency for Health Care Research and Quality, as cited by Pines et al., 2014).

The CTE structure constructed from an interpretation of the content of Pines et al.'s (2014) journal article is illustrated in Figure 5.9. The non-relational and relational propositions for each component of the CTE structure are listed in Box 5.12.

A CTE Structure for Mixed-Methods Research

Rideout's (2013) doctoral dissertation is an example of Neuman's Systems Model–guided mixed-methods research. The purpose of her research "was to explore nurses' perceptions of barriers and facilitators affecting implementation of the [shaken baby syndrome] SBS public policy in Massachusetts birthing hospitals" (Rideout, 2013, p. 1). Within the context of Neuman's Systems Model, the SBS public policy is regarded as a client system that is a social issue.

BOX 5.12 An Example of Neuman's Systems Model Experimental Research

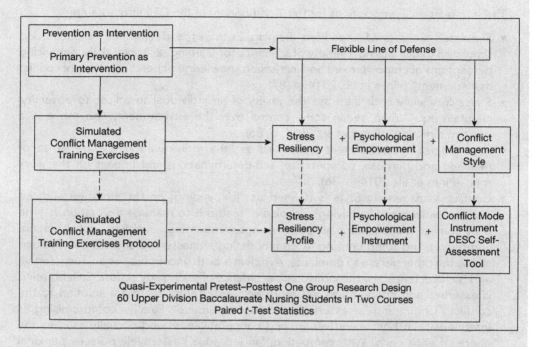

FIGURE 5.9 Conceptual–theoretical–empirical (CTE) structure for Neuman's Systems Model experimental research—theory of the effects of simulated conflict management training exercises on stress resiliency, psychological empowerment, and conflict management style.

DESC, describe the situation (D), express concerns about the action (E), suggest other alternatives (S), and consequences should be stated (C).

The *non-relational propositions* for the C *component* of the conceptual–theoretical–empirical (CTE) structure are:

- *Prevention as Intervention* is defined as the goals and outcomes components of Neuman's System Model Nursing Process Format.
- The relevant dimension of Prevention as Intervention is primary prevention as intervention.
  - o *Primary prevention as intervention* is defined as retention of wellness by increasing the strength of the flexible line of defense by means of prevention of stress and reducing risk factors (Neuman, 2011).
- *Flexible Line of Defense* is defined as the outer boundary of the client system, which is a buffer that protects the client system's normal line of defense from stressor invasion; the Flexible Line of Defense is highly dynamic in that it can rapidly expand away from the normal line of defense, offering greater protection, or rapidly draw closer to the normal line of defense, offering less protection.

(continued)

BOX 5.12   An Example of Neuman's Systems Model Experimental Research   *(continued)*

The *non-relational propositions* for the *T component* of the CTE structure are:

- *Simulated Conflict Management Training Exercises* is defined as "didactic and simulated training using a variety of scenarios for learning resiliency skills, enhancing perceptions of empowerment and increasing knowledge of personal styles of conflict management" (Pines et al., 2014, p. 87).
- *Stress Resiliency* is defined as "the ability of an individual to adjust to adversity, maintain equilibrium, retain some control over the environment, and move in a positive direction" (Pines et al., 2014, p. 86).
- *Psychological Empowerment* is defined as "the individual's perceived sense of meaning and purpose, competence, self-determination, and impact on the work role" (Pines et al., 2014, p. 86).
- *Conflict Management Style* is defined as "[depending] on the situation and the parties involved and [involving] a choice of methods to manage a situation....[The five] conflict management styles [are]: accommodating, avoiding, collaborating, competing, and compromising. Accommodating is unassertive and cooperative and allows the other person to dominate. Avoiding is both uncooperative and unassertive and is characterized by the individual's avoidance of taking any action. Collaborating is assertive and cooperative and represents an attempt to find a solution to the conflict. Competing is assertive and uncooperative. Finally, compromising is intermediate in both assertiveness and cooperativeness and partially satisfies the needs of each party. With competing, [an individual] assertively pursues personal concerns at the expense of the concerns of another. In compromising, the object is to find a mutually agreeable solution that partially satisfies both parties. Resiliency and empowerment reflect application of the appropriate strategy/style in response to the situation" (Thomas & Kilmann, as cited by Pines et al., 2014, p. 86).

The *non-relational propositions* for the *E component* of the CTE structure are:

- Simulated Conflict Management Training Exercises is operationalized by the Stimulated Conflict Management Training Exercises protocol. Pines et al. (2014) explained that the Reaching Out and Reaching In (Winder, 2006) curriculum based on the PENN Resiliency Program and TeamSTEPPS (Agency for Health Care Research and Quality, as cited by Pines et al., 2014) provided the basis of the resiliency intervention....The course content consisted of 4 modules implemented over 2 consecutive semesters of course work. Faculty presented the 1st 3 modules in the [psychiatric–mental health nursing] PMHN class in 2 weekly, 3-hour class periods. Scenarios in each session provided an opportunity for students to role play the use of problem-solving and coping skills. Module 1 focused on the principles of resiliency and behaviors of resilient nurses. Module 2 content engaged students in professional empowerment and disempowerment strategies in the workplace. Students brainstormed words they have come to associate with resilience and that reflected the characteristics of a resilient and empowered nurse who had overcome adversity and persevered with courage and strength. Module 3 focused on analyzing the advantages and disadvantages of the 5 conflict management styles. Five simulated scenarios provided students the

(continued)

BOX 5.12   An Example of Neuman's Systems Model Experimental Research   (continued)

opportunity to apply knowledge and skills to manage conflict with colleagues and clients. Each simulated activity lasted 45 minutes, with 30 minutes for simulation and a 10-minute debriefing. The 4th module used content from TeamSTEPPS, an evidence-based teamwork training system. The program included a series of interactive didactic and discussion group sessions, role playing, and videotaped scenarios. TeamSTEPPS was implemented during a 3-hour class period in the [leadership/management nursing] LMN course, with a focus on the role of manager. Students viewed the Agency for Health Care Research and Quality, TeamSTEPPS, DESC script video. This video provides a step-by-step format for managing difficult situations. The steps include describe the situation [D], express your concerns about the action [E], suggest other alternatives [S], and consequences should be stated [C]. Students then applied these principles to video scenarios from TeamSTEPPS. For example, 1 situation involved 2 nurses attending a unit meeting, 1 of whom was talking about unrelated material, whereas another nurse grows increasingly impatient to get on with the meeting (describe the situation). The charge nurse recognizes that the meeting must go on but does not want to alienate either party and suggests that they delay discussion of the unrelated material until later (express your concerns about the action). The charge nurse deflected defensiveness by keeping a positive tone in her voice and suggested that the unrelated material was not relevant but needed to be delayed to another time (suggest alternatives). The meeting proceeded as scheduled, and the involved parties did not feel slighted (consequences). During the debriefing, students completed the DESC self assessment tool to reflect on the effect of the DESC script on conflict management" (p. 87).

- Psychological Empowerment is measured by the Psychological Empowerment Instrument (PEI; Spreitzer, 1995). The PEI includes 12 items about "motivational constructs of meaning, competence, self-determination, and impact. Meaning is the perception of the individual's value of the work role; competence is the ability to perform effectively; self-determination is the perception of choice in a situation; and impact is the perception of individual ability to influence outcomes in a work environment" (Pines et al., 2014, p. 87). The PEI items are rated on a 7-point scale of "very strongly disagree" to "very strongly agree" (Pines et al., 2012).
- Stress Resiliency is measured by the Stress Resiliency Profile (Thomas & Tymon, 1992). This instrument contains 18 items about "development of effective mental habits for coping with stressors. Three interpretive habits for perceptions of stress are measured: deficiency focusing, the habit of focusing on the negatives rather than the positives in a situation; necessitating, the habit of focusing on commitment rather than choice in a situation, leading to the conclusion of no choice; and low-skill recognition, the habit of underestimating personal competence, suggesting success is due to external forces" (Pines et al., 2014, p. 87). The items are rated on a scale of 1 = strongly disagree to 7 = strongly agree (Pines et al., 2012).
- Conflict Management Style is measured by the Thomas–Kilmann Conflict Mode Instrument (TKI; Thomas & Kilmann, 2007). The TKI includes 30 forced choice items about "personal behavior along 2 dimensions: assertiveness, defined as the extent to which the individual attempts to satisfy personal concerns; and cooperativeness,

(continued)

BOX 5.12   An Example of Neuman's Systems Model
Experimental Research   *(continued)*

defined as the extent to which the individual attempts to satisfy concerns of others. Possible scores range from 0 (none) to 12 (very high) frequency of use" (Pines et al., 2014, p. 87).
- Conflict Management Style also is measured by the DESC Self-Assessment Tool (Agency for Health Care Research and Quality, as cited by Pines et al., 2014). No information about this instrument could be located.

The *relational propositions* for the *C* and *T components* of the CTE structure are:

- The primary prevention as intervention dimension of Prevention as Intervention has a positive effect on the Flexible Line of Defense, such that implementation of primary prevention as intervention strengthens the Flexible Line of Defense.
- Therefore, Simulated Conflict Management Training Exercises has a positive effect on Stress Resiliency, Psychological Empowerment, and Conflict Management Style.

The *relational propositions* for the *E component* of the CTE structure are:

- Students who participate in the Simulated Conflict Management Training Exercises protocol have higher scores on the Stress Resiliency Profile, the Psychological Empowerment Instrument, and the Conflict Mode Instrument after completing the exercises than before starting the exercises.
- Scores on the DESC Self-Assessment Tool indicate a positive effect of the DESC script component of the Simulated Conflict Management Training Exercises protocol.

Source: Pines et al. (2014).

Review of Rideout's dissertation revealed that the mixed-method research design is QUAN + QUAL (see Appendix A). The qualitative portion of the study was added to augment the findings from the quantitative portion. A correlational regression research design (see Appendix A) was used to collect data for the quantitative portion of the study using a survey completed by 155 nurses who work in birthing hospitals in Massachusetts. A simple descriptive qualitative design (see Appendix A) was used to collect data for the qualitative portion of the study using two open-ended questions on the survey from the same 155 nurses.

For the quantitative portion of the study, logistic regression statistics (see Appendix B) were used to examine the relation of barriers to and facilitators of SBS guideline implementation. For the qualitative portion of the study, data were analyzed using content analysis (see Appendix B) to identify the various responses to the open-ended questions.

The theory is SBS guidelines implementation. The conceptual model concepts are Prevention as Intervention and Optimal Client System Wellness. The relevant dimension of Prevention as Intervention is primary prevention as intervention. The theory concepts are Barriers to SBS Prevention Education, Facilitators of SBS Prevention Education, and SBS Guidelines Implementation.

The primary prevention as intervention dimension of Prevention as Intervention is represented by Barriers to SBS Prevention Education and Facilitators of SBS Prevention Education. Optimal Client System Wellness is represented by SBS Guidelines Implementation.

Barriers to SBS Prevention Education and Facilitators of SBS Prevention Education are measured by items on the investigator-developed SBS Survey for the quantitative portion of the study (Rideout, 2013). Participants' responses to two open-ended questions on the investigator-developed SBS Survey were used to generate themes for Barriers to Prevention Education and Facilitators of SBS Prevention Education for the qualitative portion of the study (Rideout, 2013). SBS Guidelines Implementation also is measured by items on the investigator-developed SBS Survey for the quantitative portion of the study (Rideout, 2013).

The CTE structure constructed from an interpretation of the content of Rideout's (2013) dissertation is illustrated in Figure 5.10. The non-relational and relational propositions for each component of the CTE structure are listed in Box 5.13.

BOX 5.13   An Example of Neuman's Systems Model Mixed-Methods Research

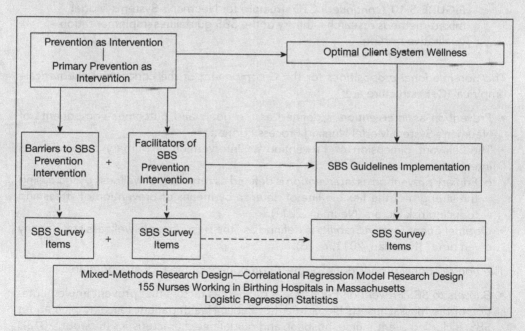

FIGURE 5.10 Conceptual–theoretical–empirical (CTE) structure for Neuman's Systems Model mixed-methods research—theory of the SBS guidelines implementation— quantitative portion.   (*continued*)

SBS, shaken baby syndrome.

(continued)

BOX 5.13   An Example of Neuman's Systems Model Mixed-Methods Research   (continued)

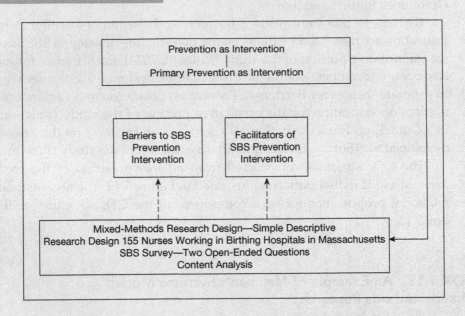

FIGURE 5.10 (continued) CTE structure for Neuman's Systems Model mixed-methods research—theory of the SBS guidelines implementation—qualitative portion.

The *non-relational propositions* for the *C component* of the conceptual–theoretical–empirical (CTE) structure are:

- *Prevention as Intervention* is defined as the goals and outcomes components of Neuman's System Model Nursing Process Format.
- The relevant dimension of Prevention as Intervention is primary prevention as intervention.
  - o *Primary prevention as intervention* is defined as retention of wellness by increasing the strength of the flexible line of defense by means of prevention of stress and reducing risk factors (Neuman, 2011).
- *Optimal Client System Stability* is defined as "the best possible wellness state at any given time" (Neuman, 2011, p. 23).

The *non-relational propositions* for the *T component* of the CTE structure are:

- *Barriers to SBS Prevention Education* is defined as factors that prevent implementation of the Massachusetts Department of Public Health patient teaching plan about SBS, including client, nurse, hospital, and guidelines characteristics (Rideout, 2013).
- *Facilitators of SBS Prevention Education* is defined as factors that support implementation of the Massachusetts Department of Public Health patient teaching plan about SBS, including client, nurse, hospital, and guidelines characteristics (Rideout, 2013).

(continued)

BOX 5.13   An Example of Neuman's Systems Model Mixed-Methods Research   *(continued)*

- *SBS Guidelines Implementation* is defined as use of the Massachusetts Department of Public Health SBS patient teaching plan, including written and oral information about SBS that is "incorporated with the teaching on newborn care currently completed by nurses with parents/guardians prior to the [client's] discharge from the hospital" (Rideout, 2013, p. 22). The specific teaching plan includes "distribution of a brochure on SBS, the provision of oral education about SBS, the provision of oral education on infant soothing methods, and documentation of SBS education in the medical record...[as well as] showing of a video on SBS" (Rideout, 2013, p. 42).

The *non-relational propositions* for the *E component* of the CTE structure for the quantitative portion of the study are:

- Barriers to SBS Prevention Education is measured by items on the investigator-developed SBS Survey.
- Facilitators of SBS Prevention Education is measured by items on the investigator-developed SBS Survey.

    The seven barriers and facilitators items on the investigator-developed SBS Survey were adapted from Peters, Harmsen, Laurant, and Wensing's (2002) Barriers and Facilitators Assessment Instrument. Six of the items are rated on a scale of 1 = strongly disagree, 2= disagree, 3 = agree, and 4 = strongly agree (Rideout, 2013), and the other item is rated as "Yes" or "No" (Rideout, 2013; p. 111). Hospital characteristics (community or teaching, number of births) were added to the SBS Survey by Rideout (2013).

- SBS Guidelines Implementation is measured by four items on the investigator-developed SBS Survey, which are rated on a scale of 0 = never, 1= sometimes, and 2 = always (Rideout, 2013).

The *non-relational proposition* for the *E component* of the CTE structure for the qualitative portion of the study is:

- Barriers to and Facilitators of SBS Prevention Education were generated from content analysis of two open-ended questions on the investigator-developed SBS Survey—"What has made implementation of the SBS guidelines easy? [and] What has made implementation of the SBS guidelines difficult?" (Rideout, 2013, pp. 52, 113).

The *relational propositions* for the *C and T components* of the CTE structure for the quantitative portion of the study are:

- Prevention as Intervention has a positive effect on Client System Stability.
- Therefore, Barriers to SBS Prevention Education has a negative effect on SBS Guidelines Implementation and Facilitators of SBS Prevention Education has a positive effect on SBS Guidelines Implementation.

(continued)

BOX 5.13   An Example of Neuman's Systems Model Mixed-Methods Research   *(continued)*

The *relational propositions* for the *E component* of the CTE structure for the qualititive portion of the study are:

- Scores for the Barriers to Prevention Education items on the SBS Survey are negatively related to scores for SBS Guidelines Implementation items on the SBS Survey.
- Scores for Facilitators of SBS Prevention Education items on the SBS Survey are positively related to SBS Guidelines Implementation items on the SBS Survey.

SBS, shaken baby syndrome.
Source: Rideout (2013).

CONCLUSION

Neuman's Systems Model is widely used as a guide for nursing practice, research, and education in the United States and other countries, especially the Netherlands and Belgium. Furthermore, Neuman's Systems Model "is congruent with the global health trends of holism and prevention. Published papers and presentations . . . document that [the model] is universally applicable [across disciplines] and culturally relevant" (Neuman & Fawcett, 2012, p. 375). International use of Neuman's Systems Model is especially exemplified by the publication of Verberk and Merks (2016). This book includes detailed explanations of the concepts of the Neuman Systems Model as well as chapters about using the model in diverse practice settings and as a guide for research.

The broad utility of Neuman's Systems Model is evident in the examples of its use as a guide for practice, quality improvement projects, and research given in this chapter.

NOTE

1. Portions of this chapter are adapted from Fawcett, J., & DeSanto-Madeya, S. (2013). *Contemporary nursing knowledge: Analysis and evaluation of nursing models and theories* (3rd ed., Chapter 7). Philadelphia, PA: F. A. Davis, with permission.

REFERENCES

American Institutes for Research (2011). *Training guide: Using simulation in TeamSTEPPS® training.* Rockville, MD: Agency for Healthcare Research and Quality. AHRQ Publication No. 11–0041EF. Retrieved from http://www.ahrq.gov/professionals/education/ curriculum-tools/teamstepps/simulation/traininggd.pdf, and from http://www.ahrq .gov/professionals/education/curriculum-tools/teamstepps/simulation/simulation slides/simslides.html

Carrigg, K. C., & Weber, R. (1997). Development of the Spiritual Care Scale. *Image: Journal of Nursing Scholarship, 29,* 293.

Cooper, H. M. (1989). *Integrating research: A guide for literature reviews* (2nd ed.). Newbury Park, CA: Sage.

Fashinpaur, D. (2002). Using the Neuman systems model to guide nursing practice in the United States: Nursing prevention interventions for postpartum mood disorders. In B. Neuman & J. Fawcett (Eds.), *The Neuman systems model* (4th ed., pp. 74–89). Upper Saddle River, NJ: Prentice Hall.

Fawcett, J. (2005). *Contemporary nursing knowledge: Analysis and evaluation of nursing models and theories* (2nd ed.). Philadelphia, PA: F. A. Davis.

Fawcett, J., & DeSanto-Madeya, S. (2013). *Contemporary nursing knowledge: Analysis and evaluation of nursing models and theories* (3rd ed.). Philadelphia, PA: F. A. Davis.

Hammonds, L. S. (2012). Implementing a distress screening instrument in a university breast cancer clinic. *Clinical Journal of Oncology Nursing, 16,* 491–494.

Kilmann, R., & Thomas, K. (1977). Developing a force-choice measure of conflict management behavior: The MODE instrument. *Education and Psychological Measures, 37,* 309–323.

Lowry, L.W. (2012). A qualitative descriptive study of spirituality guided by the Neuman systems model. *Nursing Science Quarterly, 25,* 356–361.

National Comprehensive Cancer Network. (2012). *NCCN clinical practice guidelines in oncology: Distress management* [v.1.2013]. Retrieved from http://www.nccn.org/professionals/physician_gls/pdf/distress.pdf

National Comprehensive Cancer Network. (2013). *NCCN distress thermometer for patients.* Retrieved from http://www.nccn.org/patients/resources/life_with_cancer/pdf/nccn_distress_thermometer.pdf

Neuman, B. (2002). Appendix C: Assessment and Intervention based upon the NSM. In B. Neuman & J. Fawcett (Eds.), *The Neuman systems model* (4th ed., p. 351). Upper Saddle River, NJ: Prentice Hall.

Neuman, B. (2011). The Neuman systems model. In B. Neuman & J. Fawcett (Eds.), *The Neuman systems model* (5th ed., pp. 3–33). Upper Saddle River, NJ: Pearson.

Neuman, B., & Fawcett, J. (2012). Thoughts about the Neuman Systems Model: A dialogue. *Nursing Science Quarterly, 25,* 374–376.

Neuman, B., & Young, R. J. (1972). A model for teaching total person approach to patient problems. *Nursing Research, 21,* 264–269.

Newhouse, R. P., Dearholt, S. L., Poe, S., Pugh, L. C., & White, K. M. (2007). *Johns Hopkins nursing evidence-based practice model and guidelines.* Indianapolis, IN: Sigma Theta Tau International.

Peters, M. A. J., Harmsen, M., Laurant, M. G. H., & Wensing, M. (2002). *Barriers to and facilitators for improvement of patient care.* Nijmegen, The Netherlands: Centre for Quality of Care Research (WOK), Radboud University Nijmegen Medical Centre.

Pines, E. W, Rauschhuber, M. L., Cook, J. D., Norgan, G. H., Canchosa, L., Richardson, C., & Jones, M. E. (2014). Enhancing resilience, empowerment, and conflict management among baccalaureate students: Outcomes of a pilot study. *Nurse Educator, 39,* 85–90.

Pines, E. W., Rauschhuber, M. L., Norgan, G. H., Cook, J. D., Canchola, L., Richardson, C., & Jones, M. E. (2012). Stress resiliency, psychological empowerment and conflict management styles among baccalaureate nursing students. *Journal of Advanced Nursing, 68,* 1482–1493.

Rideout, L. C. (2013). *Nurses' perceptions of barriers and facilitators affecting the shaken baby syndrome education initiative: An exploratory study of a Massachusetts public policy.* (Doctoral dissertation). Retrieved from ProQuest Dissertations and Theses Full Text (Dissertation Number 3539211; ProQuest Document ID 1095563833).

Skalski, C.A., DiGerolamo, L., & Gigliotti, E. (2006). Stressors in five client populations: Neuman systems model-based literature review. *Journal of Advanced Nursing, 56,* 69–78.

Spreitzer, G. (1995). Psychological empowerment in the workplace: Dimensions, measurement, and validation. *Academy of Management Journal, 38,* 1442–1465.

Thomas, K., & Kilmann, W. (1974). *Thomas-Kilmann Conflict Mode Instrument.* Tuxedo, NY: Xicom.

Thomas, K. W., & Kilmann, R. H. (2007). *Thomas-Kilmann Conflict Mode Instrument.* Mountain View, CA: CPP, Inc.

Thomas, K., & Tymon, W. (1992). *Stress Resiliency Profile.* Tuxedo, NY: Xicom.

van Manen, M. (2001). *Researching lived experience* (2nd ed.). London, ON, Canada: Althouse Press.

Verberk, F., & Merks, A. (2016). *Verpleegkunde volgens het Neuman Systems Model: Vertaling en bewerking voor de Nederlandse praktijk* (6th ed.). [Nursing according to the Neuman Systems Model: Translation and application for Dutch practice]. Assen, Holland: Van Gorcum.

Weber, R., & Carrigg, K. (1997). Spiritual care: Responding to an invitation. *Journal of Christian Nursing, 14*(4), 32–33.

Winder, C. (2006). *Reaching in and reaching out: Resiliency college curriculum.* Toronto, ON, Canada: George Brown College.

CHAPTER 6

OREM'S SELF-CARE FRAMEWORK[1]

Dorothea E. Orem's Self-Care Framework focuses on the actions taken by people who are considered legitimate patients to meet their own and their dependent others' therapeutic self-care demands, as well as on actions taken by nurses to effectively use nursing systems that will assist people who have limitations in their abilities to provide continuing and therapeutic self-care or care of dependent others (Orem, 2001). The goal of nursing guided by Orem's Self-Care Framework is "to compensate for or overcome patients' health-associated limitations in self-care or dependent care" (Orem, 2001, p. 289).

OREM'S SELF-CARE FRAMEWORK

This section of the chapter includes the concepts of Orem's Self-Care Framework and the definitions (non-relational propositions) of the concepts and the dimensions of the multidimensional concepts (Orem, 2001).

Patient is defined as a recipient of care from a health care professional. The two dimensions of the concept are individual and multiperson unit.
> *Individual* is defined as one person or one member of a multiperson unit who is the unit of service for nursing practice.
> *Multiperson unit* is defined as more than one person, all of whom are regarded as a whole.

Therapeutic Self-Care Demand is defined as the demand on the individual or multiperson unit for continuing effective care of self. The three dimensions of the concept are universal self-care requisites, developmental self-care requisites, and health deviation self-care requisites.
> *Universal self-care requisites* is defined as a type of self-care requisite that is common to all people at all stages of life, but adjusted for age,

developmental stage, and the environment. The eight universal self-care requisites are:

1. The maintenance of a sufficient intake of air
2. The maintenance of a sufficient intake of water
3. The maintenance of a sufficient intake of food
4. The provision of care associated with elimination processes and excrements
5. The maintenance of a balance between activity and rest
6. The maintenance of a balance between solitude and social interaction
7. The prevention of hazards to human life, human functioning, and human well-being
8. The promotion of human functioning and development within social groups in accord with human potential, known human limitations, and the human desire to be normal (Orem, 2001, p. 225)

Developmental self-care requisites is defined as requirements for self-care at each stage of development.

Health deviation self-care requisites is defined as special demands for self-care that are associated with disease, injury, disfigurement, disability, and/ or medical care interventions that physicians perform or prescribe.

Self-Care is defined as actions taken by individuals to regulate their function and development.

Self-Care Agent is defined as an individual who is able to identify his or her self-care requisites, decide what actions are needed to meet the requisites, and perform those actions.

Dependent Care is defined as actions taken by adults for dependent family members or friends who cannot perform adequate self-care.

Dependent-Care Agent is defined as an individual who provides care for children and dependent adult family members or friends.

Self-Care Agency is defined as the individual's ability to meet his or her continuing requirements for self-care, which may vary throughout the life span.

Dependent-Care Agency is defined as the individual's ability to provide care for dependent others.

Nursing Agency is defined as the power of individuals gained through education and training to master the knowledge and skills needed to practice nursing.

Basic Conditioning Factors is defined as factors that affect an individual's ability to perform required self-care. The 10 Basic Conditioning Factors are:

1. Age
2. Gender
3. Developmental state
4. Health state
5. Sociocultural orientation
6. Health care system factors, for example, medical diagnostic and treatment modalities

7. Family system factors
8. Patterns of living including activities regularly engaged in
9. Environmental factors
10. Resource availability and adequacy (Orem, 2001, p. 245).

Power Components is defined as the initiation of trains of events that enable the performance of required actions. The two dimensions of the concept are self-care agency power components and nursing agency power components.

Self-care agency power components is defined as human powers that enable the performance of actions required for self-care.

Nursing agency power components is defined as human powers that enable the performance of actions required for nursing.

Self-Care Deficit is defined as the relationship between self-care agency and therapeutic self-care demands of individuals; when therapeutic self-care demands exceed self-care agency, a self-care deficit occurs.

Dependent-Care Deficit is defined as the relationship between dependent-care agency and the therapeutic self-care demands of dependent others; when the therapeutic self-care demands of a dependent other exceed dependent-care agency, a dependent-care deficit occurs.

Environmental Features is defined as aspects of the environment that are relevant to self-care requisites. The two dimensions of the concept are physical, chemical, and biologic features; and socioeconomic–cultural features.

Physical, chemical, and biologic features is defined as the atmosphere of the earth, gaseous composition of air, solid and gaseous pollutants, smoke, weather conditions, and geologic stability of the Earth's crust, as well as pets, wild animals, and infectious organisms or agents along with their human and animal hosts.

Socioeconomic–cultural features is defined as family and community factors, such as family compositon, relationships, dynamics, and lifestyle and community composition, functions, and resourses.

Health State is defined as "the stage of an individual that reflects wholeness or soundness of the physical and mental self" (Orem, 2001, p. 186).

Well-Being is defined as the individual's perception of the condition of his or her existence, which may be characterized as feeling content, pleasure, happiness, fulfilling one's self-ideal, and having positive spiritual experiences.

Professional–Technological System of Nursing Practice is defined as the nursing process. The five dimenions of the concept are case management operations; diagnostic operations; prescriptive operations; regulatory operations—design of nursing systems for performance of regulatory opertations, planning for regulatory operations, and production of regulatory care; and control operations.

Case management operations is defined as the nurse's use of a case management approach to control, direct, and check each of the nursing diagnostic, prescriptive, regulatory, and control operations.

Diagnostic operations is defined as identification of the unit of service for nursing practice and why nursing is needed, as well as collection of demographic data and calculation of present and future therapeutic self-care demands.

Prescriptive operations is defined as specification of the means to be used to meet the therapeutic self-care demand.

Regulatory operations is defined as design and implementation of a nursing system and method(s) of helping. The subdimensions of regulatory operations are design of nursing systems for performance of regulatory operations, planning for regulatory operations, and production of regulatory care.

Design of nursing systems for performance of regulatory operations is defined as development of a nursing care plan for a wholly compensatory, partly compensatory, or supportive–educative nursing system of care and one or more methods of helping. The wholly compensatory nursing system is selected when the patient cannot or should not perform any self-care actions, and thus the nurse must perform them; the partly compensatory nursing system is selected when the patient can perform some, but not all, self-care actions; and the supportive–educative nursing system is selected when the patient can and should perform all self-care actions but requires physical, emotional, or social support and teaching. The methods of helping, which may be used with any of the three nursing systems, are acting for or doing for the patient, providing a developmental environment, supporting the patient physically or psychologically, guiding the patient, and teaching the patient.

Planning for regulatory operations is defined as specification of what is needed to produce the selected nursing system and method(s) of helping, including time, place, environmental conditions, equipment and supplies, number and qualifications of nurses and other health care providers necessary to produce the nursing system and to evaluate its effects, organization and timing of tasks to be performed, and designation of who (nurse and/or patient) is to perform the tasks.

Production of regulatory care is defined as implementation of the selected nursing system and method(s) of helping.

Control operations is defined as evaluation of the results of implementation of the selected nursing system and method(s) of helping.

OREM'S SELF-CARE FRAMEWORK: RELATIONAL PROPOSITIONS

The statements of associations (relational propositions) between concepts of Orem's Self-Care Framework are listed here.

• Basic Conditioning Factors are related to Self-Care Agency, such that the person's ability to perform self-care and the kind and amount of self-care that is required are influenced by Basic Conditioning Factors.

- The self-care agency power components dimension of the concept of Power Components is related to the concept of Self-Care Agency, such that the person's ability to perform self-care is influenced by the self-care agency power components.
- Self-Care Agency is positively related to Self-Care.
- The physical, chemical, and biologic features dimension of Environmental Features and the socioeconomic-cultural features dimension of Environmental Features are interrelated.
- Health State and Well-Being are associated. The experience of Well-Being may occur for an individual under adverse conditions, including disorders in human structure and function.
- Self-Care is positively related to Health State.
- Self-Care is positively related to Well-Being.
- Nursing Agency is related to the nursing agency power components dimension of Power Components, such that the nurse's ability to perform nursing is influenced by the nursing agency power components.
- The Professional–Technological System of Nursing Practice has a positive effect on Self-Care Agency.
- The Professional–Technological System of Nursing Practice has a positive effect on Self-Care.

OREM'S SELF-CARE FRAMEWORK: APPLICATION TO NURSING PRACTICE

The guidelines for Orem's Self-Care Framework nursing practice are listed in Box 6.1. A diagram of the practice methodology for Orem's Self-Care Framework, which is called the Professional–Technological System of Nursing Practice, is illustrated in Figure 6.1.

A practice tool that includes all aspects of the practice methodology is given in Box 6.2.

A Conceptual–Theoretical–Empirical Structure for Assessment

Fleck's (2012) journal article is an example of the use of Orem's Self-Care Framework to guide assessment of patients. Fleck developed the Nutrition Self-Care Inventory (NSCI) to assess overweight and obese young and middle-age adults' "perceived ability to make decisions regarding their nutrition practices" (p. 31).

The theory is assessment of nutrition practices. The conceptual model concept is Therapeutic Self-Care Demand. The relevant dimension is universal self-care requisites, and the relevant subdimension is "The promotion of human functioning and development within social groups in accord with human potential, known human limitations, and the human desire to be normal"

BOX 6.1 Guidelines for Orem's Self-Care Framework Nursing Practice

The distinctive purpose of Self-Care Framework–based nursing practice is to help individuals and multiperson units who seek and can benefit from nursing because of the presence of existent or predicted health-derived or health-related self-care or dependent-care deficits.

Practice problems of interest are individuals' and multiperson units' self-care deficits and dependent-care deficits. Those problems occur when the health focus is people across the life cycle, people in recovery, people with illnesses of undetermined origin, people with genetic and developmental defects or biologic immaturity, people experiencing cure or regulation of disease, people experiencing stabilization of integrated functioning, people whose quality of life is irreversibly affected, and people who have a terminal illness.

Nursing practice occurs in diverse settings, including people's homes, neighborhoods, group residential facilities, meeting places of various community-based groups, ambulatory clinics, rehabilitation and long-term care facilities, and tertiary medical centers.

An adult requires nursing when he or she does not have the ability to continuously maintain the amount and quality of self-care that is therapeutic in sustaining life and health; in recovering from disease, injury, or disability; or in coping with their effects. A child requires nursing when his or her parent or guardian cannot continuously maintain the amount and quality of care that is therapeutic.

The nursing process for the Self-Care Framework is Orem's Professional–Technological System of Nursing Practice. The components of the process are case management operations, diagnostic operations, prescriptive operations, regulatory operations, and control operations.

Self-Care Framework–based nursing practice contributes to the well-being of nursing participants by regulating self-care agency or dependent-care agency and meeting the therapeutic self-care demand.

Adapted from Fawcett and DeSanto-Madeya (2013), with permission.

(Orem, 2001, p. 225); this subdimension is henceforth referred to as desire for normalcy. Fleck (2012) explained, "Young and middle age adults often desire to lose weight. To be overweight is considered to be in the outside parameters of of normalcy" (p. 26).

The theory concept is Nutrition Decision Making, which represents the conceptual model concept subdimenion of desire for normalcy. Nutrition Decision Making is assessed by the NSCI (Fleck, 2012). The results of the NSCI are used by nurses and overweight or obese young and middle-age adults to collaborate in making individualized meal plans.

The conceptual–theoretical–empirical (CTE) structure constructed from the content of Fleck's (2012) article is illustrated in Figure 6.2. The non-relational propositions for each component of the CTE structure are listed in Box 6.3.

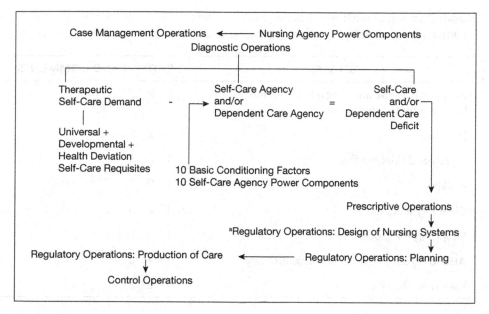

FIGURE 6.1 Orem's practice methodology: Professional–technological system of nursing practice.

[a]**Three Nursing Systems**
Wholly Compensatory
Partly Compensatory
Supportive–Educative

Five Methods of Helping
Acting for or Doing for the Patient
Guiding the Patient
Supporting the Patient
Providing a Developmental Environment
Teaching the Patient

BOX 6.2   The Orem's Self-Care Framework Practice Methodology Tool

DIAGNOSTIC OPERATIONS

Therapeutic Self-Care Demand

The nurse extracts the following information about the patient's therapeutic self-care demand from the electronic health record:

- Universal self-care demands
- Developmental self-care demands
- Health deviation self-care demands

(continued)

BOX 6.2 The Orem's Self-Care Framework Practice Methodology Tool *(continued)*

Self-Care Agency

Nurse: Please rate each of the activities I will read to you using the rating scale of 1 = I am able to do this by myself, 2 = I am able to do this with help, or 3 = I cannot do this.

ACTIVITY	RATINGS AND COMMENTS
Personal hygiene and grooming (bathing, brushing teeth, combing hair)	1 2 3
Dressing	1 2 3
Eating and drinking fluids	1 2 3
Walking	1 2 3
Climbing stairs	1 2 3
Shopping for groceries	1 2 3
Attending social events in the community	1 2 3
Taking medications	1 2 3

Power Components

Nurse: What do you know about [health condition or medical diagnosis]?
Nurse: Would you like to learn about how to care for yourself to reduce the severity of your symptoms?

Basic Conditioning Factors

The nurse extracts information about basic conditioning factors (age, gender, family system factors, sociocultural factors, health state, health care system factors) from the electronic health record.

Nursing Diagnosis

The nurse and the patient determine that his or her therapeutic self-care demand currently is (greater than/less than/equal to) his or her self-care agency due to... . The patient (agrees/does not agree) with the nurse that he or she is highly motivated to learn what is needed to increase his or her ability to take care of self.

PRESCRIPTIVE OPERATIONS AND REGULATORY OPERATIONS: DESIGN OF NURSING SYSTEMS FOR PERFORMANCE OF REGULATORY OPERATIONS

The nurse and the patient (agree/do not agree) that he or she (lacks/does not lack) knowledge of what to do to "get better." The nurse selects the (wholly compensatory/

(continued)

> ## BOX 6.2   The Orem's Self-Care Framework Practice Methodology Tool   *(continued)*
>
> partly compensatory/supportive–educative) nursing system with (indicate which one or more method[s] of helping) as the means to (increase/maintain current level of) the patient's self-care agency.
>
> ### REGULATORY OPERATIONS: PLANNING FOR REGULATORY OPERATIONS
>
> The nurse has sufficient nursing agency to implement the planned nursing system and method(s) of helping. (Add any other components of the plan.)
>
> ### REGULATORY OPERATIONS: PRODUCTION OF REGULATORY CARE
>
> The nurse and the patient carry out the plan of care (without/with) any difficulties or adjustments.
>
> ### CONTROL OPERATIONS
>
> The nurse and the patient evaluate the effectiveness of the nursing system and method(s) of helping.
>
> Adapted from Fawcett and DeSanto-Madeya (2013).

A CTE Structure for Intervention

An example of Orem's Self-Care Framework–guided nursing practice focused on intervention is found in Green's (2012) journal article. Green explained how school nurses can use Orem's Self-Care Framework to develop and implement interventions for school-age childern with special health care needs. According to the Centers for Disease Control and Prevention (as cited in Green, 2012, p. 35):

> Children with special care needs are identified as those who "have a parent-reported medical, behavioral, or other health condition that has lasted or is expected to last 12 months or longer and that has resulted in functional limitations and/or elevated use of or need for medical care, mental health or educational services, specialized therapy, or prescription medications beyond what is usual for other children of the same age."

Green (2012) discussed nursing care for a "middle school student who was born premature at 30 weeks and had been diagnosed with asthma as an infant" (p. 38). She explained that although "the school nurse was able to provide nursing care in the school clinic, . . . she could not ensure that dependent-care would continue at home" (p. 37).

BOX 6.3   An Example of a Conceptual–Theoretical–Empirical Structure for Orem's Self-Care Framework Nursing Practice: Assessment

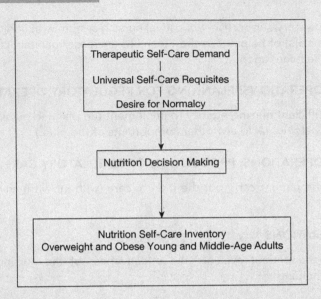

FIGURE 6.2 Conceptual–theoretical–empirical (CTE) structure for Orem's Self-Care Framework nursing practice: Assessment—theory of assessment of nutrition practices.

The *non-relational propositions* for the *C component* of the conceptual–theoretical–empirical (CTE) structure are:

- *Therapeutic Self-Care Demand* is defined as the demand on the individual or multiperson unit for continuing effective care of self.
- The relevant dimension of Therapeutic Self-Care Demand is universal self-care requisites.
  o *Universal self-care requisites* is defined as a type of self-care requisite that is common to all people at all stages of life, but adjusted for age, developmental stage, and the environment.
  o The relevant subdimension of universal self-care requisites is desire for normalcy.
    ■ *Desire for normalcy* is defined as "the human desire to be normal" (Orem, 2001, p. 225).

The *non-relational proposition* for the *T component* of the CTE structure is:

- *Nutrition Decision Making* is defined as perceived confidence in ability to make decisions about nutrition practices (Fleck, 2012).

The *non-relational proposition* for the *E component* of the CTE structure is:

- Nutrition Decision Making is assessed by the Nutrition Self-Care Inventory (NSCI; Fleck, 2012). The NSCI includes 10 items that are rated on a scale of 1 = disagree, 2 = somewhat agree, or 3 = agree.

Source: Fleck (2012).

The theory is the effect of school nursing asthma interventions on asthma self-management. One conceptual model concept is Professional–Technological System of Nursing Practice. The relevant dimension of the concept is regulatory operations, and the relevant subdimension is production of regulatory care, including wholly compensatory, partly compensatory, and supportive–educative nursing systems designed to overcome self-care and dependent-care deficits. The other conceptual model concept is Self-Care. The theory concepts are School Nursing Asthma Interventions and Asthma Self-Management.

School Nursing Asthma Interventions represents the Professional–Technological System of Nursing Practice subdimension of production of regulatory care, and Asthma Self-Management represents Self-Care. School Nursing Asthma Interventions is operationalized by the School Nursing Asthma Interventions protocol. Asthma Self-Management is measured by extent of lack of occurrence of asthma symptoms.

The CTE structure constructed from an interpretation of the content of Green's (2012) article is illustrated in Figure 6.3. The non-relational and relational propositions for each component of the CTE structure are listed in Box 6.4.

OREM'S SELF-CARE FRAMEWORK: APPLICATION TO QUALITY IMPROVEMENT PROJECTS

The guidelines for Orem's Self-Care Framework quality improvement (QI) projects are listed in Box 6.5.

A CTE Structure for a QI Project

Ryan, Aloe, and Mason-Johnson's (2009) journal article contains an example of an Orem's Self-Care Framework–guided QI project. The purpose of their project was to develop and implement a multidisciplinary group discharge teaching plan to increase patients' heart failure self-care management. Ryan et al. noted that "Group teaching is one of many patient education methods that may promote positive patient outcomes and efficient, cost-effective care" (p. 218).

The theory is the effect of group discharge teaching on heart failure self-care management. One conceptual model concept is Professional–Technological System of Nursing Practice. The relevant dimension of the concept is regulatory operations, and the relevant subdimension is production of regulatory care with emphasis on the supportive–educative nursing system directed to enhancing patients' self-care to meet their heart failure–related health deviation self-care requisites (Ryan et al., 2009). The other conceptual model concept is Self-Care.

The theory concepts are Group Discharge Teaching Plan and Heart Failure Self-Care Management. Group Discharge Teaching Plan represents the Professional–Technological System of Nursing Practice subdimension of production of regulatory care, and Heart Failure Self-Care Management represents

BOX 6.4 An Example of a Conceptual–Theoretical–Empirical Structure for Orem's Self-Care Framework Nursing Practice: Intervention

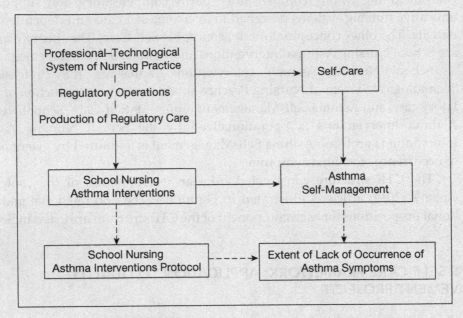

FIGURE 6.3 Conceptual–theoretical–empirical (CTE) structure for Orem's Self-Care Framework nursing practice: Intervention—theory of the effect of school nursing asthma interventions on asthma self-management.

The *non-relational propositions* for the *C component* of the conceptual–theoretical–empirical (CTE) structure are:

- *Professional–Technological System of Nursing Practice* is defined as the nursing process.
- The relevant dimension of Professional–Technological System of Nursing Practice is regulatory operations.
  - o *Regulatory operations* is defined as design and implementation of a nursing system and method(s) of helping.
  - o The relevant subdimension of regulatory operations is production of regulatory care.
    - ■ *Production of regulatory care* is defined as implementation of the selected nursing system and method(s) of helping.
- *Self-Care* is defined as actions taken by individuals to regulate their function and development.

The *non-relational propositions* for the *T component* of the CTE structure are:

- *School Nursing Asthma Interventions* is defined as nursing interventions that enhance self-management of asthma symptoms.

(continued)

BOX 6.4   An Example of a Conceptual–Theoretical–Empirical Structure for Orem's Self-Care Framework Nursing Practice: Intervention   (continued)

- *Asthma Self-Management* is defined as control of asthma symptoms.

The *non-relational propositions* for the E component of the conceptual–theoretical–empirical (CTE) structure are:

- School Nursing Asthma Interventions is operationalized by the School Nursing Asthma Interventions protocol, which includes "assisting [the student] and his [or her] family with coping strategies, and ongoing assistance through case management that involved both formal and informal networking among the family's network of community resources and support. The school nurse assumed the informal role of case manager to establish ongoing communication among a variety of providers and access to a patchwork quilt of services" (Green, 2012, p. 37).
- Asthma Self-Management is measured by the extent of the lack of occurrence of asthma symptoms (Green, 2012).

The *relational propositions* for the C and T components of the CTE structure are:

- The Professional–Technological System of Nursing Practice has a positive effect on Self-Care.
- Therefore, School Nursing Asthma Interventions have a positive effect on Asthma Self-Management.

The *relational proposition* for the E component of the CTE structure is:

- Implementation of the School Nursing Asthma Interventions protocol has a negative effect on occurrence of asthma symptoms, such that implementation of the protocol is associated with a reduction in the occurrence of asthma symptoms.

Source: Green (2012).

Self-Care. Group Discharge Teaching Plan is operationalized by the Group Discharge Teaching Plan protocol and the "Managing Your Congestive Heart Failure" booklet. Ryan et al. (2009) stated that they used the evidence-based practice approach of the PICOT (P = Patient Population, I = Intervention, C = Comparison, O = Outcome, T = Time) clinical question (Melnyk & Fineout-Overholt, 2005), which is a QI methodological theory (see Appendix A), to guide development of the protocol.

Heart Failure Self-Care Management is measured by an investigator-developed Evaluation Form (Ryan, 2009), as well as by patient readmission rates obtained from a hospital database. The differences in scores for patients who received group discharge education and those who received usual care are analyzed using descriptive statistics (numbers, percents, means; see Appendix B).

BOX 6.5   Guidelines for Orem's Self-Care Framework Quality Improvement Projects

The purpose of quality improvement (QI) projects is to test the effectiveness of nurses' use of Orem's practice methodology (Professional–Technological System of Nursing Practice) on nurses' nursing agency and/or patients' self-care agency or dependent-care agency and self-care or dependent care.

The phenomenon of interest for a QI project is the extent of nurses' use of Professional–Technological System of Nursing Practice on nurses' nursing agency and/or patients' self-care agency or dependent-care agency and self-care or dependent care.

Data for QI projects are to be collected from nurses and/or patients in various settings, such as patients' homes, nurses' private offices, ambulatory clinics, hospitals, and communities.

Any methodological theory of change or QI may be used to guide the design of the QI project and the times for data collection. Checklists, rating scales, and responses to open-ended questions may be used to determine the extent to which nurses actually implement one or more components of the Professional–Technological System of Nursing Practice. Descriptive statistics may be used to analyze data obtained from checklists or rating scales, and content analysis may be used to identify categories or themes found in responses to open-ended questions.

The results of Orem's Self-Care Framework–based QI projects enhance understanding of how using the Professional–Technological System of Nursing Practice influences nursing agency and/or self-care agency or dependent-care agency and self-care or dependent care.

The CTE structure constructed from an interpretation of the content of Ryan et al.'s (2009) article is illustrated in Figure 6.4. The non-relational and relational propositions for each component of the CTE structure are listed in Box 6.6.

OREM'S SELF-CARE FRAMEWORK: APPLICATION TO NURSING RESEARCH

The guidelines for Orem's Self-Care Framework nursing research are listed in Box 6.7.

A CTE Structure for a Systematic Literature Review

The content of Kelo, Martikaninen, and Eriksson's (2011) journal article is an example of a report of a systematic literature review guided by Orem's Self-Care Framework. The purpose of their review of literature "was to synthesize findings from empirical studies on self-care in school-age children with type 1 diabetes, thus giving insight into opportunities to develop empowering patient education" (p. 2097).

BOX 6.6   An Example of Orem's Self-Care Framework Quality Improvement Projects

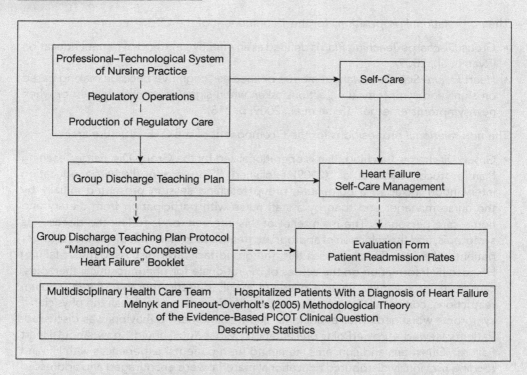

FIGURE 6.4 Conceptual–theoretical–empirical (CTE) structure for Orem's Self-Care Framework quality improvement (QI) project—theory of effects of group discharge teaching on heart failure self-care management.

PICOT, P = patient population, I = intervention, C = comparison, O = outcome, T = time.

The *non-relational propositions* for the C component of the conceptual–theoretical–empirical (CTE) structure are:

- *Professional–Technological System of Nursing Practice* is defined as the nursing process.
- The relevant dimension of Professional–Technological System of Nursing Practice is regulatory operations.
  - o *Regulatory operations* is defined as design and implementation of a nursing system and method(s) of helping.
  - o The relevant subdimension of regulatory operations is production of regulatory care.
    - ▪ *Production of regulatory care* is defined as implementation of the selected nursing system and method(s) of helping.
- *Self-Care* is defined as actions taken by individuals to regulate their function and development.

(continued)

BOX 6.6 An Example of Orem's Self-Care Framework Quality Improvement Projects *(continued)*

The *non-relational propositions* for the *T component* of the CTE structure are:

- *Group Discharge Teaching Plan* is defined as an effective method of patient education (Ryan et al., 2009).
- *Heart Failure Self-Care Management* is defined as "cognitive decision making based on signs and symptoms (i.e., actions taken when signs/symptoms worsen or when new symptoms emerge)" (Ryan et al., 2009, p. 218).

The *non-relational propositions* for the *E component* of the CTE structure are:

- Group Discharge Teaching Plan is operationalized by the Group Discharge Teaching Plan protocol. Ryan et al. (2009) explained, "The group discharge education intervention included a 60-minute, group teaching session presented initially by the nurse manager and then by a staff nurse with participation from dietary and home care personnel. The main tenet of this intervention is to link the disease, its symptoms, and the selection of appropriate treatment to skill building in critical target patient behaviors. To accomplish this, the group facilitator discussed [heart failure] HF-specific information on the causes of HF, rationale for pharmaceutical therapies, causes of intravascular volume overload in HF, diuretic therapy, dietary sodium restrictions, common HF symptoms, and instructions on when to call the physician if symptoms worsened. The rationale for self-management behaviors was discussed. Patients viewed a PowerPoint presentation, 'What You Should Know About Heart Failure.' Questions and concerns stemming from patients' experiences with HF and reading previously distributed educational material were encouraged and addressed by the group leader and participating disciplines" (p. 219). In addition, the patients received the "Managing Your Congestive Heart Failure" booklet. Development of the protocol was guided by the quality improvement methodological theory of the PICOT (P = Patient Population, I = Intervention, C = Comparison, O = Outcome, T = Time) clinical question (Melnyk & Fineout-Overholt, 2004). The clinical question for the quality improvement project is: "In adults with HF [P], does comprehensive group discharge education [I] compared with usual care [C] decrease the readmission rate [O, T]?" (Ryan et al., 2009, p. 219).
- Heart Failure Self-Care Management is measured by an investigator-developed Evaluation Form, which is made up of four items that are rated on a 5-point scale of 1 = strongly disagree to 5 = strongly agree, and that "was constructed to evaluate whether patients [thought] they had acquired information about HF and its management and if they liked learning in a group session" (Ryan et al., 2009, p. 218).
- Heart Failure Self-Care Management also is measured by patient readmission rates obtained from a hospital database (Ryan et al., 2009).

The *relational propositions* for the *C* and *T components* of the CTE structure are:

- The Professional–Technological System of Nursing Practice has a positive effect on Self-Care.

(continued)

BOX 6.6   An Example of Orem's Self-Care Framework Quality Improvement Projects   (continued)

- Therefore, Group Discharge Teaching Plan has a positive effect on Heart Failure Self-Care Management.

The *relational proposition* for the *E component* of the CTE structure is:

- Implementation of the Group Discharge Teaching Plan protocol has a positive effect on Evaluation Form scores and a negative effect on patient readmission rates, such that implementation of the protocol is associated with an increase in Evaluation Form scores and a decrease in patient readmisison rates.

Source: Ryan, Aloe, and Mason-Johnson (2009).

Kelo et al. (2011) used Whittemore and Knafl's (2005) literature review approach (see Appendix A). They searched several electronic databases (Cumulative Index to Nursing and Allied Health Literature [CINAHL], MEDLINE, PubMed, Cochrane, PsycINFO, and PsycARTICLES) using the search terms "Self-Care" AND "Self-Manage" with "Child" AND "Diabetes" OR "Diabetes Mellitus," as well as combining "Diabetes" WITH "Child" OR "Parent" AND "Experience," "Self-Report" OR "Interview." They also did manual searches of journal article reference lists. Explaining the inclusion and exclusion criteria for literature, Kelo et al. (2011) stated:

> As the treatment of diabetes has changed over the years, the search was limited to the period 01/1998–08/2010. In addition, only English-language and original research articles were accepted. An article was included if it described the self-care of school-age children with type 1 diabetes, if the mean age of the children was between 6 and 12 years and if it described children's or parents' opinions on self-care. Because technical treatment equipment was outside the scope of this review, articles focusing on evaluating the effect of a technical treatment method on self-care were excluded. (p. 2098)

The search yielded 653 articles, of which 22 were retained for the review. Twelve of the 22 articles were reports of quantitative studies, nine were reports of qualitative studies, and one was a report of a mixed-methods study.

The theory of the diabetes self-care learning process was generated from the results of the literature review. The conceptual model concept is Self-Care, which guided the search of the literature. The theory concept is Diabetes Self-Care Learning Process, which has three dimensions—related factors, content, and goals. The related factors dimension has three subdimensions—child characteristics, illness and care, and support. The content dimension has two

BOX 6.7 Guidelines for Orem's Self-Care Framework Research

The purpose of Self-Care Framework–based nursing research is to develop knowledge for the practical sciences of nursing.

Specific variables that make up nursing knowledge from the perspective of the Self-Care Framework are in the categories of the self-care requisites making up the therapeutic self-care demand, basic conditioning factors, power components, self-care agency, dependent-care agency, self-care deficits, dependent-care deficits, self-care practices, dependent-care practices, health state, health results sought, nursing requirements, nursing situations, nursing systems, nursing technologies, methods of helping, and outcomes of production of nursing systems.

The precise problems to be studied are those that reflect actual or predictable self-care deficits or dependent-care deficits.

Study participants are the individuals and multiperson units who are considered legitimate patients of nurses, that is, people with deficit relationships between their current or projected capability for providing self-care or dependent-care and the qualitative and quantitative demand for care due to the health state or health care needs of those requiring care.

Data may be collected from individuals and multiperson units in the person's home; in hospitals, clinics, and resident-care facilities; and in various other settings in which nursing occurs, using one or more Self-Care Framework–based research instruments. Descriptive, case study, correlational, and experimental research designs associated with the empiricist research paradigm are consistent with Orem's Self-Care Framework. Furthermore, ethnographic, grounded theory, and phenomenological research designs associated with the interpretive research paradigm are consistent with the Self-Care Framework, as are mixed-method designs that integrate the empiricist and interpretive paradigms. In contrast, research designs associated with the critical theory research paradigm are not consistent with Orem's Self-Care Framework, due to the focus of that paradigm on emancipation of the study participants from beliefs and values that may be oppressive, as well as to the fact that Orem did not address such major issues in the critical theory paradigm as having power over others and exercising control and domination of others.

Data analysis techniques associated with qualitative and/or quantitative data are appropriate.

Self-Care Framework–based research findings enhance understanding of patient and nurse variables that affect the performance of continuing therapeutic self-care and dependent-care.

Adapted from Fawcett and DeSanto-Madeya (2013), with permission.

subdimensions—knowledge and skills. The goals dimension has three subdimensions—normality, being able to cope, and independence. The concept of Self-Care Learning Process and its dimensions and subdimensions were generated from the integrative review of the 22 research reports.

The CTE structure constructed from the content of Kelo et al.'s (2011) article is illustrated in Figure 6.5. The non-relational propositions for each component of the CTE structure are listed in Box 6.8. The two relational propositions for the

BOX 6.8 An Example of a Conceptual–Theoretical–Empirical Structure for Orem's Self-Care Framework Literature Review

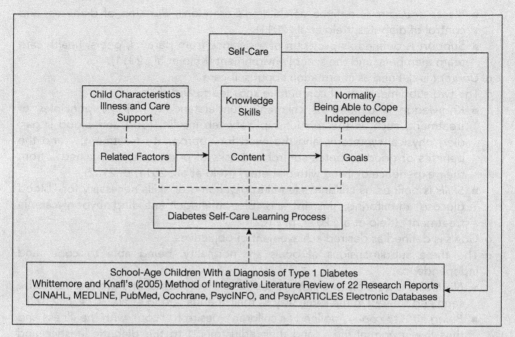

FIGURE 6.5 Conceptual–theoretical–empirical (CTE) structure for Orem's Self-Care Framework literature review—theory of the diabetes self-care learning process.

The *non-relational proposition* for the *C component* of the conceptual–theoretical–empirical (CTE) structure is:

- *Self-Care* is defined as actions taken by individuals to regulate their function and development.

The *non-relational propositions* for the *T component* of the CTE structure are:

- *Diabetes Self-Care Learning Process* is defined as learning "health-related activities required to live an everyday life" by school-age children with a diagnosis of type 1 diabetes (Kelo et al., 2011, p. 2097).
- The three dimensions of Diabetes Self-Care Learning Process are related factors, content, and goals.
  o *Related factors* is defined as variables related to self-care.
  o The three subdimensions of related factors are child characteristics, illness and care, and support.
    ▪ *Child characteristics* is defined as children's attitude, motivation, gender, and age (Kelo et al., 2011).

(continued)

BOX 6.8   An Example of a Conceptual–Theoretical–Empirical Structure for Orem's Self-Care Framework Literature Review   *(continued)*

- ■ *Illness and care* is defined as children's emotions, duration of diabetes, and control of diabetes (Kelo et al., 2011).
- ■ *Support* is defined as provision of assistance from parents, peers, health care team members, and the school environment (Kelo et al., 2011).
- o *Content* is defined as information about self-care.
- o The two subdimensions of content are knowledge and skills.
  - ■ *Knowledge* is defined as children's "understanding [of] the principles of treatment, such as the relationship between insulin, food and blood sugar; diet; physical symptoms and the need for appropriate treatment;...and the benefits of good diabetes control and risks of poor control...gained...from their experience of living with diabetes" (Kelo et al., 2011, p. 2102).
  - ■ *Skills* is defined as children's learning psychomotor skills necessary for "blood glucose monitoring, insulin and diet management and hypoglycaemia treatment" (Kelo et al., 2011, p. 2102).
- o *Goals* is defined as desired achievement of objectives.
- o The three subdimensions of goals are normality, being able to cope, and independence.
  - ■ *Normality* is defined as children's desire to "feel normal and accepted...to be seen and treated in the same way as their friends" (Kelo et al., 2011, p. 2102).
  - ■ *Being able to cope* is defined as children's desire to "cope with the illness and thus live a normal life...[and their adjustment] to the diabetic lifestyle and [accept] its demands eventually" (Kelo et al., 2011, p. 2102).
  - ■ *Independence* is defined as children's desire "to be independent in their choices and decisions concerning diabetes management" (Kelo et al., 2011, p. 2102).

The *non-relational proposition* for the *E component* of the CTE structure is:

- • The concept of Diabetes Self-Care Learning Process and its dimensions and subdimensions were extracted from an integrative literature review of 22 research reports.

The *relational propositions* for the *T component* of the CTE structure are:

- • Related factors is associated with content.
- • Content is associated with goals.

Source: Kelo, Martikaninen, and Eriksson (2011).

T component that were generated from the results of the literature review are also included in Box 6.8; these propositions state the relations among the three dimensions of Diabetes Self-Care Learning Process.

A CTE Structure for Instrument Development

The journal article by Srikan and Phillips (2014) presents an example of a report of development of an instrument derived from Orem's Self-Care Framework.

They explained that they developed the Dietary Salt Reduction Self-Care Behavior (DSR-SCB) Scale "to acquire a comprehensive understanding of hypertensive older adults' perceptions toward their behavior in managing salt reduction in daily life" (p. 235).

The theory is dietary salt reduction behavior. The conceptual model concept is Self-Care, which is represented by the theory concept of Dietary Salt Reduction Behavior. The DSR-SCB Scale measures Dietary Salt Reduction Behavior. Srikan and Phillips (2014) reported that estimates of the psychometric properties of the DSR-SCB Scale are adequate. They estimated internal consistency reliability with Cronbach's alpha. Construct validity was estimated with principal components factor analysis, which yielded one factor, indicating that the theory concept of Dietary Salt Reduction Behavior is unidimensional. Validity also was estimated with Rasch analysis (see Appendix B).

The CTE structure constructed from the content of Srikan and Phillips's (2014) article is illustrated in Figure 6.6. The non-relational propositions for each component of the CTE structure are listed in Box 6.9.

A CTE Structure for Descriptive Qualitative Research

A journal article by Fex, Flensner, Ek, and Söderhamn (2011) is an example of a report of descriptive qualitative research guided by Orem's Self-Care Framework. The purpose of Fex et al.'s study was to "gain a deeper understanding of the meaning of living with an adult family member using advanced medical technology at home" (p. 338). They used a hermeneutic research design developed by Fleming, Gaidys, and Robb (2003; see Appendix A).

The theory of the meaning of living with an adult family member using advanced medical technology at home was generated from the study data. The conceptual model concept is Dependent-Care. The theory concept is Meaning of Living With an Adult Family Member Using Advanced Medical Technology at Home. The theory concept has 10 dimensions—focusing on the patient, supporting practically and psychologically and being constantly there, favoring and learning to deal with technology, adjusting home and means of transport, being autonomous and changing roles, regretting life as having changed and worrying about the future, seeking explanation, getting used to and making the best of the situation, needing support from health care professionals, and needing support from significant others.

Dependent-Care guided the selection of research methods and overall interpretation of the data. The theory concept and its dimensions were discovered in the responses of 11 family member caregivers of persons requiring home-based advanced medical technology to an open-ended interview question and follow-up questions to clarify responses to the open-ended question (Fex et al.,

BOX 6.9   An Example of a Conceptual–Theoretical–Empirical Structure for Orem's Self-Care Framework Instrument Development

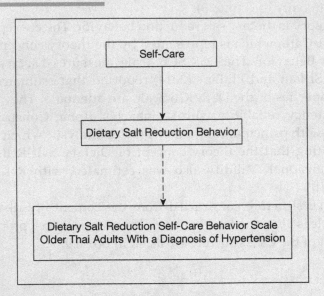

FIGURE 6.6 Conceptual–theoretical–empirical (CTE) structure for Orem's Self-Care Framework instrument development research—theory of dietary salt reduction behavior.

The *non-relational proposition* for the *C component* of the conceptual–theoretical–empirical (CTE) structure is:

- *Self-Care* is defined as actions taken by individuals to regulate their function and development.

The *non-relational proposition* for the *T component* of the CTE structure is:

- *Dietary Salt Reduction Behavior* is defined as "hypertensive older adults' perceptions toward their behavior in managing salt reduction in daily life" (Srikan & Phillips, 2014, p. 235).

The *non-relational proposition* for the *E component* of the CTE structure is:

- Dietary Salt Reduction Behavior is measured by the Dietary Salt Reduction Self-Care Behavior (DSR-SCB) Scale. Srikan and Phillips (2014) explained that they generated an initial pool of 58 items—which was eventually reduced to nine items—for the DSR-SCB Scale from a review of "research related to salt reduction behavior, hypertension, and health behavior in a variety of topics, including dietary sources of salt, effects of excessive salt consumption on blood pressure, daily salt recommendations, checking food labels for sodium, initiating strategies to reduce daily salt consumption, and other factors influencing salt consumption" (p. 235). The items are rated on a 5-point scale of 1 = never, 2 = seldom, 3 = sometimes, 4 = often, and 5 = always. An English-language version and a Thai-language version of the DSR-SCB Scale are available.

Source: Srikan and Phillips (2014).

2011). The caregivers' responses to the interview question are analyzed using a hermeneutic method of data analysis (see Appendix B).

The CTE structure constructed from the content of Fex et al.'s (2011) research report is illustrated in Figure 6.7. The non-relational propositions for each component of the CTE structure are listed in Box 6.10.

A CTE Structure for Correlational Research

White's (2013) journal article is an example of Orem's Self-Care Framework-guided correlational research (see Appendix A). The purpose of her study was to test an expansion of Orem's framework by adding spiritual self-care as a mediator of the relation between self-care and well-being.

The theory is the relation of heart failure self-care practices, spiritual self-care practices, and quality of life. White (2013) tested the theory with a sample of "142 African American patients diagnosed with heart failure who were being treated in two outpatient clinics associated with a large medical center in a major urban area" (p. 26).

The conceptual model concepts are Self-Care, Spiritual Self-Care, and Well-Being. White (2013) explained that she added Spiritual Self-Care Practices to Orem's Self-Care Framework as a conceptual model concept that is distinct from Self-Care.

The theory concepts are Heart Failure Self-Care Practices, Spiritual Self-Care Practices, and Quality of Life. Heart Failure Self-Care Practices represents Self-Care, Spiritual Self-Care Practices represents Spiritual Care, and Quality of Life represents Well-Being. Heart Failure Self-Care Practices is measured by the Heart Failure Self-Care Behavior Scale (HFSCBS; Artinian, Magnan, Sloan, & Lange, 2002). Spiritual Self-Care Practices is measured by the Spiritual Self-Care Practices Scale (SSCPS; White, 2010). Quality of Life is measured by the World Health Organization—Quality of Life-Brief (WHOQOL-BREF; World Health Organization, 1996).

The CTE structure constructed from the content of White's (2103) research report is illustrated in Figure 6.8, as is the mediation method of correlational data analysis (Baron & Kenny, 1986; Kenny, 2012/2016; see Appendix B). The non-relational and relational propositions for each component of the CTE structure are listed in Box 6.11.

A CTE Structure for Experimental Research

Nazik and Eryilmaz's (2013) journal article is an example of a report of experimental research guided by Orem's Self-Care Framework. The purpose of their study was to examine the effects of Orem's Self-Care Framework–based home care on problems and complications experienced by women following birth of their first child and on the women's care of themselves.

BOX 6.10   An Example of a Conceptual–Theoretical–Empirical Structure for Orem's Self-Care Framework Descriptive Qualitative Research

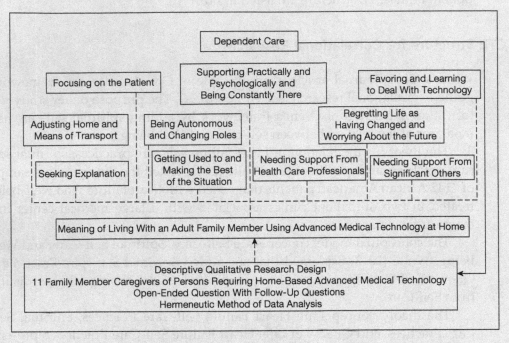

FIGURE 6.7 Conceptual–theoretical–empirical (CTE) structure for Orem's Self-Care Framework descriptive qualitative research—theory of the meaning of living with an adult family member using advanced medical technology at home.

The *non-relational proposition* for the *C component* of the conceptual–theoretical–empirical (CTE) structure is:

- *Dependent-Care* is defined as actions taken by adults for dependent family members or friends who cannot perform adequate self-care.

The *non-relational propositions* for the *T component* of the CTE structure are:

- *Meaning of Living With an Adult Family Member Using Advanced Medical Technology at Home* is defined as "being closely connected to, but on the other hand also being separated from, him or her. It means sorrow, but there is also reconciliation. Further, dependence on others is shown in the need for support from healthcare professionals and significant others" (Fex et al., 2011, p. 346).
- Meaning of Living With an Adult Family Member Using Advanced Medical Technology at Home has 10 dimensions—focusing on the patient, supporting practically and psychologically and being constantly there, favoring and learning to deal with technology, adjusting home and means of transport, being autonomous and changing roles, regretting life as having changed and worrying about the future,

(continued)

BOX 6.10   An Example of a Conceptual–Theoretical–Empirical Structure for Orem's Self-Care Framework Descriptive Qualitative Research   *(continued)*

seeking explanation, getting used to and making the best of the situation, needing support from health care professionals, and needing support from significant others.

o *Focusing on the patient* is defined as focusing "on the patient's needs, even when the patient was away" (Fex et al., 2011, p. 340).

o *Supporting practically and psychologically and being constantly there* is defined as "bringing various things when the patient was in treatment" (practical support) and "being someone who listens and is engaged, and a source of security" (psychological support and being constantly there) (Fex et al., 2011, p. 342).

o *Favoring and learning to deal with technology* is defined as supporting the person's decision to use health-related technology at home and learning how to manage the technology, frequently from health care professionals, as well as learning to recognize signs and symptoms of illness (Fex et al., 2011).

o *Adjusting home and means of transport* is defined as adapting the home and car or van to accommodate the demands of the technology (Fex et al., 2011).

o *Being autonomous and changing roles* is defined as "switching the focus from the patients' needs to the participants' [needs, while] sometimes disregarding interests was a learning process of letting go....[and taking] responsibility for more demanding domestic duties while the patients performed the less strenuous ones, like cooking" (Fex et al., 2011, p. 343).

o *Regretting life as having changed and worrying about the future* is defined as "sorrow to realize that earlier hopes for their old age, like frequent trips to distant countries, were unattainable...[and worrying] about what might happen the day their strength lessened: where would they live, and how would they manage daily life activities" (Fex et al., 2011, p. 343).

o *Seeking explanation* is defined as finding "explanations for the disease and the need for technology" (Fex et al., 2011, p. 343).

o *Getting used to and making the best of the situation* is defined as "a learning process to get used to the patient's impaired strength and daily life with technology...[and striving to not] let technology restrict their activities and to have an eventful life" (Fex et al., 2011, p. 343).

o *Needing support from health care professionals* is defined as receiving support "from healthcare professionals by telephone whenever a question arose [which] was considered vital. Just knowing that expert advice was always available meant security, allowing the participants to become confident in solving problems themselves" (Fex et al., 2011, p. 343).

o *Needing support from significant others* is defined as having "a social network of family and friends to confide in, and who understood and accepted the situation concerning the technology" (Fex et al., 2011, p. 343).

The *non-relational proposition* for the *E* component of the CTE structure is:

• Meaning of Living With an Adult Family Member Using Advanced Medical Technology at Home and its dimensions were discovered in responses of 11 family member caregivers to an open-ended question—"What [is] the meaning of living with someone who is using advanced medical technology at home?" (Fex et al., 2011, p. 339)—and follow up elucidating questions.

Source: Fex, Flensner, Ek, and Söderhamn (2011).

BOX 6.11 An Example of a Conceptual–Theoretical–Empirical Structure for Orem's Self-Care Framework Correlational Research

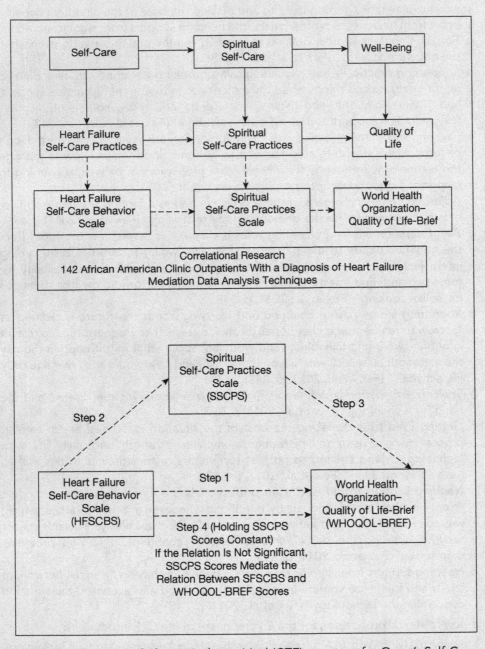

FIGURE 6.8 Conceptual–theoretical–empirical (CTE) structure for Orem's Self-Care Framework correlational research—theory of the relations of heart failure self-care practice, spiritual self-care practices, and quality of life.

(continued)

BOX 6.11   An Example of a Conceptual–Theoretical–Empirical Structure for Orem's Self-Care Framework Correlational Research   *(continued)*

The *non-relational propositions* for the C component of the conceptual–theoretical–empirical (CTE) structure are:

- *Self-Care* is defined as actions taken by individuals to regulate their function and development.
- *Spiritual Self-Care* "is defined as the set of spiritually-based practices in which people engage to promote continued personal development and well-being in times of health and illness" (White, 2013, p. 24).
- *Well-Being* is defined as the individual's perception of the condition of his or her existence, which may be characterized as feeling content, pleasure, happiness, fulfilling one's self-ideal, and having positive spiritual experiences.

The *non-relational propositions* for the T component of the CTE structure are:

- *Heart Failure Self-Care Practices* is defined as focusing primarily on health deviation self-care requisites, specifically "those activities that persons engage [in] to manage ongoing limitations in structural or functional integrity" (Freitas & Mendes, as cited in White, 2013, p. 25). "Health care practitioners (HCPs) routinely advise patients diagnosed with [heart failure] HF about obtaining daily weights, monitoring swelling, taking medications, eating a low-sodium diet, obtaining routine vaccinations (e.g., yearly flu vaccine), exercising daily, and seeing their HCP regularly" (White, 2013, pp. 25–26).
- *Spiritual Self-Care Practices* is defined as focusing on developmental self-care requisites "based on an individual's mind/spirit/body connection, upbringing, moral and religious background, and life experiences that originate from faith, feelings, and emotions. Examples of spiritual self-care can include building social networks or volunteering…listening to inspirational music…meditation…and developing a sense of inner peace and quiet…Other examples of spiritual self-care include practicing yoga or Tai Chi, attending religious services, reading sacred or inspirational texts, prayer or [meditation], hiking, walking or otherwise enjoying nature, and developing or mending personal relationships" (White, 2013, p. 26).
- *Quality of Life* is defined as "an individually defined and perceived state of well-being…'[individuals'] perception of their position in life in the context of the culture and value system in which they live and in relation to their goals, expectations, standards, and concerns' (World Health Organization, as cited in White, 2013, p. 25) [that includes] physical, emotional, and social effects on the individual's perception of daily life" (White, 2013, p. 25).

The *non-relational propositions* for the E component of the CTE structure are:

- Heart Failure Self-Care Practices is measured by the Heart Failure Self-Care Behavior Scale (HFSCBS; Artinian, Magnan, Sloan, & Lange, 2002). The HFSCBS contains 29 heart failure behaviors that are rated on a 6-point scale of 0 = none of the time to 5 = all of the time.

(continued)

BOX 6.11   An Example of a Conceptual–Theoretical–Empirical Structure for Orem's Self-Care Framework Correlational Research   (continued)

- Spiritual Self-Care Practices is measured by the Spiritual Self-Care Practices Scale (SSCPS; White, 2010). The SSCPS includes 36 spiritual self-care actions that are rated on a 4-point scale of 1 = not a spiritual practice to 4 = very much a spiritual practice.
- Quality of Life is measured by the World Health Organization—Quality of Life-Brief (WHOQOL-BREF; World Health Organization, 1996). The WHOQOL-BREF contains 26 questions about physical capacity, psychological state, social relationships, and the environment that are rated on a 5-point scale of 1 = not at all to 5 = extremely.

The *relational propositions* for the C and T components of the CTE structure are:

- Self-Care is positively related to Well-Being.
- Spiritual Self-Care mediates the relation between Self-Care and Well-Being (White, 2013).
- Therefore, Spiritual Care Practices mediates the relation between Heart Failure Self-Care Practices and Quality of Life, such that Heart Failure Self-Care Practices is positively related to Spiritual Self-Care, which is positively related to Quality of Life.

The *relational proposition* for the E component of the CTE structure is:

- Scores on the SSCPS mediate the relation between scores on the HFSCBS and the WHOQOL-BREF, such that scores on the HFSCBS are related to the scores on the SSCPS, and scores on the SSCPS are related to the scores on the WHOQOL-BREF.

Source: White (2013).

The theory is the effects of home care on postpartum problems and complications and on care of self. Nazik and Eryilmaz (2013) used a quasi-experimental one group pretest–posttest research design (see Appendix A) to test the theory with 63 randomly selected primiparous women residing in Turkey. Each woman had a normal vaginal delivery of one infant and was discharged from the hospital 8 to 12 hours following delivery of the infant.

One conceptual model concept is Professional–Technological System of Nursing Practice. The relevant dimension of the concept is regulatory operations, and the relevant subdimension is production of regulatory care, focusing on the supportive–educative nursing system. The other conceptual model concepts are Self-Care Agency and Self-Care. The theory concepts are Home Care

Visits, Care of Self, and Postpartum Problems and Complications. The production of regulatory care subdimension of the Professional–Technological System of Nursing Practice is represented by Home Care Visits. Self-Care Agency is represented by Care of Self, and Self-Care is represented by Postpartum Problems and Complications.

Home Care Visits is operationalized by the Home Care Visits protocol. Care of Self is measured by the Self-Care Agency Scale (Nahcivan, 2004). Problems and Complications are measured by the investigator-developed Maternity Follow-Up Form (Nazik & Eryilmaz, 2013). t-test and McNemar statistics (see Appendix B) were used to test the differences in care of self and in the number and type of postpartum problems and complications between the first and seventh week postpartum.

The CTE structure constructed from the content of Nazik and Eryilmaz's (2013) research report is illustrated in Figure 6.9. The non-relational propositions for each component of the CTE structure are listed in Box 6.12.

A CTE Structure for Mixed-Methods Research

Burdette's (2012) journal article is an example of a report of mixed-methods (QUAN + qual) research (see Appendix A) guided by Orem's Self-Care Framework. The purpose of the QUAN portion of her study was to examine the relations of education, age, number of chronic conditions, distance from health care provider, body mass index, and self-care power to self-care activities. The purpose of the QUAL portion of her study was to "illuminate the experience of rural midlife women" (p. 8).

For the QUAN portion of the study, Burdette (2012) used a correlational path model research design (see Appendix A) to test the theory with 224 midlife women residing in a rural area of the upper midwestern United States. For the qual portion of the study, she used a simple descriptive qualitative research design (see Appendix A).

The theory is the relations of education, age, number of chronic conditions, distance from health care provider, body mass index, and self-care power to self-care activities. The conceptual model concepts are Basic Conditioning Factors, Self-Care Agency, Self-Care, and Health Status. The theory concepts are Education, Age, Number of Chronic Conditions, Distance From Health Care Provider, Body Mass Index, Self-Care Power, Self-Care Activities, Meaning of Self-Care, and Meaning of Health.

Basic Conditioning Factors is represented by Education, Age, Number of Chronic Conditions, Distance From Health Care Provider, and Body Mass Index. Self-Care Agency is represented by Self-Care Power, and Self-Care is represented by Self-Care Activities.

Burdette (2012) developed the Demographic Data Instrument to measure Education, Age, Number of Chronic Conditions, and Distance From Health Care Provider. Body Mass Index is measured by a mathematical calculation of anthropomorphic measurements (height and weight). Self-Care Power is measured by

BOX 6.12   An Example of a Conceptual–Theoretical–Empirical Structure for Orem's Self-Care Framework–Guided Experimental Research

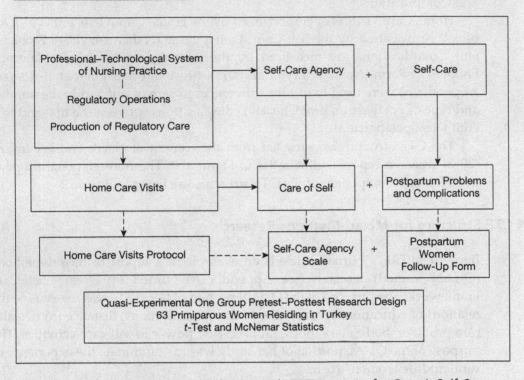

FIGURE 6.9 Conceptual–theoretical–empirical (CTE) structure for Orem's Self-Care Framework experimental research—theory of the effects of home care visits on postpartum problems and complications and on care of self.

The *non-relational propositions* for the *C component* of the conceptual–theoretical–empirical (CTE) structure are:

- *Professional–Technological System of Nursing Practice* is defined as the nursing process.
- The relevant dimension of Professional–Technological System of Nursing Practice is regulatory operations.
  - o *Regulatory operations* is defined as design and implementation of a nursing system and method(s) of helping.
  - o The relevant subdimension of regulatory operations is production of regulatory care.
    - ■ *Production of regulatory care* is defined as implementation of the selected nursing system and method(s) of helping.
- *Self-Care Agency* is defined as the individual's ability to meet his or her continuing requirements for self-care, which may vary throughout the life span.

(continued)

BOX 6.12   An Example of a Conceptual–Theoretical–Empirical Structure for Orem's Self-Care Framework–Guided Experimental Research   (continued)

- *Self-Care* is defined as actions taken by individuals to regulate their function and development.

The *non-relational propositions* for the *T* component of the CTE structure are:

- *Home Care Visits* is defined as nursing care provided to women in their homes for 7 weeks following childbirth.
- *Care of Self* is defined as actions taken by women to care for themselves during the postpartum.
- *Postpartum Problems and Complications* is defined as occurrence following childbirth of inadequate nutrition, inadequate intake of fluids, sleep disturbances, fatigue, loneliness, inadequate hygiene, infections, inadequate breastfeeding, hemorrhoids, discomfort, pain, and inadequate knowledge of family planning (Nazik & Eryilmaz, 2013).

The *non-relational propositions* for the *E* component of the CTE structure are:

- Home Care Visits is operationalized by the Home Care Visits protocol, which stipulates that "The Postpartum Women Follow-Up Form and Self-Care Agency Scale were given to postpartum women, and the pretest data were collected just before the women were discharged from the hospital. Women who were given care using Orem's Self-Care [Framework] were evaluated on the basis of the North American Nursing Diagnosis Association (NANDA) nursing diagnoses and necessary nursing interventions were undertaken. After women were discharged from the hospital, the women were visited at their homes [eight] times (twice in the first week, then once a week). New nursing diagnoses were identified with the Postpartum Women Follow-Up Form and also old diagnoses were assessed at every home visit. Nursing care was given for the new diagnoses. Care results were evaluated and the Self-Care Agency Scale was completed with the Postpartum Women Follow-Up Form again, and posttest data were obtained at the end of the postpartum period (7 weeks). An appointment was made for the next meeting after each visit, and the researcher's phone number was given to women if they needed to make contact" (Nazik & Eryilmaz, 2013, p. 362).
- Care of Self is measured by the Self-Care Agency Scale (Nahcivan, 2004). The Self-Care Agency Scale, which is the Turkish version of the Exercise of Self-Care Agency scale developed by Kearney and Fleischer (1979), includes 35 items that are rated on a 5-point scale of 0 = it never defines me, 1 = it does not define me, 2 = I have no idea, 3 = it defines me little, and 4 = it defines me much, for positively worded items; negatively worded items are reverse scored (Nazik & Eryilmaz, 2013).
- Postpartum Problems and Complications is measured by the investigator-developed Postpartum Women Follow-Up Form, which includes questions about "Orem's universal self-care needs, developmental self-care needs, and health deviations relevant to nursing diagnoses" (Nazik & Eryilmaz, 2013, p. 361).

(continued)

BOX 6.12   An Example of a Conceptual–Theoretical–
Empirical Structure for Orem's Self-Care Framework–Guided
Experimental Research   (continued)

The *relational propositions* for the *C* and *T components* of the CTE structure are:

- The Professional–Technological System of Nursing Practice has a positive effect on Self-Care Agency.
- Therefore, Home Care Visits have a positive effect on Care of Self, such that Home Care Visits increase Care of Self.
- The Professional–Technological System of Nursing Practice has a positive effect on Self-Care.
- Therefore, Home Care Visits have a positive effect on Postpartum Problems and Complications such that Home Care Visits prevent the occurrence of Postpartum Problems and Complications.

The *relational propositions* for the *E component* of the CTE structure are:

- Implementation of the Home Care Visits protocol results in higher scores on the Self-Care Agency Scale.
- Implementation of the Home Care Visits protocol results in lower scores on the Postpartum Women Follow-Up Form.

Source: Nazik and Eyilmaz (2013).

the Denyes Self-Care Agency Instrument (DSCAI-90; Denyes, 1988, 1990a), and Self-Care Activities is measured by the Denyes Self-Care Practice Instrument (DSCPI-90; Denyes, 1988, 1990b). The conceptual model concepts Self Care and Health Status guided the QUAL portion of the study.

Burdette (2012) analyzed the number data using path analysis with hierarchical regression analysis (see Appendix B). Meaning of Self-Care and Meaning of Health were discovered in the responses of the women to open-ended questions on the investigator-developed Demographic Data Instrument. Burdette (2012) analyzed the word data using content analysis (see Appendix B).

The CTE structure constructed from the content of Burdette's (2012) research report is illustrated in Figure 6.10. The non-relational and relational propositions for each component of the CTE structure are listed in Box 6.13.

CONCLUSION

Orem's Self-Care Framework represents a substantial contribution to nursing knowledge by providing an explicit and specific focus for nursing actions that is different from that of other health care professions. Orem fulfilled her goal of identifying the domain and boundaries of nursing as a science and an art. The Self-Care Framework has, as Orem (2001) pointed out, been widely accepted "by

BOX 6.13   An Example of a Conceptual–Theoretical–
Empirical Structure for Orem's Self-Care Framework–Guided
Mixed-Methods Research

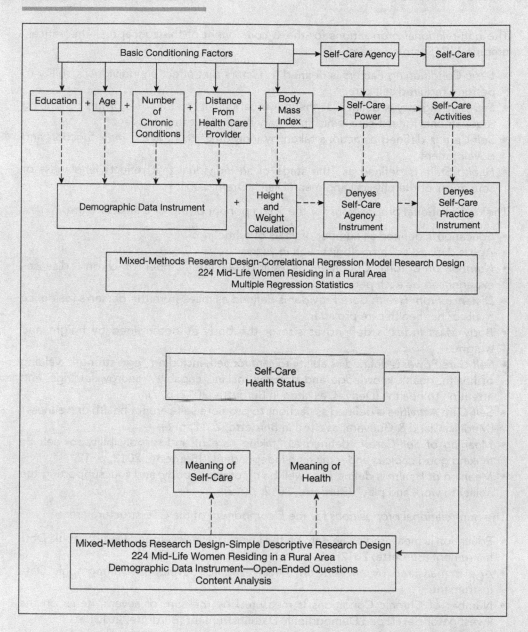

FIGURE 6.10 Conceptual–theoretical–empirical (CTE) structure for Orem's Self-Care Framework mixed-methods research—theory of the relations of education, age, number of chronic conditions, distance from health care provider, body mass index, and self-care power to self-care activities—quantitative and qualitative portions.

(continued)

BOX 6.13 An Example of a Conceptual–Theoretical–Empirical Structure for Orem's Self-Care Framework–Guided Mixed-Methods Research *(continued)*

The *non-relational propositions* for the *C component* of the conceptual–theoretical–empirical (CTE) structure are:

- *Basic Conditioning Factors* is defined as factors that affect an individual's ability to perform required self-care.
- *Self-Care Agency* is defined as the individual's ability to meet his or her continuing requirements for self-care, which may vary throughout the life span.
- *Self-Care* is defined as actions taken by individuals to regulate their function and development.
- *Health State* is defined as "the stage of an individual that reflects wholeness or soundness of the physical and mental self" (Orem, 2001, p. 186).

The *non-relational propositions* for the *T component* of the CTE structure are:

- *Education* is defined as number of years of schooling.
- *Age* is defined as chronological age in years.
- *Number of Chronic Conditions* is defined as the number of chronic diseases experienced by each person.
- *Distance From Health Care Provider* is defined as miles from the person's residence to his or her health care provider.
- *Body Mass Index* is defined as size of the body as determined by height and weight.
- *Self-Care Power* is defined as ability to care for self, including "ego strength, valuing of health, health knowledge and decision-making capabilty, energy, feelings, and attention to health" (Denyes, as cited in Burdette, 2012, p. 7).
- *Self-Care Activities* is defined as "actions to promote self-care for health or wellness" (Medias, Clark, & Guevara, as cited in Burdette, 2012, p. 6).
- *Meaning of Self-Care* is defined as "taking care of and responsibility for self by making good choices and remaining independent" (Burdette, 2012, p. 12).
- *Meaning of Health* is defined as "well-being of mind, body, and soul supporting the ability to work and play" (Burdette, 2012, p. 12).

The *non-relational propositions* for the *E component* of the CTE structure are:

- Education is measured by an item on the investigator-developed Demographic Data Instrument (Burdette, 2012).
- Age is measured by an item on the investigator-developed Demographic Data Instrument.
- Number of Chronic Conditions is measured by the sum of several items on the investigator-developed Demographic Data Instrument (Burdette, 2012).
- Distance From Health Care Provider is measured by an item on the investigator-developed Demographic Data Instrument (Burdette, 2012).
- Body Mass Index is measured by a mathmatical calculation of anthropomorphic measurements—weight (in kilograms) divided by height (in meters, squared).

(continued)

BOX 6.13   An Example of a Conceptual–Theoretical–Empirical Structure for Orem's Self-Care Framework–Guided Mixed-Methods Research   *(continued)*

- Self-Care Power is measured by the Denyes Self-Care Agency Instrument (DSCAI-90; Denyes, 1988, 1990a). The DSCAI-90 includes 24 items arranged in six subscales—"ego strength, valuing of health, health knowledge and decisicon-making capabilty, energy, feelings, and attention to health" (Denyes as cited in Burdette, 2012, p. 7). Items are rated on a ratio scale that yields a score ranging from 0% to 100%. Total and subscale scores can be calculated.
- Self-Care Activities is measured by the Denyes Self-Care Practice Instrument (DSCPI-90; Denyes, 1988, 1990b). The DSCPI-90 is made up of 18 items, which are rated on a ratio scale that yields a score ranging from 0% to 100%.
- Meaning of Self-Care was extracted by content analysis of responses to an open-ended question—"What does self-care mean to you?"—on the investigator-developed Demographic Data Instrument (Burdette, 2012, p. 12).
- Meaning of Health is extracted by content analysis of responses to an open-ended question on the investigator-developed Demographic Data Instrument asking for the definition of health (Burdette, 2012).

For the quantitative portion of the study, the *relational propositions* for the C and *T components* of the CTE structure are:

- Basic Conditioning Factors are related to Self-Care Agency, such that the person's ability to perform self-care and the kind and amount of self-care that is required are influenced by the Basic Conditioning Factors.
- Therefore, Education, Age, Number of Chronic Conditions, Distance From Health Care Provider, and Body Mass Index are related to Self-Care Power.
- Self-Care Agency is positively related to Self-Care.
- Therefore, Self-Care Power is positively related to Self-Care Activities.

For the quantitative portion of the study, the *relational propositions* for the E component of the CTE structure are:

- Scores for the Demographic Data Instrument items are related to scores on the DSCAI-90.
- Scores on the Denyes Self-Care Agency Instrument are related to scores on the DSCPI-90.

Source: Burdette (2012).

nursing practitioners, by nursing curriculum designers, by teachers of nursing, by nursing researchers and scholars as a valid general comprehensive [nursing conceptual model]" (p. 420). It is noteworthy that the Self-Care Framework presents an optimistic view of patients' contributions to their health care that is in keeping with contemporary social values.

Perhaps, the most important contribution of the Self-Care Framework is its explicit focus on what matters to nurses and how that focus helps nurses to retain a nursing perspective in the multidisciplinary milieu of health care. Dodd (1997) explained,

> Orem's [framework] provides a nursing-based focus and systematic guidelines for examining the balance between a person's needs, capabilities, and limitations in exercising self-care actions to enhance personal health....Although we have incorporated knowledge from other disciplines (e.g., physiology, pharmacology, dentistry), Orem's [framework] assisted us in maintaining a focus on issues salient to nursing practice. (p. 987)

The wide acceptance and application of Orem's Self-Care Framework is evident in the examples of its use as a guide for practice, quality improvement projects, and research given in this chapter.

NOTE

1. Portions of this chapter are adapted from Fawcett, J., & DeSanto-Madeya, S. (2013). *Contemporary nursing knowledge: Analysis and evaluation of nursing models and theories* (3rd ed., Chapter 8). Philadelphia, PA: F. A. Davis, with permission.

REFERENCES

Artinian, N. T., Magnan, M., Sloan, M., & Lange, M. P. (2002). Self-care behaviors among patients with heart failure. *Heart & Lung, 31*, 161–172.

Baron, R. M., & Kenny, D. A. (1986). The moderator-mediator variable distinction in social psychological research: Conceptual, strategic and statistical considerations. *Journal of Personality and Social Psychology, 51*, 1173–1182.

Burdette, L. (2012). Relationship between self-care agency, self-care practices, and obesity among rural midlife women. *Self-Care, Dependent-Care and Nursing, 19*(1), 5–14.

Denyes, M. (1988). Orem's model used for health promotion: Directions from research. *Advances in Nursing Science, 11*(1), 13–21.

Denyes, M. (1990a). Denyes Self-Care Agency Instrument. Available from M. J. Denyes, College of Nursing, Wayne State University, Detroit, MI. Retired; retrieved from http://wayne.edu/search-advanced/?first_name=Mary+&last_name=Denyes&accessid=&email=&phone=&department=&title=&advanced_search=Search

Denyes, M. (1990b). Denyes Self-Care Practice Instrument. Available from M. J. Denyes, College of Nursing, Wayne State University, Detroit, MI. Retired; retrieved from http://wayne.edu/search-advanced/?first_name=Mary+&last_name=Denyes&accessid=&email=&phone=&department=&title=&advanced_search=Search

Dodd, M. J. (1997). Self-care: Ready or not! *Oncology Nursing Forum, 24*, 981–990.

Fawcett, J., & DeSanto-Madeya, S. (2013). *Contemporary nursing knowledge: Analysis and evaluation of nursing models and theories* (3rd ed.). Philadelphia, PA: F. A. Davis.

Fex, A., Flensner, G., Ek, A-C., & Söderhamn, O. (2011). Living with an adult family member using advanced medical technology at home. *Nursing Inquiry, 18*, 336–347.

Fleck, L. M. (2012). The Nutrition Self-Care Inventory. *Self-Care, Dependent-Care & Nursing, 19*(1), 26–34.

Fleming, V., Gaidys, U., & Robb, Y. (2003). Hermeneutic research in nursing: Developing a Gadamerian-based research method. *Nursing Inquiry, 10*, 113–120.

Green, R. (2012). Application of the self care deficit nursing theory to the care of children with special needs in the school setting. *Self-Care, Dependent-Care & Nursing, 19*(1), 35–40.

Kearney, H. P., & Fleischer, B. J. (1979). Development of an instrument to measure exercise of self-care agency. *Research in Nursing and Health, 2,* 25–34.

Kelo, M., Martikaninen, M., & Eriksson, E. (2011). Self-care of school-age children with diabetes: An integrative review. *Journal of Advanced Nursing, 67,* 2096–2108.

Kenny, D. A. (2012/2016). *Mediation.* Retrieved from http://davidakenny.net/cm/mediate .htm

Melnyk, B. M., & Fineout-Overholt, E. (2005). *Evidence-based practice in nursing and healthcare: A guide to best practice.* Philadelphia, PA: Lippincott Williams and Wilkins.

Nahcivan, N. Ö. (2004). A Turkish language equivalence of the exercise of self-care agency scale. *Western Journal of Nursing Research, 26,* 813–824.

Nazik, E., & Eyilmaz, G. (2013). The prevention and reduction of postpartum complications: Orem's model. *Nursing Science Quarterly, 26,* 360–364.

Orem, D. E. (2001). *Nursing: Concepts of practice* (6th ed.). St. Louis, MO: Mosby.

Ryan, M., Aloe, K., & Mason-Johnson, J. (2009). Improving self-management and reducing hospital readmission in heart failure patients. *Clinical Nurse Specialist: The Journal of Advanced Nursing Practice, 23,* 216–223.

Smith, P., & Phillips, K. D. (2013). Development and validation of the Dietary Sodium Restriction Self-Care Agency Scale. *Research in Gerontological Nursing, 6,* 139–147.

Srikan, P., & Phillips, K. D. (2014). Psychometric properties of the Dietary Salt Reduction Self-Care Behavior Scale. *Nursing Science Quarterly, 27,* 234–241.

White, M. L. (2010). *Spirituality and spiritual self care: Expanding self-care deficit nursing theory* (Dissertation). Wayne State University, Detroit, MI.

White, M. L. (2013). Spirituality self-care effects on quality of life for patients diagnosed with chronic illness. *Self-Care, Dependent-Care & Nursing, 20*(1), 23–32.

Whittemore, R., & Knafl, K. (2005). The integrative review: Updated methodology. *Journal of Advanced Nursing 52,* 546–553.

World Health Organization. (1996). *WHOQOL-BREF: Introduction, administration, scoring and generic version of the assessment.* Geneva: Author. Retrieved from http://www.who.int/ mental_health/media/en/76.pdf

CHAPTER 7

ROGERS'S SCIENCE OF UNITARY HUMAN BEINGS[1]

Martha E. Rogers's conceptual system, the Science of Unitary Human Beings, focuses on "unitary, irreducible human beings and their respective environments" (Rogers, 1990, p. 108). Rogers (1992) explained that "the irreducible nature of individuals is different from the sum of their parts" (p. 28). The goal of nursing is "to promote human betterment wherever people are, on planet earth or in outer space" (Rogers, 1992, p. 33).

ROGERS'S SCIENCE OF UNITARY HUMAN BEINGS: CONCEPTS AND NON-RELATIONAL PROPOSITIONS

This section of the chapter includes the concepts of Rogers's Science of Unitary Human Beings and the definitions (non-relational propositions) of the concepts and the dimensions of the multidimensional concepts (Rogers, 1990, 1992, 1994).

Energy Field is defined by two words: "Field...is a unifying concept and energy signifies the dynamic nature of the field. Energy fields are infinite and pandimensional; they are in continuous motion" (Rogers, 1992, p. 30). The two dimensions of the concept are human energy field and environmental energy field.

Human energy field is defined as a unitary human being who is irreducible and indivisible into parts, and who is "identified by pattern and manifesting characteristics that are specific to the whole and which cannot be predicted from knowledge of the parts" (Rogers, 1992, p. 29). Human energy fields are individuals and groups.

Environmental energy field is defined as "an irreducible, [indivisible]...energy field identified by pattern and integral with the human [energy] field" (Rogers, 1992, p. 29).

Openness is defined as a characteristic of human energy fields and environmental energy fields, which "are open, not a little bit or sometimes, but continuously" (Rogers, 1992, p. 30).

Pattern is defined as a unique "abstraction, [the nature of which] changes continuously, and [that] gives identity to the [energy] field" (Rogers, 1992, p. 30). Energy field patterns are not directly observable, although manifestations of energy field patterning are observable as experiences, perceptions, expressions, situations, and events.

Pandimensionality is defined as "a nonlinear domain without spatial or temporal attributes" (Rogers, 1992, p. 29).

Homeodynamics is defined as principles that characterize changes in human energy field and environmental energy field patterns. The three dimensions of the concept are resonancy, helicy, and integrality.

Resonancy is defined as the "continuous change from lower to higher frequency wave patterns in human and environmental [energy] fields" (Rogers, 1990, p. 8) that delineates the direction of evolutionary change in energy field patterns.

Helicy is defined as the "continuous, innovative, unpredictable, increasing diversity of human and environmental [energy] field patterns" (Rogers, 1990, p. 8) that characterizes human and environmental field patterns.

Integrality is defined as the "continuous mutual human [energy] field and environmental [energy] field process" (Rogers, 1990, p. 8) that characterizes the nature of the integral and indivisible relationship between the human and environmental energy fields.

Well-Being is defined as a value that expresses the life process; its meaning is defined by each society—thus, what is wellness and what is illness or disease is defined by each society.

Health Patterning Practice Method is defined as the nursing process. The three dimensions of the concept are pattern manifestation knowing and appraisal—assessment, voluntary mutual patterning, and pattern manifestation knowing and appraisal—evaluation (Barrett, 1998; Cowling, 1990, 1997).

Pattern manifestation knowing and appraisal—assessment is defined as the continuous process of apprehending and identifying manifestations of human energy field and environmental energy field patterns that relate to current health events.

Voluntary mutual patterning is defined as the continuous process whereby the nurse with the client patterns the environmental energy field to promote harmony related to health events. Voluntary mutual patterning processes that are most consistent with Rogers's Science of Unitary Human Beings are noninvasive modalities.

Pattern manifestation knowing and appraisal—evaluation is defined as evaluation of voluntary mutual patterning by means of pattern manifestation knowing and appraisal.

ROGERS'S SCIENCE OF UNITARY HUMAN BEINGS: RELATIONAL PROPOSITIONS

The statements of associations (relational propositions) between concepts of Rogers's Science of Unitary Human Beings are listed here. Given Rogers's (1990, 1992) rejection of causality, causal terms such as effects are not used in relational propositions.

- Human energy fields and environmental energy fields are integral.
- Manifestations of Pattern are interrelated.
- Well-Being values are interrelated.
- Health Patterning Practice Method is associated with Pattern.
- Health Patterning Practice Method is associated with Well-Being.

ROGERS'S SCIENCE OF UNITARY HUMAN BEINGS: APPLICATION TO NURSING PRACTICE

The guidelines for Rogers's Science of Unitary Human Beings nursing practice are listed in Box 7.1. A diagram of the practice methodology for Rogers's Science of Unitary Human Beings, which is called the Health Patterning Practice Method, is illustrated in Figure 7.1. The diagram reflects the nonlinear nature of the practice methodology.

A practice tool that includes all aspects of the practice methodology is given in Box 7.2.

A Conceptual–Theoretical–Empirical Structure for Assessment

One section of Barrett's (2010) practice exemplar focuses on use of Rogers's Science of Unitary Human Beings to guide assessment. Barrett (2010) described a 37-year-old man who sought nursing in her health patterning private nursing practice. The man, whom Barrett referred to as a "healing partner" (p. 271), explained that he had not maintained organized billing records. He stated,

> I'm desperate. I need your help with this mess....I'm afraid I'm going to be fired from my job as a saleman. I haven't kept clear records and now my boss is claiming I haven't billed customers for many orders that have been delivered. These papers are all mixed up and I can't make heads or tails out of them. (Barrett, 2010, p. 270)

The theory used to guide practice is assesment of power. The conceptual model concept is Health Patterning Practice Method. The relevant dimension of the concept is pattern manifestation knowing and appraisal—assessment. The theory concept is Power. The pattern manifestation knowing and

BOX 7.1 Guidelines for Rogers's Science of Unitary Human Beings Practice

The primary purpose of Science of Unitary Human Beings–based nursing practice is to promote well-being for all human beings, wherever they are. Another purpose of Science of Unitary Human Beings–based nursing practice is to assist both patients and nurses to increase their awareness of their own rhythms and to make choices among a range of options congruent with their perceptions of well-being.

Practice problems of interest are those manifestations of human and environmental energy field patterns that nursing as a discipline and society as a whole deem relevant for nursing; pattern manifestations include experiences, perceptions, expressions, situations, and events.

Nursing may be practiced in any setting in which nurses encounter people, ranging from hospitals to the community to outer space.

Legitimate participants in nursing practice encompass all people of all ages, both as individual human energy fields and as group energy fields.

The nursing process for the Science of Unitary Human Beings is the Health Patterning Practice Method. The components of the method are pattern manifestation knowing and appreciation—assessment, voluntary mutual patterning, and pattern manifestation knowing and appreciation—evaluation.

Science of Unitary Human Beings–based nursing practice contributes to human betterment; however, human betterment is defined by a society, and leads to acceptance of diversity as the norm and of the integral connectedness of human and environmental energy fields, as well as to viewing change as positive.

Adapted from Fawcett and DeSanto-Madeya (2013), with permission.

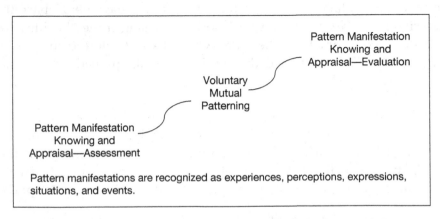

FIGURE 7.1 Rogers's Science of Unitary Human Beings practice methodology.

BOX 7.2 The Rogers's Science of Unitary Human Beings Practice Methodology Tool

PATTERN MANIFESTATION KNOWING AND APPRECIATION—ASSESSMENT

Nurse: Please tell me what you have been thinking about and feeling recently.
Patient:
Nurse: Please tell me more about what you mean by...
Patient:
Nurse: Do you remember feeling this way at other times?
Patient:
Nurse: What have you done at those other times?
Patient:

VOLUNTARY MUTUAL PATTERNING

Nurse: Would you like to try [a noninvasive modality] to...?
Patient:
If the patient indicated interest in the noninvasive modality, the nurse helps the patient to learn how to do (the name of the noninvasive modality) and gives the patient a "prescription" for the amount of time for each session and the number of times to use the modality each day.

PATTERN MANIFESTATION KNOWING AND APPRECIATION—EVALUATION

The patient returns to see the nurse (approximately) 1 week later.

Nurse: How are you feeling now?
Patient:

Adapted from Fawcett and DeSanto-Madeya (2013), with permission.

appraisal—assessment dimension of Health Patterning Practice Method is represented by Power, which is assessed by the Power as Knowing Participation in Change Tool, Version II (PKPCT, Version II; Barrett & Caroselli, 1998).

The conceptual–theoretical–empirical (CTE) structure that was constructed from an interpretation of the assessment content of Barrett's (2010) practice exemplar is illustrated in Figure 7.2. The non-relational propositions for each component of the CTE structure are listed in Box 7.3.

A CTE Structure for Intervention

Another section of Barrett's (2010) practice exemplar focuses on use of Rogers's Science of Unitary Human Beings to guide intervention. Barrett (2010) described

BOX 7.3 An Example of a Conceptual–Theoretical–Empirical Structure for Rogers's Science of Unitary Human Beings Nursing Practice: Assessment

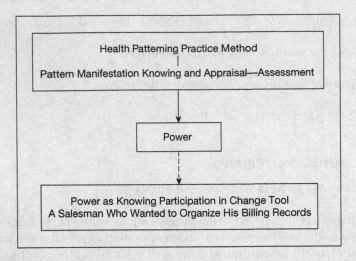

FIGURE 7.2 Conceptual–theoretical–empirical (CTE) structure for Rogers's Science of Unitary Human Beings nursing practice: assessment—theory of assessment of power.

The *non-relational propositions* for the *C component* of the conceptual–theoretical–empirical (CTE) structure are:

- *Health Patterning Practice Method* is defined as the nursing process.
- The relevant dimension of the concept is pattern manifestation knowing and appraisal—assessment.
  - o *Pattern manifestation knowing and appraisal—assessment* is defined as the continuous process of apprehending and identifying manifestations of human energy field and environmental energy field patterns that relate to current health events.

The *non-relational propositions* for the *T component* of the CTE structure are:

- *Power* is defined as "the capacity to participate knowingly in the nature of change characterizing continuous patterning of the human and environment [energy] fields. The observable, measureable manifestations of power are awarenss (A), choices (C), freedom to act intentionally (F), and involvement in creating change (I)" (Caroselli & Barrett, 1998, p. 9).

(continued)

BOX 7.3 An Example of a Conceptual–Theoretical–Empirical Structure for Rogers's Science of Unitary Human Beings Nursing Practice: Assessment (continued)

The *non-relational propositions* for the *E component* of the CTE structure are:

- Power is assessed by the Power as Knowing Participation in Change Tool, Version II (PKPCT, Version II; Barrett & Caroselli, 1998). The PKPCT, Version II includes four subscales—awareness, choices, freedom to act intentionally, and involvement in creating change—each of which is rated on 12 opposite adjective pairs, and each adjective pair is rated on a 1- to 7-point semantic differential scale (Barrett, 1990; see Appendix B). The adjective pairs are profound/superficial, seeking/avoiding, valuable/worthless, assertive/timid, leading/following, orderly/chaotic, expanding/shrinking, pleasant/unpleasant, informed/uninformed, free/constrained, important/unimportant. The adjective pairs are listed in random order for each subscale, and the positive and negative adjectives are randomly reversed.

Source: Barrett (2010).

---

how noninvasive modalities were used with a 37-year-old man who was a healing partner in her health patterning private nursing practice.

The theory used to guide practice is association of a power prescription plan with power. One conceptual model concept is Health Pattern Practice Method; the relevant dimension of the concept is voluntary mutual patterning. The other conceptual model concept is Pattern. The theory concepts are Power Prescription Plan and Power.

The voluntary mutual patterning dimension of Health Patterning Practice Method is represented by Power Prescription Plan, which is operationalized by the Power Prescription Plan protocol. Pattern is represented by Power, which is measured by the PKPCT, Version II (Barrett & Caroselli, 1998).

The CTE structure that was constructed from an interpretation of the intervention content of Barrett's (2010) practice exemplar is illustrated in Figure 7.3. The non-relational and relational propositions for each component of the CTE structure are listed in Box 7.4.

ROGERS'S SCIENCE OF UNITARY HUMAN BEINGS: APPLICATION TO QUALITY IMPROVEMENT PROJECTS

The guidelines for Rogers's Science of Unitary Human Beings quality improvement (QI) projects are listed in Box 7.5.

BOX 7.4   An Example of a Conceptual–Theoretical–Empirical Structure for Rogers's Science of Unitary Human Beings Nursing Practice: Intervention

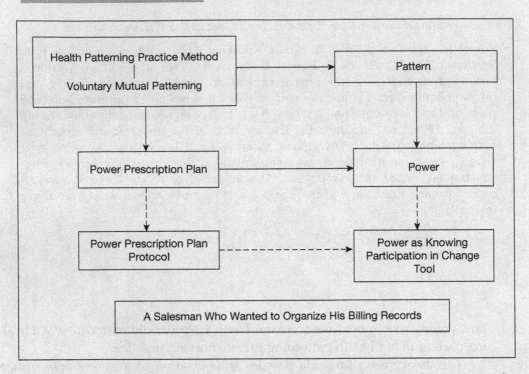

FIGURE 7.3 Conceptual–theoretical–empirical (CTE) structure for Rogers's Science of Unitary Human Beings nursing practice: Assessment—theory of association of a power prescription plan with power.

The *non-relational propositions* for the *C component* of the conceptual–theoretical–empirical (CTE) structure are:

- *Health Patterning Practice Method* is defined as the nursing process.
- The relevant dimension of Health Patterning Practice Method is voluntary mutual patterning.
  o *Voluntary mutual patterning* is defined as the continuous process whereby the nurse with the client patterns the environmental energy field to promote harmony related to health events. Voluntary mutual patterning processes that are most consistent with Rogers's Science of Unitary Human Beings are noninvasive modalities.
- *Pattern* is defined as a unique "abstraction, [the nature of which] changes continuously, and [that] gives identity to the [energy] field" (Rogers, 1992, p. 30). Energy field patterns are not directly observable, although manifestations of energy field patterning are observable as experiences, perceptions, expressions, situations, and events.

(continued)

BOX 7.4   An Example of a Conceptual–Theoretical–Empirical Structure for Rogers's Science of Unitary Human Beings Nursing Practice: Intervention   *(continued)*

The *non-relational propositions* for the *T component* of the CTE structure are:

- *Power Prescription Plan* is defined as health patterning modalities that are specifically selected for a particular healing partner (Barrett, 2010).
- *Power* is defined as "the capacity to participate knowingly in the nature of change characterizing continuous patterning of the human and environment [energy] fields. The observable, measureable manifestations of power are awarenss (A), choices (C), freedom to act intentionally (F), and involvement in creating change (I)" (Caroselli & Barrett, 1998, p. 9).

The *non-relational propositions* for the *E component* of the CTE structure are:

- Power Prescription Plan is operationalized by the specific Power Prescription Plan protocol for the healing partner, a 37-year-old salesman. This protocol includes discussion of "giving [the healing partner] the freedom to act on his intention to straighten out his life by beginning with straightening out his papers...[and] suggestions as to how he could organize his paperwork." The specific power prescription, written on a card, is "I am free to chose with awareness how I participate in changes I intend to create" (Barrett, 2010, p. 271). The protocol also includes a short "imagery exercise that incorporate[s] color, sound, light, and motion" (p. 271), which is used as a noninvasive relaxation modality. Barrett (2010) explained that she "suggested [the healing partner] tape record the [imagery] exercise and that hearing his own voice could reinforce his confidence to believe that he was taking charge of his life" (p. 271).
- Power is measured by the Power as Knowing Participation in Change Tool, Version II (PKPCT, Version II; Barrett & Caroselli, 1998). The PKPCT, Version II includes four subscales—awareness, choices, freedom to act intentionally, and involvement in creating change—each of which is rated on 12 opposite adjective pairs, and each adjective pair is rated on a 1- to 7-point semantic differential scale (Barrett, 1990; see Appendix B). The adjective pairs are profound/superficial, seeking/avoiding, valuable/worthless, assertive/timid, leading/following, orderly/chaotic, expanding/shrinking, pleasant/unpleasant, informed/uninformed, free/constrained, important/unimportant. The adjective pairs are listed in random order for each subscale, and the positive and negative adjectives are randomly reversed.

The *relational propositions* for the *C and T components* of the CTE structure are:

- Health Patterning Practice Method is associated with Pattern.
- Therefore, Power Prescription Plan is associated with Power.

The *relational proposition* for the *E component* of the CTE structure is:

- Implementation of the Power Prescription Plan protocol is associated with scores on the PKPCT, Version II.

Source: Barrett (2010).

BOX 7.5   Guidelines for Rogers's Science of Unitary Human Beings Quality Improvement Projects

The purpose of quality improvement (QI) projects is to test the association of nurses' use of Rogers's practice methodology (Health Patterning Practice Method) with nurse and/or patient energy field pattern manifestations.

The phenomenon of interest for QI projects is the extent of nurses' use of the Health Patterning Practice Method on changes in nurse and/or patient energy field pattern manifestations.

Data for QI projects are to be collected from nurses and/or patients in various settings, such as patients' homes, nurses' private offices, ambulatory clinics, hospitals, and communities, as well as (potentially) in outer space.

Any methodological theory of change or QI may be used to guide the design of the QI project and the times for data collection. Checklists, rating scales, and responses to open-ended questions may be used to determine the extent to which nurses actually implement one or more components of the Health Patterning Practice Method—pattern manifestation knowing and appreciation—assessment, voluntary mutual patterning, and pattern manifestation knowing and appreciation—evaluation.

Descriptive statistics may be used to analyze data obtained from checklists or rating scales, and content analysis may be used to identify categories or themes found in responses to open-ended questions.

The results of Rogers's Science of Unitary Human Beings–based QI projects enhance understanding of how using the Health Patterning Practice Method is associated with changes in nurse and/or patient energy field pattern manifestations.

A CTE Structure for a QI Project

A journal article by Kim, Smith, and West (2012) is an example of a QI project guided by Rogers's Science of Unitary Human Beings. The purpose of their project, which they referred to as a program evaluation, was

> (1) To evaluate the effectiveness of a breast health education program to increase the participation of women employees [working at the corporate level of a healthcare system] with regard to screening mammogram and (2) to examine how employee participation with [a] breast health education program relates to power. (Kim et al., 2012, p. 26)

The theory is association of an educational program with power and screening mammography rate. The conceptual model concepts are Health Patterning Practice Method and Well-Being. The relevant dimension of Health Patterning Practice Method is voluntary mutual patterning. The theory concepts are Screening Mammography Educational Program, Power, and Screening Mammography Rate.

The voluntary mutual patterning dimension of Health Patterning Practice Method is represented by Screening Mammography Educational Program, and Well-Being is represented by Power and Screening Mammography Rate. Screening Mammography Educational Program is operationalized by the My Health: A Female Focus Program protocol. Kim et al. (2012) did not explicitly identify a methodological theory of change or quality improvement as a guide for development of the protocol. However, the objectives of the project, which "were to increase knowledge and motivation, overcome fears, and provide tools to ensure convenient access to services including screening mammogram" (Kim et al., 2012, p. 28), are similar to the three stages of change of Lewin's (1951) methodological theory of change—unfreezing, moving, and refreezing (see Appendix A).

Power is measured by the PKPCT, Version II (Barrett, 1990). Screening Mammography Rate is measured by items on an online survey. Kim et al. (2012) used descriptive (numbers, percents, means, and standard deviations), Chi-square, t-test, and correlational statistics (see Appendix B) to analyze the data.

The CTE structure that was constructed from an interpretation of the content of Kim et al.'s (2012) journal article is illustrated in Figure 7.4. The nonrelational and relational propositions for each component of the CTE structure are listed in Box 7.6.

APPLICATION TO NURSING RESEARCH

The guidelines for Rogers's Science of Unitary Human Beings nursing research are listed in Box 7.7.

A CTE Structure for a Systematic Literature Review

Kim's (2009) journal article is an example of a report of a literature review guided by Rogers's Science of Unitary Human Beings. She conducted a review of literature about Barrett's Theory of Power as Knowing Participation in Change and Barrett's PKPCT that encompassed and extended an earlier 15-year review by Caroselli and Barrett (1998). Kim (2009) indicated that she reviewed the literature from 1983, which was when Barrett introduced her power theory, which she derived directly from Rogers's Science of Unitary Human Beings, and the PKPCT. Barrett (1983, 1990) defined power as "the capacity to participate knowingly in the nature of change characterizing the continuous patterning of the human and environmental fields as manifested by awareness, choices, freedom to act intentionally, and involvement in creating changes" (1990, p. 159).

Kim (2009) began her search of literature by sending a survey questionnaire to "96 individuals who had requested permission from Dr. Barrett to use Power as Knowing Participation in Change [Tool] (PKPCT)" (p. 19). This part of the search yielded 36 reports of use of the PKPCT. For her literature review, Kim (2009) included the 27 research reports that had been reviewed by

BOX 7.6   An Example of a Conceptual–Theoretical–Empirical Structure for Rogers's Science of Unitary Human Beings Quality Improvement Project

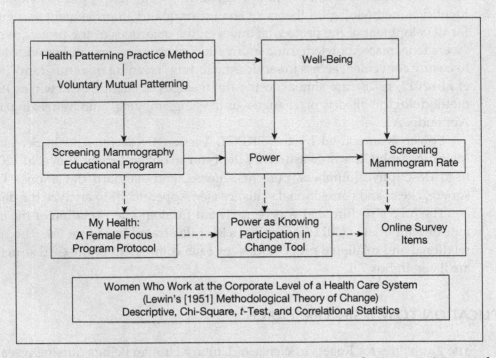

FIGURE 7.4 Conceptual–theoretical–empirical (CTE) structure for Rogers's Science of Unitary Human Beings quality improvement (QI) project—theory of association of an educational program with power and screening mammography rate.

The *non-relational propositions* for the *C component* of the conceptual–theoretical–empirical (CTE) structure are:

- *Health Patterning Practice Method* is defined as the nursing process.
- The relevant dimension of Health Patterning Practice Method is voluntary mutual patterning.
  - o *Voluntary mutual patterning* is defined as the continuous process whereby the nurse with the client patterns the environmental energy field to promote harmony related to health events. Voluntary mutual patterning processes that are most consistent with Rogers's Science of Unitary Human Beings are noninvasive modalities.
- *Well-Being* is defined as a value that expresses the life process; its meaning is defined by each society—thus, what is wellness and what is illness or disease is defined by each society.

(continued)

BOX 7.6 An Example of a Conceptual–Theoretical–Empirical Structure for Rogers's Science of Unitary Human Beings Quality Improvement Project *(continued)*

The *non-relational propositions* for the *T component* of the CTE structure are:

- *Screening Mammography Educational Program* is defined as "a health patterning modality" (Kim et al., 2012, p. 28) focused on breast cancer prevention.
- *Power* is defined as "the capacity to participate knowingly in the nature of change characterizing continuous patterning of the human and environment [energy] fields. The observable, measureable manifestations of power are awarenss (A), choices (C), freedom to act intentionally (F), and involvement in creating change (I)" (Caroselli & Barrett, 1998, p. 9).
- *Screening Mammogram Rate* is defined as frequency of screening mammograms.

The *non-relational propositions* for the *E component* of the CTE structure are:

- The Screening Mammogram Educational Program is operationalized by the *My Health: A Female Focus Program* protocol. The protocol, which was based on evidence from the literature and national organization web sites (National Cancer Institute, Centers for Disease Control and Prevention, National Women's Health Research Center) included "practical tips centered around women's wellness with [a] specific focus on breast health.... Three core educational activities having the largest influence on motivating annual mammogram screening were designed first. They were 'Breast Health: Throughout Your Life,' 'Family History: It's Important to Your Health,' and 'Breast Care Center Tour.' Four additional educational classes developed included 'Lifestyle Choices and Cancer Prevention,' 'Family History: Computer Lab,' 'Feeding the Body and Soul,' and 'Reading E-Mails or Online Articles.' The three core educational activities and 'Lifestyle Choices and Cancer Prevention' were offered both in-person/class and online. Each of the educational sessions averaged one hour in length" (Kim et al., 2012, pp. 28–29). The overall project objectives are to "increase knowledge and motivation, overcome fears, and provide tools to ensure convenient access to services including screening mammogram" (Kim et al., 2012, p. 28). Although the methodological theory is not explicit, these project objectives are consistent with Lewin's (1951) theory of change, which includes three stages—unfreezing, moving, and refreezing. Accordingly, the *My Health: A Female Focus Program* protocol focuses on increasing women's knowledge about and motivation for screening mammograms (unfreezing), overcoming fears by encouraging the women to participate in the educational program (moving), and institutionalizing annual screening mammograms by providing easy access to screening mammogram (refreezing).
- Power is measured by the Power as Knowing Participation in Change Tool, Version II (PKPCT, Version II; Barrett & Caroselli, 1998). The PKPCT, Version II includes four subscales—awareness, choices, freedom to act intentionally, and involvement in creating change—each of which is rated on 12 opposite adjective pairs, and each adjective pair is rated on a 1- to 7-point semantic differential scale (Barrett, 1990; see Appendix B). The adjective pairs are profound/superficial, seeking/avoiding, valuable/worthless, assertive/timid, leading/following, orderly/chaotic, expanding/

(continued)

BOX 7.6   An Example of a Conceptual–Theoretical–Empirical Structure for Rogers's Science of Unitary Human Beings Quality Improvement Project   (continued)

---

shrinking, pleasant/unpleasant, informed/uninformed, free/constrained, important/unimportant. The adjective pairs are listed in random order for each subscale, and the positive and negative adjectives are randomly reversed.

- Mammogram Screening Rate is measured by online survey items asking if the woman had obtained "a mammogram in the last 13 months...or [planned to schedule a] mammogram in the next few weeks" (Kim et al, 2012, pp. 28, 32).

The *relational propositions* for the *C* and *T components* of the CTE structure are:

- Health Patterning Practice Method is associated with Well-Being.
- Well-Being values are interrelated.
- Therefore, Screening Mammogram Educational Program is associated with Power, and Power is associated with Screening Mammogram Rate.

The *relational proposition* for the *E component* of the CTE structure is:

- Implementation of the *My Health: A Female Focus Program* protocol is associated with high scores on the PKPCT, Version II, which are associated with scores on the online survey indicating a high rate of screening mammograms.

Source: Kim, Smith, and West (2012).

Caroselli and Barrett (1998). In addition, her search of the Cumulative Index to Nursing and Allied Health Literature (CINAHL) and Dissertation Abstracts International (DAI) electronic databases using the search terms "Barrett's power," and "knowing participation and change" yielded 18 research reports. An additional research report (a master's thesis) was obtained from Barrett. When duplicates were eliminated, a total of 46 research reports was included in the final literature review ([36+ 27 + 18 + 1] – 36 duplicates = 46).

Kim (2009) categorized the research reports by "design and methods, population and sample, concepts/interventions[,] reliability, and major findings" (p. 20). She reported that the PKPCT was used as an instrument in all of the studies included in the review. However, "several researchers used the PKPCT to measure concepts other than power" (p. 22), including empowerment, health empowerment, and purposeful participation.

The theory of correlates of power was generated from the literature review. The conceptual model concept is Homeodynamics. The theory concept is Power Correlates. The two dimensions of Power Correlates are concept correlates and intervention correlates. Power Correlates and its dimensions were extracted from the review of the 46 research reports.

BOX 7.7   Guidelines for Rogers's Science of Unitary Human Beings Research

The purpose of Science of Unitary Human Beings–based basic research is to develop new theoretical knowledge about unitary human energy fields in mutual process with environmental energy fields. The goal of basic nursing research is pattern seeing. The purpose of Science of Unitary Human Beings–based applied research is to test already available knowledge in practice situations.

The phenomena to be studied are those that are central to nursing—pattern manifestations of human and environmental energy fields.

The problems to be studied are the manifestations of human energy field patterns and environmental energy field patterns, especially pattern profiles, which are clusters of related pattern manifestations.

Inasmuch as nursing is a service to all people, wherever they may be, virtually any human being or group in its natural setting would be appropriate for study, with the proviso that both human being or group and environment are taken into account.

A variety of qualitative, quantitative, and/or mixed-methods research methods currently are regarded as appropriate designs for Science of Unitary Human Beings–based research, although qualitative methods are more congruent with the Science of Unitary Human Beings than are quantitative methods. Although descriptive and correlational designs are regarded as consistent with the Science of Unitary Human Beings, strict experimental designs are of questionable value because of Rogers's rejection of the notion of causality. However, in the absence of new methods, some researchers continue to conduct experimental research. Specific existing methodologies that are used across disciplines but currently are regarded as appropriate include Husserlian phenomenology; existentialism; rational interpretive hermeneutics; interpretive evaluation methods, such as Fourth Generation Evaluation; participatory action and cooperative inquiry; focus groups; ecological thinking; dialectical thinking; and historical inquiries, as well as methods that focus on the uniqueness of each human being, such as imagery, direct questioning, personal structural analysis, and the Q-sort. Science of Unitary Human Beings–specific methodologies include the unitary pattern appreciation case method, unitary appreciative inquiry, the Rogerian process of inquiry method, the unitary field pattern portrait research method, and the photo-disclosure methodology. Case studies and longitudinal research designs that focus on the identification of manifestations of human and environmental energy field patterns are more appropriate than cross-sectional designs, given the emphasis in the Science of Unitary Human Beings on the uniqueness of the unitary human being. Research instruments that are directly derived from the Science of Unitary Human Beings should be used. Inclusion of study participants in the process of inquiry enhances mutual exploration, discovery, and knowing participation in change.

Synthesis rather than an analysis that separates parts is the goal of data analysis. Ideally, data analysis techniques should take the unitary nature of human beings and the integrality of the human and environmental energy fields into account.

(continued)

> **BOX 7.7   Guidelines for Rogers's Science of Unitary Human Beings Research   (continued)**
>
> Consequently, the use of standard data analysis techniques that employ the components of variance model of statistics is questionable, inasmuch as this statistical model is logically inconsistent with the assumption of holism stating that the whole is greater than the sum of parts. Multivariate analysis procedures, particularly canonical correlation, are useful techniques for generating a constellation of variables representing human field pattern properties. However, canonical correlation is a component of variance procedure, as are all parametric correlational techniques. New data analysis techniques that permit examination of the integrality of human and environmental energy fields must be developed so that the ongoing testing of the Science of Unitary Human Beings does not have to be done through the logical empiricist criterion of meaning, testing the hypodeductive system for consistency, and then testing correspondence to the world. Note that in the absence of new data analysis techniques that focus on unitary wholes, most researchers continue to use statistical techniques that focus on parts. Bracketing and objectivity are not possible given the integral nature of the researcher and the study participants as energy fields in mutual process.
>
> Science of Unitary Human Beings–based research enhances understanding of the continuous mutual process of human and environmental energy fields and manifestations of changes in energy field patterns. Ultimately, Science of Unitary Human Beings–based research will yield a body of nursing discipline-specific knowledge.
>
> Adapted from Fawcett and DeSanto-Madeya (2013), with permission.

The CTE structure that was constructed from an interpretation of the content of Kim's (2009) journal article is illustrated in Figure 7.5. The non-relational propositions for each component of the CTE structure are listed in Box 7.8.

A CTE Structure for Instrument Development

Gueldner et al.'s (2005) journal article is an example of a report of development of an instrument derived from Rogers's Science of Unitary Human Beings. They developed the Well-Being Picture Scale (WPS) to measure general well-being of unitary human beings based on an individual's energy pattern. Gueldner et al. explained that the WPS "is a shorter, refined version of the 18-item Index of Field Energy (IFE)" (p. 42) and provided a detailed description of development and psychometric testing of both the IFE and the WPS. The initial description of the IFE was published by Gueldner, Bramlett, Johnston, and Guillory (1996).

The theory is general well-being. The conceptual model concept is Homeodynamics. The three dimensions of the concept are resonancy, helicy, and integrality. The theory concept is General Well-Being, which has four dimensions—frequency, awareness, action, and power.

BOX 7.8 An Example of a Conceptual–Theoretical–Empirical Structure for Rogers's Science of Unitary Human Beings Literature Review

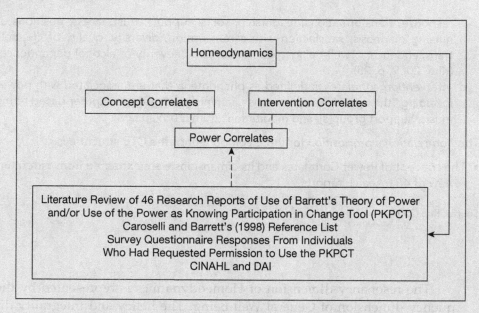

FIGURE 7.5 Conceptual–theoretical–empirical (CTE) structure for Rogers's Science of Unitary Human Beings literature review—theory of correlates of power.

CINAHL, Cumulative Index to Nursing and Allied Health Literature; DAI, Dissertation Abstracts International.

The *non-relational proposition* for the *C component* of the conceptual–theoretical–empirical (CTE) structure is:

- *Homeodynamics* is defined as principles that characterize changes in human energy field and environmental energy field patterns.

The *non-relational propositions* for the *T component* of the CTE structure are:

- *Power Correlates* is defined as phenomena that are associated with power. Power is defined as "the capacity to participate knowingly in the nature of change characterizing the continuous patterning of the human and environmental [energy] fields as manifested by awareness, choices, freedom to act intentionally, and involvement in creating changes" (Barrett, 1990, p. 159).
- The two dimensions of Power Correlates are concept correlates and intervention correlates.
  o *Concept correlates* is defined as phenomena that are associated with power, including "empathy, job satisfaction, decision making, organizational commitment, self-esteem, professionally inviting teaching behaviors, overall satisfaction with previous health care experience, satisfaction with current health care encounter, spirituality, hope, perception of self, choosing the best practice

(continued)

BOX 7.8 An Example of a Conceptual–Theoretical–Empirical Structure for Rogers's Science of Unitary Human Beings Literature Review *(continued)*

response, transformational leadership, social support, trust, stress, positions on nursing diagnosis, satisfaction with career option, diversity, quality of life, self-transcendence,...well-being...depression, and severity of alcohol dependence" (Kim, 2009, p. 25).

 o *Intervention correlates* is defined as phenomena that are associated with power, including "therapeutic touch, exercise, feminist pedagogy, computer-based terms, music, support group[s], and meditation" (Kim, 2009, p. 25).

The *non-relational proposition* for the *E component* of the CTE structure is:

• The concept of Power Correlates and its dimensions were extracted from a literature review of 46 research reports.

Source: Kim (2009).

The resonancy dimension of Homeodynamics is represented by the frequency dimension of General Well-Being. The helicy and integrality dimensions of Homeodynamics are represented by the awareness dimension of General Well-Being. The integrality dimension of Homeodynamics is represented by the action dimension of General Well-Being. The helicy dimension of Homeodynamics is represented by the power dimension of General Well-Being.

General Well-Being, with its four dimensions, is measured by the WPS. Gueldner et al. (2005) reported acceptable estimates of internal consistency reliability using Cronbach's alpha and item analysis, as well as construct validity using a confirmatory factor analysis approach (see Appendix B). They explained that although a confirmatory factor analysis of the WPS revealed four factors corresponding to the four dimensions of General Well-Being, the "scoring of the WPS was not designed with subscales in mind" (p. 48). Therefore, the scores for all 10 WPS items are summed for a single score.

The CTE structure that was constructed from the content of Gueldner et al.'s (2005) journal article is illustrated in Figure 7.6. The non-relational propositions for each component of the CTE structure are listed in Box 7.9.

A CTE Structure for Descriptive Qualitative Research

A research report published as a journal article by Fuller, Davis, Servonsky, and Butcher (2012) is an example of descriptive qualitative research guided by Rogers's Science of Unitary Human Beings. The purpose of their study was "to enhance understanding of the experience of substance abuse by illuminating

BOX 7.9   An Example of a Conceptual–Theoretical–Empirical Structure for Rogers's Science of Unitary Human Beings Instrument Development

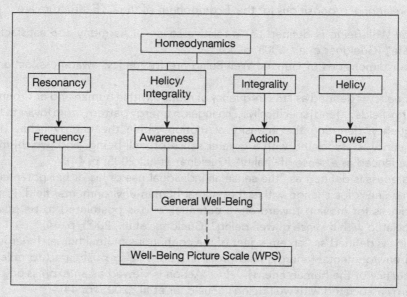

FIGURE 7.6 Conceptual–theoretical–empirical (CTE) structure for Rogers's Science of Unitary Human Beings instrument development—theory of general well-being.

The *non-relational propositions* for the *C component* of the conceptual–theoretical–empirical (CTE) structure are:

- *Homeodynamics* is defined as principles that characterize changes in human energy field and environmental energy field patterns.
- The three dimensions of Homeodynamics are resonancy, helicy, and integrality.
  - o *Resonancy* is defined as the "continuous change from lower to higher frequency wave patterns in human and environmental [energy] fields" (Rogers, 1990, p. 8) that delineates the direction of evolutionary change in energy field pattern.
  - o *Helicy* is defined as the "continuous, innovative, unpredictable, increasing diversity of human and environmental [energy] field patterns" (Rogers, 1990, p. 8) that characterizes human and environmental field patterns.
  - o *Integrality* is defined as the "continuous mutual human [energy] field and environmental [energy] field process" (Rogers, 1990, p. 8) that characterizes the nature of the integral and indivisible relationship between the human and environmental energy fields.

(continued)

BOX 7.9   An Example of a Conceptual–Theoretical–Empirical Structure for Rogers's Science of Unitary Human Beings Instrument Development   (continued)

The *non-relational propositions* for the *T component* of the CTE structure are:

- *General Well-Being* is defined as "a relative sense of harmony and satisfaction in one's life" (Gueldner et al., 2005, p. 43).
- The four dimensions of General Well-Being are frequency, awareness, action, and power.
  - *Frequency* is defined as "the frequency of motion within human and environmental energy fields...[and] specifically...changes in energy pattern, from lower to higher frequency, denoting the intensity of motion within the energy field....higher frequency is associated with a greater sense of well-being, and [which] may be experienced as a sense of vitality" (Gueldner et al., 2005, p. 44).
  - *Awareness* is defined as "the sense an individual has of his or her potential and/or readiness for change within the mutual human-environmental field. It signals readiness for moving toward one's potential, and is postulated to be positively associated with a sense of well-being" (Gueldner et al., 2005, p. 44).
  - *Action* is defined as "an emergent of the continuous mutual human [energy] field and environmental [energy] field process...but is also postulated to reflect the frequency of the human energy field...Action is viewed as an expression of field energy associated with well-being" (Gueldner et al., 2005, p. 44).
  - *Power* is defined as "the capacity of an individual to engage knowingly in change....the degree to which an individual is able to express energy as power to create desired change within [the] human-environmental energy field process" (Gueldner et al., 2005, p. 44).

The *non-relational proposition* for the *E component* of the CTE structure is:

- General Well-Being, with its four dimensions—frequency, awareness, action, and power—is measured by the Well-Being Picture Scale (WPS; Gueldner et al., 2005), which has no subscales. The WPS is made up of 10 professionally drawn pictures, each of which is rated on a 7-point semantic differential scale (see Appendix B). The 10 pictures are "eyes open/closed, shoes passive/active, butterfly/turtle, candle lit/not lit, faucet running full/dripping, puzzle pieces together/separated, pencil sharp/dull, sun full/partially cloud covered, balloons inflated/partially deflated, and lion/mouse" (Gueldner et al., 2005, p. 47).

Source: Gueldner et al. (2005).

the patterns of adult substance users and their family while they are in rehabilitation" (p. 44).

The theory is unitary field pattern. The conceptual model concept that guided the study is Pattern. The theory concept is Unitary Field Pattern Portrait, which has five dimensions—being content with ever changing emotions, living patterns of recovery while resisting temptation, the power to control today's choices, being in an environment where change is possible, and enhanced by supportive guidance in changing family patterns (Fuller et al., 2012). The theory concept and its dimensions are generated from application of the Unitary Field Pattern Portrait (UFPP) Research Method (Butcher, 1998, 2005; see Appendix A). Data were collected by interviews and participants' journals from three females and eight males who were participating in a drug rehabilitation program. Data analysis was consistent with the UFPP Research Method (see Appendix B).

The CTE structure that was constructed from the content of Fuller et al.'s (2005) journal article is illustrated in Figure 7.7. The non-relational propositions for each component of the CTE structure are listed in Box 7.10.

A CTE Structure for Correlational Research

A journal article by Hindman (2011) is an example of a report of correlational research guided by Rogers's Science of Unitary Human Beings. The purpose of her study "was to investigate the relationship between humor and field energy" (p. 47). A bivariate correlational research design was used (see Appendix A). Study participants were 80 older adults, 40 of whom lived independently in a community and attended regional senior centers and 40 of whom resided in nursing homes.

The theory is the association of humor and field energy. The conceptual model concept is Pattern. The theory concepts are Humor and Field Energy, both of which represent Pattern.

Humor is measured by the Situational Humor Response Questionnaire (SHRQ; Lefcourt & Martin, 1986). Field Energy is measured by the Index of Field Energy (IFE; Gueldner, Bramlett, Johnston, & Guillory, 1996). Hindman (2011) tested the association between scores for the SHRQ and the IFE using the Pearson product moment coefficient of correlation (r; see Appendix B).

The CTE structure that was constructed from the content of Hindman's (2011) journal article is illustrated in Figure 7.8. The non-relational and relational propositions for each component of the CTE structure are listed in Box 7.11.

A CTE Structure for Experimental Research

Reis and Alligood's (2014) journal article is a report of experimental research guided by Rogers's Science of Unitary Human Beings. The purpose of their study was "to explore human-environmental field patterning changes in optimism, power, and well-being over time, in women during the second and third trimesters of pregnancy and upon completion of a six-week prenatal yoga program" (p. 31).

The study is a quasi-experimental one group pretest–posttest research design (see Appendix A). Twenty-seven pregnant women volunteered to participate in the study. Inclusion criteria for participation were women who were "(a) in the second and third trimesters of pregnancy between 20 to 32 weeks gestation;

BOX 7.10   An Example of a Conceptual–Theoretical–Empirical Structure for Rogers's Science of Unitary Human Beings Descriptive Qualitative Research

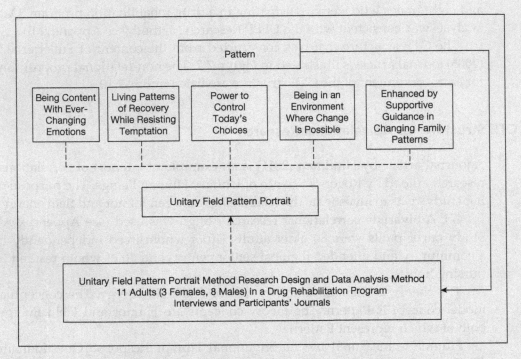

FIGURE 7.7 Conceptual–theoretical–empirical (CTE) structure for Rogers's Science of Unitary Human Beings descriptive qualitative research—theory of unitary field pattern.

The *non-relational proposition* for the *C component* of the conceptual–theoretical–empirical (CTE) structure is:

- *Pattern* is defined as a unique "abstraction, [the nature of which] changes continuously, and [that] gives identity to the [energy] field" (Rogers, 1992, p. 30). Energy field patterns are not directly observable, although manifestations of energy field patterning are observable as experiences, perceptions, expressions, situations, and events.

The *non-relational propositions* for the *T component* of the CTE structure are:

- *Unitary Field Pattern Portrait* is defined "resonating themes that included the experiences, perceptions, and expressions of adult substance users and family pattern in rehabilitation" (Fuller et al., 2012, p. 56). The Unitary Field Pattern Portrait discovered in Fuller et al.'s (2012) study is "Being content with ever changing emotions and living patterns of recovery while resisting temptation and the power

(continued)

BOX 7.10 An Example of a Conceptual–Theoretical–Empirical Structure for Rogers's Science of Unitary Human Beings Descriptive Qualitative Research (continued)

to control today's choices while being in an environment where change is possible which is enhanced by supportive guidance in changing family patterns" (p. 59).

o The five dimensions of Unitary Field Pattern Portrait are being content with ever-changing emotions, living patterns of recovery while resisting temptation, the power to control today's choices, being in an environment where change is possible, and enhanced by supportive guidance in changing family patterns.

o *Being content with ever-changing emotions* is defined as participants' "descriptions of their emotional awareness" (Fuller et al., 2012, p. 56).

o *Living patterns of recovery while resisting temptation* is defined as participants' "descriptions of their past and current life patterns" (Fuller et al., 2012, p. 57).

o *The power to control today's choices* is defined as "participants' statements about believing they have the power to change" (Fuller et al., 2012, p. 57).

o *Being in an environment where change is possible* is defined as participants' affirmative response to being asked "if they could change" (Fuller et al., 2012, p. 57).

o *Enhanced by supportive guidance in changing family patterns* is defined as participants' discussion of "their family pattern and family influences on their recovery" (Fuller et al., 2012, p. 58).

The *non-relational proposition* for the *E component* of the CTE structure is:

• Unitary Field Pattern Portrait and its five dimensions were discovered in interview data and journals from 11 adults (three females, eight males) participating in a drug rehabiliation program.

Source: Fuller, Davis, Servonsky, and Butcher (2012).

(b) 18 years old and above; (c) able to speak, read, and write in English; and (d) experiencing an uncomplicated, low-risk pregnancy" (Reis & Alligood, 2014, p. 32).

The theory is the association of prenatal yoga with optimism, power, and unitary well-being. One conceptual model concept is Health Patterning Practice Method; the relevant dimension is voluntary mutual patterning. The other conceptual model concept is Pattern. The theory concepts are Prenatal Yoga, Optimism, Power, and Unitary Well-Being.

The voluntary mutual patterning dimension of Health Patterning Practice Method is represented by Prenatal Yoga. Pattern is represented by Optimism, Power, and Unitary Well-Being. Prenatal Yoga is operationalized by the Healthy Moms® Prenatal Yoga Class protocol. Optimism is measured by the Life Orientation Test-Revised (LOT-R; Scheier, Carver, & Bridges, 1994). Power is measured by the PKPCT, Version II (Barrett, 2010). Unitary Well-Being is measured by the WPS (Gueldner et al., 2005) and the Short-Form 12 Version 2.0

BOX 7.11   An Example of a Conceptual–Theoretical–Empirical Structure for Rogers's Science of Unitary Human Beings Correlational Research

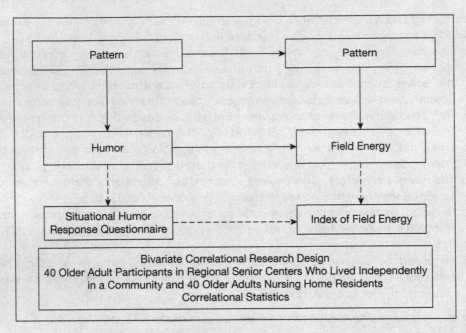

FIGURE 7.8 Conceptual–theoretical–empirical (CTE) structure for Rogers's Science of Unitary Human Beings correlational research—theory of the association of humor and field energy.

The *non-relational proposition* for the *C component* of the conceptual–theoretical–empirical (CTE) structure is:

- *Pattern* is defined as a unique "abstraction, [the nature of which] changes continuously, and [that] gives identity to the [energy] field" (Rogers, 1992, p. 30). Energy field patterns are not directly observable, although manifestations of field patterning are observable as experiences, perceptions, expressions, situations, and events.

The *non-relational propositions* for the *T component* of the CTE structure are:

- *Humor* is defined as "spontaneous and incongruent, involving a change of mind...the quality in individuals that mediates the amusing, the comic, the laughable, the ludicrous, the witty, and the funny...an expression that [is] produced when an individual cognitively perceives amusement stimulated by an incongruence or absurdity in the ordinary pattern of life" (Hindman, 2011 p. 48).

(continued)

BOX 7.11   An Example of a Conceptual–Theoretical–Empirical Structure for Rogers's Science of Unitary Human Beings Correlational Research   (continued)

- *Field Energy* is defined as "an intense absorption and awareness of self without regard to time or space...[which may range from] a sense of exuberance, sometimes associated with a relaxed and revitalized feeling...[and] an inward sense of wellbeing or vitality for life...[to feeling] lackluster" (Hindman, 2011, p. 49).

The *non-relational propositions* for the *E component* of the CTE structure are:

- Humor is measured by the Situational Humor Response Questionnaire (SHRQ; Lefcourt & Martin, 1986). The SHRQ is made up of 21 items about "the frequency of smiles, laughter, and other mirthful behaviors in a variety of situations....[The SHRQ includes] 18 situational items, and 3 generalized self-report items. The situational items describe a particular situation, such as meeting an old acquaintance while shopping, followed by 5 response options, ranging from 1 ('I would not have been particularly amused') to 5 ('I would have laughed heartily'). The 3 general self-report items ask [people] to rate their overall amusement in a variety of situations, the degree to which their amusement varies from situation to situation, and the desirability of choosing friends who are easily amused" (Lebowitz, Suh, Diaz, & Emery, 2011, p. 313). The items are rated on a Guttman-like scale (see Appendix B).
- Field Energy is measured by the Index of Field Energy (IFE; Gueldner, Bramlett, Johnston, & Guillory, 1996). The IFE includes 18 pictures, each of which is rated on a 7-point semantic differential scale (see Appendix B). The 18 pictures are "lock/shooting stars, fence/kite, flat tire/hot air balloon, brick wall/musical note, stop sign/rainbow, ball and chain/fireworks, snail/sea gull in flight, and shuttle/cane, eyes open/closed, shoes passive/active, butterfly/turtle, candle lit/not lit, faucet running full/dripping, puzzle pieces together/separated, pencil sharp/dull, sun full/partially cloud covered, balloons inflated/partially deflated, and lion/mouse" (Gueldner et al., 2005, p. 47).

The *relational propositions* for the *C* and *T* components of the CTE structure are:

- Manifestations of Pattern are interrelated.
- Therefore, Humor is associated with Field Energy.

The *relational proposition* for the *E* components of the CTE structure is:

- Scores on the Situational Humor Response Questionnaire are associated with scores on the Index of Field Energy.

Source: Hindman (2011).

(SF-12v2; Ware, Kosinski, Turner-Bowker, & Gandek, 2009). Reis and Alligood (2014) used paired-samples two-tailed *t*-tests and Mann–Whitney U test statistics (see Appendix B) to analyze the data.

The CTE structure that was constructed from the content of Reis and Alligood's (2014) journal article is illustrated in Figure 7.9. The non-relational and relational propositions for each component of the CTE structure are listed in Box 7.12.

A CTE Structure for Mixed-Methods Research

Malinski and Todaro-Franceschi's (2011) journal article is an example of mixed-methods (QUAN + QUAL) research (see Appendix A) guided by Rogers's Science of Unitary Human Beings. The purpose of the QUAN portion of their study was to examine the association of co-meditation with state anxiety, trait anxiety, systolic blood pressure, diastolic blood pressure, pulse rate, and respiratory rate. The QUAN portion of the study was conducted using a quasi-experimental pretest–posttest research design, with the 23 participants used as their own controls (see Appendix A). Data were collected prior to beginning co-meditation and 1 month later.

Malinski and Todaro-Franceschi (2011) explained that they added the QUAL portion of their study "to capture the essence of the experience from the perspective of participants themselves" (p. 244). Within the context of Rogers's Science of Unitary Human Beings, "descriptive data from participants are invaluable in grounding [numerical] measures in the overall patterning context, reflecting experiences and awareness of [the pattern of] their unique human–environmental mutual process" (Malinski & Todaro-Franceschi, 2011, p. 244). The QUAL portion of the study was conducted with 14 of the 23 participants 1 month after beginning co-meditation, using a simple descriptive qualitative design (see Appendix A).

The theory is the association of co-meditation with anxiety and vital signs. One conceptual model concept is Health Patterning Practice Method; the relevant dimension is voluntary mutual patterning. The other conceptual model concept is Pattern. The theory concepts are Co-Meditation, Anxiety, Vital Signs, and Experience of Co-Meditation. The two dimension of Anxiety are state anxiety and trait anxiety. The four dimensions of Vital Signs are systolic blood pressure, diastolic blood pressure, pulse rate, and respiratory rate. The two dimensions of Experience of Co-Meditation are practice frequency and feelings. The subdimensions of feelings are calmer, more relaxed, balanced, and centered.

Co-Meditation represents the voluntary mutual patterning dimension of Health Patterning Practice Method. Anxiety and its dimensions, Vital Signs and its dimensions, and Experience of Co-Meditation and its dimensions and subdimensions represent Pattern.

Co-Meditation is operationalized by the Co-Meditation protocol. The state anxiety dimension of Anxiety is measured by the State Anxiety Inventory (Self-Evaluation Questionnaire, STAI Form Y-1; Spielberger, 1983), and the trait anxiety dimension of Anxiety is measured by the Trait Anxiety Inventory (Self-Evaluation Questionnaire, STAI Form Y-2; Spielberger, 1983). The systolic blood pressure and the diastolic blood pressure dimensions of Vital Signs are measured by readings from a wall-mounted blood pressure machine. Malinski and Todaro-Franceschi (2011) did not indicate how the pulse rate and respiratory

BOX 7.12   An Example of a Conceptual–Theoretical–Empirical Structure for Rogers's Science of Unitary Human Beings Experimental Research

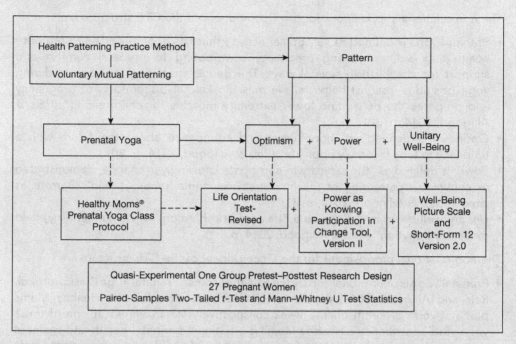

FIGURE 7.9 Conceptual–theoretical–empirical (CTE) structure for Rogers's Science of Unitary Human Beings experimental research—theory of association of prenatal yoga with optimism, power, and well-being.

The *non-relational propositions* for the *C component* of the conceptual–theoretical–empirical (CTE) structure are:

- *Health Patterning Practice Method* is defined as the nursing process.
- The relevant dimension of the Health Patterning Practice Method is voluntary mutual patterning.
  - *Voluntary mutual patterning* is defined as the continuous process whereby the nurse with the client patterns the environmental energy field to promote harmony related to health events. Voluntary mutual patterning processes that are most consistent with Rogers's Science of Unitary Human Beings are noninvasive modalities.
- *Pattern* is defined as a unique "abstraction, [the nature of which] changes continuously, and [that] gives identity to the [energy] field" (Rogers, 1992, p. 30). Energy field patterns are not directly observable, although manifestations of energy field patterning are observable as experiences, perceptions, expressions, situations, and events.

(continued)

BOX 7.12   An Example of a Conceptual–Theoretical–Empirical Structure for Rogers's Science of Unitary Human Beings Experimental Research   *(continued)*

The *non-relational propositions* for the *T component* of the CTE structure are:

- *Prenatal Yoga* is defined as "a popular activity that has been reported to promote health and wellness during pregnancy contributing to prenatal comfort and support for childbirth in several ways. The gentle stretching that occurs during yoga positions (asanas) helps relieve musculoskeletal discomforts of pregnancy and prepares the pelvic and lower extremity muscles for childbearing" (Reis & Alligood, 2014, p. 30).
- *Optimism* is defined as "hopefulness and confidence about the future with a tendency to look favorably upon life" (Reis & Alligood, 2014, p. 30).
- *Power* is defined as "the capacity to participate knowingly in change, demonstrated as continuous patterning of the human-environmental [energy] field" (Barrett, as cited in Reis & Alligood, 2014, p. 31).
- *Unitary well-being* is defined as a "balance and harmony of human [energy] field motion and rhythm" (Reis & Alligood, 2014, p. 31).

The *non-relational propositions* for the *E component* of the CTE structure are:

- Prenatal Yoga is operationalized by the Healthy Moms® Prenatal Yoga Class protocol. Reis and Alligood (2014) explained, "Participants attended the Healthy Moms prenatal yoga program once a week consecutively for six weeks at one of three yoga studio locations....Healthy Moms is a national perinatal health and wellness company that is 'dedicated to promoting successful health and wellness programs to new expectant moms...before, during and after pregnancy' " (Healthy Moms, as cited in Reis & Alligood, 2014, p. 33). The standard Healthy Moms prenatal yoga 60-minute class format includes checking in, centering, warm-up, flow (specific standing positions), other standing positions, mat work (seated positions and hip rotations), left side-lying positon, and meditation (Reis & Alligood, 2014).
- Optimism is measured by the Life Orientation Test-Revised (LOT-R; Scheier, Carver, & Bridges, 1994). The LOT-R is made up of 10 items—six items about optimism and four other items that are not included in the scoring; each item is rated on a 5-point Likert scale (see Appendix B) of 0 = strongly disagree; 1 = disagree; 2 = neutral; 3 = agree; and 4 = strongly agree.
- Power is measured by the Power as Knowing Participation in Change Tool, Version II (PKPCT, Version II; Barrett, 2010). The PKPCT, Version II includes four subscales—awareness, choices, freedom to act intentionally, and involvement in creating change—each of which is rated on 12 opposite adjective pairs, and each adjective pair is rated on a 1- to 7-point semantic differential scale (Barrett, 1990; see Appendix B). The adjective pairs are profound/superficial, seeking/avoiding, valuable/worthless, assertive/ timid, leading/following, orderly/chaotic, expanding/shrinking, pleasant/unpleasant, informed/uninformed, free/constrained, important/unimportant. The adjective pairs are listed in random order for each subscale, and the positive and negative adjectives are randomly reversed.

(continued)

BOX 7.12   An Example of a Conceptual–Theoretical–Empirical Structure for Rogers's Science of Unitary Human Beings Experimental Research   (continued)

- Unitary Well-Being is measured by the Well-Being Picture Scale (WPS; Gueldner et al., 2005). The WPS is made up of 10 professionally drawn pictures, each of which is rated on a 7-point semantic differential scale (see Appendix B). The 10 pictures are "eyes open/closed, shoes passive/active, butterfly/turtle, candle lit/not lit, faucet running full/dripping, puzzle pieces together/separated, pencil sharp/dull, sun full/partially cloud covered, balloons inflated/partially deflated, and lion/mouse" (Gueldner et al., 2005, p. 47).
- Unitary Well-Being also is measured by the Short-Form 12 Version 2.0 (SF-12v2; Ware, Kosinski, Turner-Bowker, & Gandek, 2009). The SF-12v2 includes 12 items that are scored as a total health-related quality of life score or as a Physical Component Summary (PCS) and a Mental Component Summary (MCS). "The PCS score addresses [the] physical functioning, role physical, bodily pain, and general health [domains of the SF-12v2] and the MCS score addresses [the] vitality, social functioning, role emotional, and mental health domains of the SF-12v2" (Reis & Alligood, 2014, p. 33). Various rating scales are used for the 12 items. Specifically, Item 1 is rated on a 5-point scale of "excellent," "very good," "good," "fair," or "poor." Items 2 and 3 are rated on a 3-point scale of "yes, liked a lot," "yes, liked a little," or "no, not liked at all." Items 3, 4, 5, and 6 are rated as "yes" or "no." Item 7 is rated on a 5-point scale of "not at all," "a little bit," "moderately," "quite a lot," or "extremely." Items 8, 9, 10, and 11 are rated on a 6-point scale of "all of the time," "most of the time," "a good bit of the time," "some of the time," "a little of the time," or "none of the time." Item 12 is rated on a 5-point scale of "all of the time," "most of the time," "some of the time," "a little of the time," or "none of the time" (Ware, Kosinski, & Keller, 1996, p. 225).

The *relational propositions* for the *C* and *T components* of the CTE structure are:

- Health Patterning Practice Method is associated with Pattern.
- Therefore, Prenatal Yoga is associated with Optimism, Power, and Unitary Well-Being.

The *relational proposition* for the *E components* of the CTE structure is:

- Participation in the Healthy Moms Prenatal Class is associated with changes in scores for the LOT-R; the PKPCT, Version II; the WPS; and the SF-12v2, from prior to beginning until completion of the Healthy Moms Prenatal Classes.

Source: Reis and Alligood (2014).

rate dimensions of Vital Signs are measured. Experience of Co-Meditation and its dimensions and subdimensions were generated from responses from 14 of the 23 participants in the QUAN portion of the study to an interview guide that included four open-ended questions.

The quantitative data were analyzed with the linear mixed model approach to repeated measures analysis of variance (see Appendix B). Content analysis was used to extract themes from the participants' responses to three of the four open-ended questions, and descriptive statistics (mean, range; see Appendix B) were used to analyze the data for the other open-ended question.

The CTE structure that was constructed from the content of Malinski and Todaro-Franceschi's (2011) journal article is illustrated in Figure 7.10. The non-relational and relational propositions for each component of the CTE structure are listed in Box 7.13.

BOX 7.13   An Example of a Conceptual–Theoretical–Empirical Structure for Rogers's Science of Unitary Human Beings Mixed-Methods Research

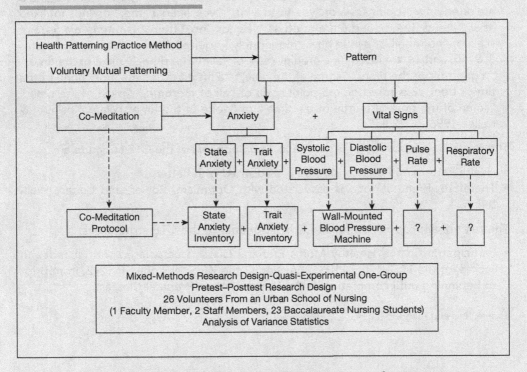

FIGURE 7.10 Conceptual–theoretical–empirical (CTE) structure for Rogers's Science of Unitary Human Beings mixed-methods research—theory of association of co-meditation with anxiety and vital signs—quantitative portion. (*continued*)

(continued)

BOX 7.13   An Example of a Conceptual–Theoretical–Empirical Structure for Rogers's Science of Unitary Human Beings Mixed-Methods Research   *(continued)*

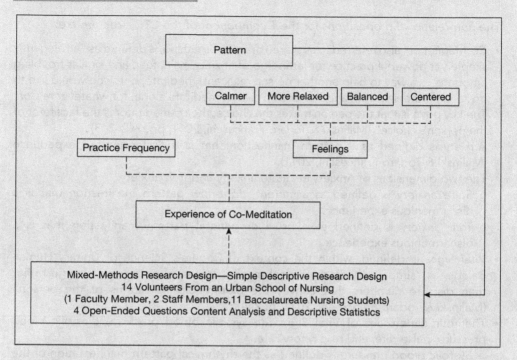

FIGURE 7.10 —Qualitative portion.   *(continued)*

The *non-relational propositions* for the *C component* of the conceptual–theoretical–empirical (CTE) structure are:

- *Health Patterning Practice Method* is defined as the nursing process.
- The relevant dimension of the Health Patterning Practice Method is voluntary mutual patterning.
  o *Voluntary mutual patterning* is defined as the continuous process whereby the nurse with the client patterns the environmental energy field to promote harmony related to health events. Voluntary mutual patterning processes that are most consistent with Rogers's Science of Unitary Human Beings are noninvasive modalities.
- *Pattern* is defined as a unique "abstraction, [the nature of which] changes continuously, and [that] gives identity to the [energy] field" (Rogers, 1992, p. 30). Energy field patterns are not directly observable, although manifestations of energy field patterning are observable as experiences, perceptions, expressions, situations, and events.

(continued)

BOX 7.13   An Example of a Conceptual–Theoretical–Empirical Structure for Rogers's Science of Unitary Human Beings Mixed-Methods Research *(continued)*

The *non-relational propositions* for the *T component* of the CTE structure are:

- *Co-Meditation*, also referred to as shared or cross-breathing, is defined as "an elegantly simple yet powerful practice for letting go of anxiety, pain, fear, and similar troubling emotions....a way to help another person relax and meditate, one who would like to do so in partnership with another or who cannot meditate alone, for whatever reason. The key point is that the person makes the choice; the co-meditator is the facilitator of the person's choice" (Malinski & Todaro-Franceschi, 2011, pp. 242–243).
- *Anxiety* is defined as a pattern manifestion that is a disharmonious experience (Malinski & Todaro-Franceschi, 2011).
- The two dimensions of Anxiety are state anxiety and trait anxiety.
  - *State anxiety* is defined as a current, right-now pattern manifestion that is a disharmonious experience.
  - *Trait anxiety* is defined as a usual or general pattern manifestion that is a disharmonious experience.
- *Vital Signs* is defined, within the context of Rogers's Science of Unitary Human Beings, as "simply varying rhythmical manifestations of patterning change rather than discrete numbers that convey the biophysiological status of the person" (Malinski & Todaro-Franceschi, 2011, p. 244).
- The four dimensions of Vital Signs are systolic blood pressure, diastolic blood pressure, pulse rate, and respiratory rate.
  - *Systolic blood pressure* is defined as the rhythmical pattern manifestation of the pressure of the blood on the walls of the arteries during contraction of the cardiac ventricles.
  - *Diastolic blood pressure* is defined as the rhythmical pattern manifestation of the pressure of the blood on the walls of the arteries when the cardiac ventricles are filling.
  - *Pulse rate* is defined as the rhythmical pattern manifestation of heart beats.
  - *Respiratory rate* is defined as the rhythmical pattern manifestation of breathing.
- Experience of Co-Meditation is defined as participants' reports of what they experienced as they participated with a partner in the co-meditation procedure.
- The two dimensions of Experience of Co-Meditation are practice frequency and feelings.
  - *Practice frequency* is defined as the number of times each participant practiced co-meditation.
  - *Feelings* is defined as the participants' expressions of how they felt during co-meditation.
  - The four subdimensions of feelings are calmer, more relaxed, balanced, and centered.
    - *Calmer* is defined as a feeling of quiet, serenity, and tranquility.
    - *More relaxed* is defined as a feeling of being rested.
    - *Balanced* is defined as a feeling of being in equality with the environmental energy field.
    - *Centered* is defined as a feeling of inner peace.

(continued)

BOX 7.13 An Example of a Conceptual–Theoretical–Empirical Structure for Rogers's Science of Unitary Human Beings Mixed-Methods Research *(continued)*

The *non-relational propositions* for the *E component* of the CTE structure are:

- Co-Meditation is operationalized by the Co-Meditation protocol. Malinski and Todaro-Franceschi (2011) explained that the participants chose "partners and then select[ed] a cubicle, with one lying on the bed and the other seated in the chair next to the bed. The researchers then demonstrated the relaxation process and the steps of the co-meditation process. The entire procedure was described as taking 20 to 30 minutes, with one person lying down and one seated near that person's head with enough light to observe the rise and fall of the chest/abdomen as the person breathes. The relaxation phase started with, 'Let attention focus on each part of your body and feel it relaxing....Your scalp is relaxing....' through 'Your feet and toes are relaxing...' with 5- to 10-second pauses between each phrase. This phase ended with, 'Let any remaining tension or discomfort melt away, feeling your body becoming softer....' Phase 1 of the co-meditation sequence involved the facilitator making the softly extended 'AAAHHH' sound, the universal sound of letting go, with each exhalation of the person lying down. This went on for approximately 5 minutes. Phase 2 involved softly drawing out the numbers 1 through 10 on each exhalation, then starting from 1 to 10 again for about 5 minutes. In Phase 3, the facilitator, having already asked the person if she or he had a favorite word or short phrase [he or she] would like to hear, softly verbalized that word or phrase for the person as she or he exhaled. If no word or phrase had been chosen, the facilitator returned to the 'AAAHHH' sound for another 5 minutes. The sequence concluded with the facilitator addressing the person by name, saying something like, 'Realize the comfort and peace you feel now,' and asking the person to slowly come back into awareness of the room and to sit up slowly when ready. Working in pairs, each member served as facilitator for the other until everyone had experienced co-meditation....The participants were given a one-page copy of the relaxation exercise and co-meditation sequence that could be used by a partner of their choice once the participants explained and demonstrated the process to them. They were asked to practice, with a partner and setting of their choice, a minimum of two times weekly for a month and then to return for a brief one-to-one interview with one of the researchers. At that time, they were given a copy of the book by Boerstler and Kornfeld (1995), *Life to Death*" (p. 245).
- The state anxiety dimension of Anxiety is measured by the State Anxiety Inventory (Self-Evaluation Questionnaire, STAI Form Y-1; Spielberger, 1983). The STAI Form Y-1 includes 20 items that are rated on a 4-point scale of 1 = not at all, 2 = somewhat, 3 = moderately so, and 4 = very much so.
- The trait anxiety dimension of Anxiety is measured by the Trait Anxiety Inventory (Self-Evaluation Questionnaire, STAI Form Y-2; Spielberger, 1983). The STAI Form Y-2 includes 20 items that are rated on a 4-point scale of 1 = almost never, 2 = sometimes, 3 = often, and 4 = almost always.
- The systolic blood pressure and diastolic blood pressure dimensions of Vital Signs are measured by a wall-mounted blood pressure machine (Malinski & Todaro-Franceschi, 2011).

(continued)

BOX 7.13 An Example of a Conceptual–Theoretical–Empirical Structure for Rogers's Science of Unitary Human Beings Mixed-Methods Research *(continued)*

- Malinski and Todaro-Franceschi (2011) did not indicate how the pulse rate and respiratory rate dimensions of Vital Signs are measured.
- The practice frequency dimension of Experience of Co-Meditation was discovered in and is measured by responses to an open-ended question on an interview guide. The question is: "Having learned co-meditation, how often have you practiced it?" (Malinski & Todaro-Franceschi, 2011, p. 246).
- The feelings dimension of Experience of Co-Meditation and its subdimensions were discovered in responses to three open-ended questions on an interview guide. The questions are: "Has it helped you to relax and diminish feelings of anxiety? How did you feel in relation to your partner having performed this exercise with him or her? How did your partner feel, having performed this exercise with you?" (Malinski & Todaro-Franceschi, 2011, p. 246).

For the quantitative portion of the sudy, the *relational propositions* for the *C and T components* of the CTE structure are:

- Health Patterning Practice Method is associated with Pattern.
- Therefore, Co-Meditation is associated with Anxiety and Vital Signs.

For the quantitative portion of the sudy, the *relational proposition* for the *E components* of the CTE structure is:

- Use of the Co-Meditation protocol is associated with changes in scores for the STAI Form Y-1, the STAI Form Y-2, and in scores for systolic blood pressure, diastolic blood pressure, pulse rate, and respiratory rate from before to after 1 month of using the protocol.

Source: Malinski and Todaro-Franceschi (2011).

CONCLUSION

Rogers was one of the first nurse scholars to explicitly identify the human being as the central phenomenon of nursing's concern. Although other conceptual models of nursing consider human beings in a holistic manner, Rogers's view of human beings as unitary is distinctive in that no parts or components or subsystems of the human being are delineated—each human being is a unified whole energy field. Furthermore, although other conceptual models consider the environment and its relationship with human beings, Rogers's view of human beings and environment as integral energy fields is unique and visionary.

Commenting on the contributions of her model, Rogers (as cited in Safier, 1977) stated,

> The conceptual system...provides for a substantive body of knowledge in nursing that will have relevance for all workers concerned with people, but with special relevance for nurses, not

because it matters to nurses per se, but because it matters to human beings, and consequently to nurses. (p. 320)

Moreover, Rogers (1986) pointed out that "the Science of Unitary Human Beings identifies nursing's uniqueness and signifies the potential of nurses to fulfill their social responsibility in human service" (p. 8).

The distinctive focus of applications of Rogers's Science of Unitary Human Beings is evident in the examples of its use as a guide for practice, QI projects, and research given in this chapter.

NOTE

1. Portions of this chapter are adapted from Fawcett, J., & DeSanto-Madeya, S. (2013). *Contemporary nursing knowledge: Analysis and evaluation of nursing models and theories* (3rd ed., Chapter 9). Philadelphia: F. A. Davis, with permission.

REFERENCES

Barrett, E. A. M. (1983). *An empirical investigation of Martha E. Rogers' principle of helicy: The relationship of human field motion and power.* (Doctoral dissertation). Retrieved from ProQuest Dissertations and Theses Full Text (Dissertation number 8406278; ProQuest document ID 303172899).

Barrett, E. A. M. (1990). A measure of power as knowing participation in change. In O. Strickland & C. Waltz (Eds.), *The measurement of nursing outcomes: Measuring client self-care and coping skills* (Vol. 4, pp. 159–180). New York: Springer Publishing.

Barrett, E. A .M. (1998). A Rogerian practice methodology for health patterning. *Nursing Science Quarterly, 11*, 136–138.

Barrett, E. A. M. (2010). Practice exemplar. In M. E. Parker & M. C. Smith (Eds.), *Nursing theories and nursing practice* (3rd ed., pp. 270–271). Philadelphia, PA: F. A. Davis.

Barrett, E. A. M., & Caroselli, C. (1998). Methodological pondering related to the power as knowing participation in change tool. *Nursing Science Quarterly, 11*, 17–22.

Boerstler, R. W., & Kornfeld, H. S. (1995). *Life to death: Harmonizing the transition, a holistic and meditative approach for caregivers and the dying.* Rochester, VT: Healing Arts Press.

Butcher, H. K. (1998). Crystallizing the processes of the unitary field pattern portrait research method. *Visions: The Journal of Rogerian Nursing Science, 6*, 13–26.

Butcher, H. K. (2005). The unitary field pattern portrait research method: Facets, processes, and findings. *Nursing Science Quarterly, 18*, 293–297.

Caroselli, C., & Barrett, E. A. M. (1998). A review of the power as knowing participation in change literature. *Nursing Science Quarterly, 11*, 9–16.

Cowling, W. R., III (1990). A template for unitary pattern-based nursing practice. In E. A. M. Barrett (Ed.), *Visions of Rogers' science-based nursing* (pp. 45–65). New York, NY: National League for Nursing Press.

Cowling, W. R., III. (1997). Pattern appreciation: The unitary science/practice of reaching for essence. In M. Madrid (Ed.), *Patterns of Rogerian knowing* (pp. 129–142). New York, NY: National League for Nursing Press.

Fawcett, J., & DeSanto-Madeya, S. (2013). *Contemporary nursing knowledge: Analysis and evaluation of nursing models and theories* (3rd ed.). Philadelphia, PA: F. A. Davis.

Fuller, J. M., Davis, B. L., Servonsky, E. J., & Butcher, H. K. (2012). A family field pattern portrait of adult substance users in rehabilitation. *Visions: The Journal of Rogerian Nursing Science, 19*, 42–64.

Gueldner, S. H., Bramlett, M. H., Johnston, L. W., & Guillory, J. A. (1996). Index of Field Energy. *Rogerian Nursing Science News, 8*(4), 6.

Gueldner, S. H., Michel, Y., Bramlett, M. H., Liu, C-F., Johnston, L. W.,....Carlyle, M. S. (2005). The Well-Being Picture Scale: A revision of the Index of Field Energy. *Nursing Science Quarterly, 18*, 42–50.

Hindman, M. E. (2011). Humor and field energy in older adults. *Visions: The Journal of Rogerian Nursing Science, 18*, 47–58.

Kim, T. S. (2009). The theory of power as knowing participation in change: A literature review update. *Visions: The Journal of Rogerian Nursing Science, 16*, 19–39.

Kim, T. S., Smith, A. S., & West, L. (2012). Educational interventions to enhance employee breast health: A program evaluation using the Barrett power theory. *Visions: The Journal of Rogerian Nursing Science, 19*, 26–41.

Lebowitz, K. R., Suh, S., Diaz, P. T., & Emery, C. F. (2011). Effects of humor and laughter on psychological functioning, quality of life, health status, and pulmonary functioning among patients with chronic obstructive pulmonary disease: A preliminary investigation. *Heart & Lung, 40*, 310–319.

Lefcourt, H. M., & Martin, R. A. (1986). *Humor and life stress: Antidote to adversity.* New York, NY: Springer-Verlag.

Lewin, K. (1951). *Field theory in social science.* London, UK: Tavistock Publications.

Malinski, V. M., & Todaro-Franceschi, V. (2011). Exploring co-meditation as a means of reducing anxiety and facilitating relaxation in a nursing school setting. *Journal of Holistic Nursing, 29*, 242–248.

Reis, P. J., & Alligood, M. R. (2014). Prenatal yoga in late pregnancy and optimism, power, and well-being. *Nursing Science Quarterly, 27*, 30–36.

Rogers, M. E. (1986). Science of unitary human beings. In V. M. Malinski (Ed.), *Explorations on Martha Rogers' science of unitary human beings* (pp. 3–8). Norwalk, CT: Appleton-Century-Crofts.

Rogers, M. E. (1990). Space-age paradigm for new frontiers in nursing. In M. E. Parker (Ed.), *Nursing theories in practice* (pp. 105–113). New York, NY: National League for Nursing Press.

Rogers, M. E. (1992). Nursing science and the space age. *Nursing Science Quarterly, 5*, 27–34.

Rogers, M. E. (1994). The science of unitary human beings: Current perspectives. *Nursing Science Quarterly, 7*, 33–35.

Safier, G. (1977). *Contemporary American leaders: An oral history.* New York, NY: McGraw-Hill.

Scheier, M. F., Carver, C. S., & Bridges, M. W. (1994). Distinguishing optimism from neuroticism (and trait anxiety, self-mastery, and self-esteem): A reevaluation of the Life Orientation Test. *Journal of Personality and Social Psychology, 67*, 1063–1078.

Spielberger, C. D. (1983). *State-Trait Anxiety Inventory (Form Y).* Redwood City, CA: Mind Garden.

Ware, J. E., Kosinski, M., & Keller, S. (1996). A 12-item Short-Form Health Survey: Construction of scales and preliminary tests of reliability and validity. *Medical Care, 34*, 220–223.

Ware, J. E., Kosinski, M., Turner-Bowker, D. M., & Gandek, B. (2009). *Users' manual for the SF-12v2® health survey.* Lincoln, RI: QualityMetric Incorporated.

CHAPTER 8

ROY'S ADAPTATION MODEL[1]

Sister Callista Roy's Adaptation Model focuses on changes experienced by human beings as they respond to environmental stimuli to maintain their integrity (Roy, 2009). The goal of Roy's Adaptation Model nursing is promotion of an integrated level of adaptation for individuals and groups that will advance wellness, the quality of life, and death with dignity (Roy, 2009).

ROY'S ADAPTATION MODEL: CONCEPTS AND NON-RELATIONAL PROPOSITIONS

This section of the chapter includes the concepts of Roy's Adaptation Model and the definitions (non-relational propositions) of the concepts and the dimensions of the multidimensional concepts (Roy, 2009).

Human Adaptive System is defined as a unified whole made up of parts (Roy, 2009). The two dimensions of the concept are individual persons and groups or relational persons.

Individual persons is defined as a single person.

Groups or relational persons is defined as a collective or aggregate who relate within the context of the collective, such as families, organizations, communities, nations, and society as a whole.

Coping Processes is defined as "innate coping processes [that] are genetically determined or common to the species and are generally viewed as automatic process; people do not have to think about them...[and] acquired coping processes [that] are developed through strategies such as learning" (Roy, 2009, p. 41). The two dimensions of the concept that pertain to individual persons are regulator coping subsystem and cognator coping subsystem. The two dimensions that pertain to groups or relational persons are stabilizer subsystem control process and innovator subsystem control process.

Regulator coping subsystem, which pertains to individuals, is defined as a major coping process that "responds through neural, chemical, and endocrine coping channels" (Roy, 2009, p. 41).

Cognator coping subsystem, which pertains to individuals, is defined as a second major coping process that involves "four cognitive-emotive channels: perceptual and information processing, learning, judgment, and emotion" (Roy, 2009, p. 41).

Stabilizer subsystem control process, which pertains to groups, is defined as "the established structure, values, and daily activities whereby participants accomplish the primary purpose of the group and contribute to common purposes of society" (Roy, 2009, p. 42).

Innovator subsystem control process, which pertains to groups, is defined as "the internal subsystem that involves structures and processes for change and growth in human social systems" (Roy, 2009, p. 43).

Behavior is defined as "All [observable and nonobservable] responses of the human adaptive system including capacities, assets, knowledge, skills, abilities, and commitments" (Roy, 2009, p. 39). The two dimensions of the concept are adaptive responses and ineffective responses.

Adaptive responses is defined as responses that promote "integrity of the human adaptive system in terms of the goals of survival, growth, reproduction, mastery, and human and environment transformations" (Roy, 2009, p. 58).

Ineffective responses is defined as responses that "can, in the immediate situation or if continued over a long time, threaten the human system's survival, growth, reproduction, mastery, or people and environment transformations" (Roy, 2009, p.40).

Adaptive Modes is defined as ways in which human adaptive systems respond to stimuli from the environment that are processed through the coping processes. The four dimensions of the concept are physiological/physical mode, self-concept/group identity mode, role function mode, and interdependence mode.

Physiologic Mode, which pertains to individuals, is defined as "the manifestation of the physiologic activities of all the cells, tissues, organs, and systems comprising the human body" (Roy, 2009, p. 90). The nine subdimensions of Physiological Mode are oxygenation; nutrition; elimination; activity and rest; protection; senses; fluid, electrolyte, and acid–base balance; neurological function; and endocrine function.

Oxygenation is defined as "The processes (ventilation, gas exchange, and transport of gases [to and from the tissues]) by which cellular oxygen supply is maintained in the body" (Roy, 2009, p. 111).

Nutrition is defined as "The series of processes by which a person takes in nutrients and assimilates and uses them to maintain body tissue, promote growth, and provide energy" (Roy, 2009, p. 130).

Elimination is defined as a life process that concerns elimination of waste products from the body, including intestinal elimination and urinary elimination (Roy, 2009).

Activity and rest is defined as "body movement and serves various purposes such as carrying out daily living chores and protecting self or others from bodily injuries…Rest…involves changes in activity in which energy requirements are minimal" (Roy, 2009, p. 166).

Protection is defined as "two basic life processes: nonspecific defense processes and specific defense processes. Together these two functional defense systems work to protect the body from 'foreign' substances such as bacteria, viruses, parasites, and abnormal body cells" (Roy, 2009, p. 200).

Senses is defined as "seeing [vision], hearing, and feeling, [which] are processes by which an individual receives and exchanges information needed for the activities of life, including relating to others" (Roy, 2009, p. 224).

Fluid, electrolyte, and acid–base balance is defined as "Fluid balance [refers to the balance of fluids] between intracellular and extracellular compartments.…Electrolyte balance addresses concentrations of salts within the body.…[Acid-base balance refers to the] status of body fluids[,] is related to the concentration of hydrogen ions and is described in terms of pH" (Roy, 2009, pp. 256, 257, 258).

Neurological function is defined as the components of the central nervous system (brain and spinal cord) and the peripheral nervous system (cranial and spinal nerves) (Roy, 2009).

Endocrine function is defined as integration and maintenance of "all the body's physiologic processes to promote normal growth, development, and maintenance of structure and function" (Roy, 2009, p. 302).

Physical Mode, which pertains to people interacting in groups, is defined as the "way in which the group adaptive system manifests adaptation concerning basic operating resources" (Roy, 2009, p. 91).

Self-Concept Mode, which pertains to individuals, is defined as behavior "pertaining to the personal aspect of human systems" (Roy, 2009, p. 95). The two subdimensions of self-concept mode are physical self and personal self.

Physical self is defined as "appraisal of one's own physical being, including physical attributes, functioning, sexuality, health and illness states, and appearance [that encompasses] body sensation and body image.…Body sensation [refers to] how one feels and experiences the self as a physical being.…Body image [refers to] how one views oneself physically and one's view of personal appearance" (Roy, 2009, pp. 322, 323).

Personal self is defined as "appraisal of one's own characteristics, expectations, values, and worth, including self-consistency, self-ideal, and the moral-ethical-spiritual self.…Self-consistency [refers to] that part of the personal self…which strives to maintain a consistent self-organization and to avoid disequilibrium; an organized system of ideas about self. . . . Self-ideal [refers to] that aspect of the personal self that relates to what the person would like to be or is capable of doing. . . . Moral-ethical-spiritual self [refers to] that aspect of the personal self which includes a belief system and an evaluation of who one is in relation to the universe" (Roy, 2009, p. 323).

Group Identity Mode, which pertains to groups, is defined as referring to "shared relations, goals, and values, which act within and create a social milieu and culture, a group self-image, and coresponsibility for goal achievement" (Roy, 2009, p. 433). The four subdimensions of group identity mode are interpersonal relationships, group self-image, social milieu, and group culture.

Interpersonal relationships is defined as a component of the group identity mode.

Group self-image is defined as a component of the group identity mode.

Social milieu is defined as a component of the group identity mode that is the "total human-made environment that suurounds the group in which it is embedded" (Roy, 2009, p. 433).

Group culture is defined as a component of the group identity mode that addresses the "group's agreed upon expectations, including values, goals, and norms for relating" (Roy, 2009, p.433).

Role Function Mode, which pertains to both individuals and groups, is defined as behaviors—or activities—that are associated with ascribed and acquired roles (Roy, 2009). The seven subdimensions of the role function mode are primary role, secondary role, tertiary role, instrumental behavior, expressive behavior, role-taking, and integrating roles.

Primary role is defined as an "ascribed role based on age, sex, and developmental stage; it determines the majority of behaviors engaged in by a person during a particular growth period of life" (Roy, 2009, p. 359).

Secondary role is defined as a "role that a person assumes to complete the tasks associated with a developmental stage and primary role" (Roy, 2009, p. 359).

Tertiary role is defined as a "role that is freely chosen by a person, temporary in nature, and often associated with the accomplishment of a minor task in a person's current development" (Roy, 2009, p. 360).

Instrumental behavior is defined as "goal-oriented behavior; role activities the person performs" (Roy, 2009, p. 359).

Expressive behavior is defined as the "feelings and attitudes held by the person about role performance" (Roy, 2009, p. 359).

Role-taking is defined as a "process of looking at or anticipating another person's behavior by viewing it within a role attributed to the other" (Roy, 2009, p. 359).

Integrating roles is defined as the "process of managing different roles and their expectations" (Roy, 2009, p. 466).

Interdependence Mode, which pertains to individuals and groups, is defined as "interactions related to the giving and receiving of love, respect, and value" (Roy, 2009, p. 45). The eight subdimensions of the interdependence mode are affectional adequacy, developmental adequacy, resource adequacy, significant others, support systems, context, infrastructure, and resources.

> *Affectional adequacy*, which pertains to both individuals and groups, is defined as the "need to give and receive love, respect, and value satisfied through effective relations and communication" (Roy, 2009, p. 385).

> *Developmental adequacy*, which pertains to both individuals and groups, is defined as "learning and maturation in relationships achieved through developmental processes" (Roy, 2009, p. 385).

> *Resource adequacy*, which pertains to both individuals and groups, is defined as the "need for food, clothing, shelter, health, and security achieved through interdependent processes" (Roy, 2009, p. 485).

> *Significant others* pertaining to individuals is defined as the "individuals to whom the most meaning or importance is given [by a person]" (Roy, 2009, p. 385).

> *Significant others* pertaining to groups is defined as "other groups to whom the most meaning or importance is given [by the group]" (Roy, 2009, p. 485).

> *Support systems* pertaining to individuals is defined as the "persons, groups, [and] organizations with whom one associates in order to achieve affectional, developmental, and resources requirements" (Roy & Andrews, 1999, p. 475).

> *Support systems* pertaining to groups is defined as "persons, groups, [and] organizations with which a group associates in order to achieve affectional, developmental, and resources requirements" (Roy, 2009, p. 485).

> *Context*, which pertains to groups, is defined as "external (economic, social, political, cultural, belief, family systems) and internal (mission, vision, values, principles, goals, plans) influences within relationships" (Roy & Andrews, 1999, p. 474).

> *Infrastructure*, which pertains to groups, is defined as the "affectional, resource, and developmental processes that exist within a relationship" (Roy & Andrews, 1999, p. 474).

> *Resources*, which pertains to groups, is defined as food, clothing, shelter, meeting places, physical facilities for organizations, supplies, equipment, technology, and finances (Roy & Andrews, 1999).

Stimuli is defined as "factor[s] in the internal … and external environment … that provoke a response, or more generally, the point of interaction of the human system and the environment" (Roy, 2009, p. 27). The three dimensions of the concept are focal stimulus, contextual stimuli, and residual stimuli.

> *Focal stimulus* is defined as the internal or external environmental stimulus most immediately confronting the adaptive system (Roy, 2009, p. 63).

Contextual stimuli is defined as other than the focal stimulus, "all other internal or external [environmental] stimuli affecting the situation" (Roy, 2009, p. 63).

Residual stimuli is defined as "those stimuli having an indeterminate effect on the behavior of the individual or group adaptive system" (Roy, 2009, p. 64).

Adaptation is defined as the "process and outcome whereby thinking and feeling persons, as individuals or in groups, use conscious awareness and choice to create human and environmental integration" (Roy, 2009, p. 26). The five dimensions of the concept are survival, growth, reproduction, mastery, and person and environment transformations.

Survival is defined as a goal of adaptation.

Growth is defined as a goal of adaptation.

Reproduction is defined as a goal of adaptation that includes "the continuation of the human species by having children, but it also involves the many ways that people extend themselves in time and space by creative works and moral presence" (Roy, 2009, p. 39).

Mastery is defined as a goal of adaptation.

Person and environment transformations is defined as a goal of adaptation.

Adaptation Level is defined as the "condition of the life processes as a significant focal, contextual, or residual stimulus in a situation.... The pooled effect of focal, contextual, and residual stimuli determines the adaptation level" (Roy, 2009, pp. 33, 38). The three dimensions of the concept are integrated life process, compensatory life process, and compromised life process.

Integrated life process is defined as the "Adaptation level at which the structures and functions of a life process are working as a whole to meet human needs" (Roy, 2009, p. 27).

Compensatory life process is defined as the "Adaptation level at which the cognator and regulator [or stabilizer and innovator] have been activated by a challenge to the integrated life processes" (Roy, 2009, p. 26).

Compromised life process is defined as the "Adaptation level resulting from inadequate integrated and compensatory life process; an adaptation problem" (Roy, 2009, p. 26).

Health is defined as a "state and process of being and becoming an integrated and whole human being" (Roy, 2009, p. 48).

Roy's Adaptation Model Nursing process is defined as the nursing process. The six dimensions of the concept are assessment of behaviors, assessment of stimuli, nursing diagnosis, goal setting, intervention, and evaluation.

Assessment of behaviors is defined as systematic collection of data about the behavior of the human adaptive system and judgment about the current state of the coping process and of adaptation in each adaptive mode—physiological/physical mode, self-concept/group identity mode, role function mode, and interdependence mode.

Assessment of stimuli is defined as identification of the internal and external focal and contextual stimuli that are influencing the behaviors of particular interest, in the order of priority established at the end of the assessment of behaviors dimension of Roy's Adaptation Model Nursing Process.

Nursing diagnosis is defined as a statement conveying the adaptation status of the human adaptive system of interest, specifically a statement about the behaviors of interest together with the most relevant influencing stimuli.

Goal setting is defined as a clear statement of the desired behavioral outcomes in response to nursing provided for the human adaptive system.

Intervention is defined as management of stimuli using nursing approaches that have a high probability of changing stimuli or strengthening adaptive processes. Stimuli may be altered, increased, decreased, removed, or maintained.

Evaluation is defined as judgment about the effectiveness of nursing interventions in relation to the behaviors of the human adaptive system.

ROY'S ADAPTATION MODEL: RELATIONAL PROPOSITIONS

The statements of associations (relational propositions) between concepts of the Roy Adaptation Model are listed here.

- Stimuli are related to Coping Processes.
- Coping Processes are related to Adaptive Modes.
- Stimuli are related to Adaptive Modes.
- Roy's Adaptation Model Nursing Process has an effect on Adaptive Modes.
- The four dimensions of Adaptive Modes—physiological/physical mode, self-concept/group identity mode, role function mode, and interdependence mode—are interrelated.

ROY'S ADAPTATION MODEL: APPLICATION TO NURSING PRACTICE

The guidelines for Roy's Adaptation Model nursing practice are listed in Box 8.1. A diagram of the practice methodology for Roy's Adaptation Model, which is called the Roy Adaptation Model Nursing Process, is illustrated in Figure 8.1.

A practice tool that includes all aspects of the practice methodology is given in Box 8.2.

A Conceptual–Theoretical–Empirical Structure for Assessment

Roy and Zhan's (2010) book chapter includes a practice exemplar, one section of which focuses on assessment. They described the use of Roy's Adaptation Model Nursing Process with three generations of a Chinese American family. The family members are a 50-year-old man, his wife, and their 7-year-old daughter, the man's uncle, the man's 32-year-old cousin and her husband and 5-year-old son, and the man's 75-year-old mother, who has a medical diagnosis

BOX 8.1 Guidelines for Roy's Adaptation Model Practice

The broad purpose of Roy's Adaptation Model–based nursing practice is to promote the ability of human adaptive systems to adjust effectively to changes in the environment and also to create changes in the environment. The more specific purpose of Roy's Adaptation Model–based nursing practice is to promote the human adaptive system's adaptation in the physiological/physical, self-concept/group identity, role function, and interdependence modes.

Practice problems of interest encompass adaptive and ineffective behavioral responses of human adaptive systems in the physiological/physical, self-concept/group identity, role function, and interdependence adaptive modes.

Nursing may be practiced in any setting in which nurses encounter individuals and groups, ranging from virtually every type of health care institution to people's homes and the community at large.

Legitimate participants in nursing practice are human adaptive systems—including individuals, families, and other groups, communities, and society—considered sick or well. Those adaptive systems may or may not manifest specific adaptation problems and ineffective behavioral responses.

The practice methodology is Roy's Adaptation Model Nursing Process. The components of the process are assessment of behaviors, assessment of stimuli, nursing diagnosis, goal setting, intervention, and evaluation.

Roy's Adaptation Model–based nursing practice contributes to the well-being of human adaptive systems by maintaining or enhancing the adaptation level and adaptive behavioral responses.

Adapted from Fawcett and DeSanto-Madeya (2013).

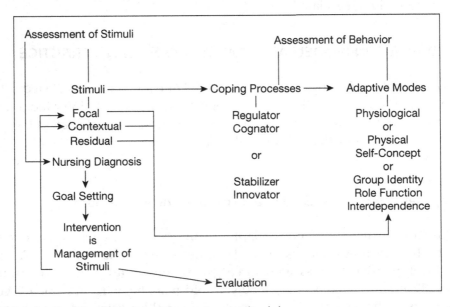

FIGURE 8.1 Roy's Adaptation Model practice methodology: Roy's Adaptation Model nursing process.

BOX 8.2   The Roy's Adaptation Model Practice Methodology Tool for Individuals or Groups

ASSESSMENT OF BEHAVIORS AND STIMULI

Physiological/Physical Mode Assessment

Note: Physiological mode assessment may also include the patient's vital signs, results of laboratory tests, and other physiological parameters.

Nurse: On a scale of 0 to 10, with 0 indicating "very sick" and 10 indicating "very well," how do you feel physically?

Patient:

Nurse: What is happening right now to make you feel that way? [Asking about focal and contextual stimuli]

Patient:

Self-Concept/Group Identity Mode Assessment

Nurse: On a scale of 0 to 10, with 0 indicating "very sad" and 10 indicating "very excited," how do you feel emotionally?

Patient:

Nurse: What is happening right now to make you feel that way? [Asking about focal and contextual stimuli]

Patient:

Role Function Mode Assessment

Nurse: On a scale of 0 to 10, with 0 indicating "not at all" and 10 indicating "totally," to what extent do you think you will maintain your usual activities when you have recovered from [the health condition]?

Patient:

Nurse: What do you think will happen to help you or hinder you in doing your usual activities? [Asking about focal and contextual stimuli]

Patient:

Interdependence Mode Assessment

Nurse: On a scale of 0 to 10, with 0 indicating "none" and 10 indicating "a lot," to what extent are you receiving help from your family and friends?

Patient:

Nurse: In what areas do you need more help? [Asking about focal and contextual stimuli]

Patient:

Regulator Coping Processes

Assessment of regulator coping processes requires information for autonomic nervous system activity evident in tests for fluid, electrolyte, and acid–base balance and hormones.

(continued)

BOX 8.2   The Roy's Adaptation Model Practice Methodology Tool for Individuals or Groups   *(continued)*

Cognator Coping Processes/Stabilizer and Innovator Subsystem Control Processes

Nurse: On a scale of 0 to 10, with 0 indicating "not well" and 10 indicating "very well," to what extent are you managing to cope with all that is happening right now?

Patient:

NURSING DIAGNOSIS

Note: Adaptive behaviors are those indicating the patient's goals for survival, growth, mastery, and person–environmental transformation have been achieved, that is, the patient's needs have been met. Ineffective behaviors are those indicating that the goals have not been achieved, that is, that the patient's needs have not been met and that nursing intervention is required.

The nursing diagnosis is stated as behaviors of interest with the most relevant influencing focal and/or contextual stimuli.

Physiologic Mode: Physiologic mode behaviors are (adaptive or ineffective) due to the environmental stimulus/stimuli of . . .
Self-Concept Mode: Self-concept mode behaviors are (adaptive or ineffective) due to the environmental stimulus/stimuli of . . .
Role Function Mode: Role function mode behaviors are (adaptive or ineffective) due to the environmental stimulus/stimuli of . . .
Interdependence Mode: Interdependence mode behaviors are (adaptive or ineffective) due to the environmental stimulus/stimuli of . . .

GOAL SETTING

Goals are established in collaboration between the nurse and the patient and are stated as objectives to be achieved within a specific time frame.

INTERVENTION

The nurse and the patient discuss and select one or more interventions to be used to meet the goals.

EVALUATION

The nurse and the patient determine the extent to which the goals were met and the effectiveness of the interventions.

Adapted from Fawcett and DeSanto-Madeya (2013).

of dementia. Roy and Zhan explained, "As [the man's] mother's cognitive function deteriorated, [he] was virtually overwhelmed by caring for his mother [in his home] while keeping his responsibility of managing the [family's Chinese] restaurant" (pp. 176–177).

The theory used to guide practice is assesment of family coherence. The conceptual model concept is Roy's Adaptation Model Nursing Process. The relevant dimensions of the concept are assessment of behavior and assessment of stimuli. The theory concept is Family Coherence. One dimension of Family Coherence is family structure, function, relationships, and consistency. The other two dimensions are demands and problems.

The assessment of behaviors dimension of Roy's Adaptation Model Nursing Process is represented by the family structure, function, relationships, and consistency dimension of Family Coherence. The assessment of stimuli dimension of Roy's Adaptation Model Nursing Process is represented by the demands and problems dimensions of Family Coherence. Roy and Zhan (2010) used the assessment of behavior and assessment of stimuli sections of Roy's Adaptation Model Practice Methodology to assess Family Coherence and its dimensions.

The conceptual–theoretical–empirical (CTE) structure that was constructed from the assessment content of Roy and Zhan's (2010) practice exemplar is illustrated in Figure 8.2. The non-relational propositions for each component of the CTE structure are listed in Box 8.3.

BOX 8.3   An Example of a Conceptual–Theoretical–Empirical Structure for Roy's Adaptation Model Nursing Practice: Assessment

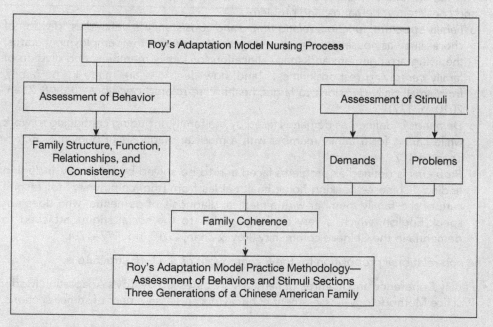

FIGURE 8.2 Conceptual–theoretical–empirical (CTE) structure for Roy's Adaptation Model nursing practice: Assessment—theory of family coherence.

(continued)

BOX 8.3   An Example of a Conceptual–Theoretical–Empirical Structure for Roy's Adaptation Model Nursing Practice: Assessment *(continued)*

The *non-relational propositions* for the *C component* of the conceptual–theoretical–empirical (CTE) structure are:

- *Roy's Adaptation Model Nursing Process* is defined as the nursing process.
- The relevant dimensions of Roy's Adaptation Model Nursing Process are assessment of behaviors and assessment of stimuli.
  o *Assessment of behaviors* is defined as systematic collection of data about the behavior of the human adaptive system and judgment about the current state of the coping processes and of adaptation in each adaptive mode—physiological/physical mode, self-concept/group identity mode, role function mode, and interdependence mode.
  o *Assessment of stimuli* is defined as identification of the internal and external focal and contextual stimuli that are influencing the behaviors of particular interest, in the order of priority established at the end of the assessment of behaviors dimension of the Roy's Adaptation Model Nursing Process.

The *non-relational propositions* for the *T component* of the CTE structure are:

- *Family Coherence* is defined as "an indicator of positive adaptation [that] refers to a state of unity or a consistent sequence of thoughts that connects family members who share group identity, goals, and values" (Roy & Zhan, 2010, p. 176).
- The dimensions of Family Coherence are family structure, function, relationships, and consistency; demands; and problems.
  o *Family structure, function, relationships, and consistency* is defined as "division of chores such as housekeeping, shopping, and/or repairs; their employment status; the living arrangement and space allocation for family members; and division of family caregiving responsibilities...[and] how decisions are made in the family, from small daily decisions to larger, health care-related decisions" (Roy & Zhan, 2010, p. 177).
  o *Demands* is defined as demands faced by the family, including continuing to work while caring for a family member with a medical diagnosis of dementia (Roy & Zhan, 2010).
  o *Problems* is defined as problems faced and to be solved by the family, including finding "Chinese-speaking home health aides from [the] community" for respite care of the family member with a medical diagnosis of dementia, who does not speak English, which is very challenging due to the social stigma attached to dementia in the Chinese community (Roy & Zhan, 2010, pp. 177–178).

The *non-relational proposition* for the *E component* of the CTE structure is:

- Family Coherence and its three dimensions are assessed by Roy's Adaptation Model Practice Methodology—assessment of behaviors and assessment of stimuli sections.

Source: Roy and Zhan (2010).

A CTE Structure for Intervention

Another section of Roy and Zhan's (2010) practice exemplar focuses on use of Roy's Adaptation Model to guide intervention. They described how strategies to manage stimuli were used with the members of a three-generation Chinese American family; details about the family are given in the "An Example of a Conceptual–Theoretical–Empirical Structure for Roy's Adaptation Model Nursing Practice: Assessment" section of this chapter.

The theory used to guide practice is effects of focusing on stimuli on family coping strategies and family resources. One conceptual model concept is Roy's Adaptation Model Nursing Process. The relevant dimension of the concept is intervention. The other conceptual model concepts are Coping Processes and Adaptive Modes. The relevant dimension of Coping Processes is stabilizer subsystem control process, and the relevant dimension of Adaptive Modes is role function mode.

The theory concepts are Focus on Stimuli, Family Coping Strategies, and Family Resources. The intervention dimension of Roy's Adaptation Model Nursing Process is represented by Focus on Stimuli. The stabilizer subsystem control process dimension of Coping Processes is represented by Family Coping Strategies. The role function mode dimension of Adaptive Modes is represented by Family Resources.

Focus on Stimuli is operationalized by the intervention section of Roy's Adaptation Model Nursing Process. Family Coping Strategies is measured by data from evaluation of the Coping Processes–stabilizer subsystem control process section of Roy's Adaptation Model Practice Methodology. Family Resources is measured by data from evaluation of the adaptive modes–role function mode section of Roy's Adaptation Model Practice Methodology.

The CTE structure that was constructed from an interpretation of the intervention content of Roy and Zhan's (2010) practice exemplar is illustrated in Figure 8.3. The non-relational and relational propositions for each component of the CTE structure are listed in Box 8.4.

APPLICATION TO QUALITY IMPROVEMENT PROJECTS

The guidelines for Roy's Adaptation Model quality improvement (QI) projects are listed in Box 8.5.

A CTE Structure for a QI Project

Kaur and Mahal's (2012) journal article is an example of a report of Roy's Adaptation Model QI project. The purpose of their project was to determine "the acceptability for utilization of [the] Roy Adaptation [Model] based nursing assessment tool" (p. 133).

The theory is the effect of an educational program on utilization of Roy's Adaptation Model Assessment Tool. One conceptual model concept is Roy's

BOX 8.4   An Example of a Conceptual–Theoretical–Empirical Structure for Roy's Adaptation Model Nursing Practice: Intervention

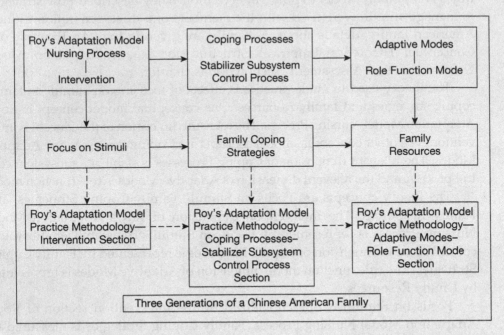

FIGURE 8.3 Conceptual–theoretical–empirical (CTE) structure for Roy's Adaptation Model nursing practice: Intervention—theory of effects of focus on stimuli on family coping strategies and family resources.

The *non-relational propositions* for the *C component* of the conceptual–theoretical–empirical (CTE) structure are:

- *Roy's Adaptation Model Nursing Process* is defined as the nursing process.
- The relevant dimension of Roy's Adaptation Model Nursing Process is intervention.
  - *Intervention* is defined as management of stimuli using nursing approaches that have a high probability of changing stimuli or strengthening adaptive processes. Stimuli may be altered, increased, decreased, removed, or maintained.
- *Coping Processes* is defined as "innate coping processes [that] are genetically determined or common to the species and are generally viewed as automatic process; people do not have to think about them...[and] acquired coping processes [that] are developed through strategies such as learning" (Roy, 2009, p. 41).
- The relevant dimension of Coping Process is stabilizer subsystem control process.
  - *Stabilizer subsystem control process* is defined as "the established structure, values, and daily activities whereby participants accomplish the primary purpose of the group and contribute to common purposes of society" (Roy, 2009, p. 42).
- *Adaptive Modes* is defined as ways in which human adaptive systems respond to stimuli from the environment that are processed through the coping processes.
- The relevant dimension of Adaptive Modes is role function mode.

(continued)

BOX 8.4   An Example of a Conceptual–Theoretical–Empirical Structure for Roy's Adaptation Model Nursing Practice: Intervention (continued)

o *Role function mode* is defined as behaviors—or activities—that are associated with ascribed and acquired roles (Roy, 2009).

The *non-relational propositions* for the *T component* of the CTE structure are:

- *Focus on Stimuli* is defined as "focusing on the stimuli affecting the behaviors and managing the stimuli by altering, increasing, or decreasing, removing, or maintaining stimuli as proposed by the Roy Adaptation Model" (Roy & Zhan, 2010, p. 179).
- *Family Coping Strategies* is defined as "use [of] effective coping strategies to strengthen compensatory processes by acknowledging how good the family is at transcending the crisis" (Roy & Zhan, 2010, p. 179).
- *Family Resources* is defined as "working with the family to identify additional resources in support of family caregiving and by reinforcing their shared goals, values, relations, and group identity" (Roy & Zhan, 2010, p. 179).

The *non-relational propositions* for the *E component* of the CTE structure are:

- Focus on Stimuli is operationalized by the intervention section of Roy's Adaptation Model Practice Methodology.
- Family Coping Strategies is measured by the Coping Processes–stabilizer subsystem control processes section of Roy's Adaptation Model Practice Methodology.
- Family Resources is measured by the Adaptive Modes–role function mode section of Roy's Adaptation Model Practice Methodology.

The *relational propositions* for the *C* and *T components* of the CTE structure are:

- Stimuli are related to Coping Processes.
- Therefore, Focus on Stimuli is related to Family Coping Strategies.
- Coping Processes are related to Adaptive Modes.
- Therefore, Family Coping Strategies are related to Family Resources.

The *relational propositions* for the *E component* of the CTE structure are:

- Implementation of the intervention section of Roy's Adaptation Model Practice Methodology is related to data from evaluation of the Coping Processes–stabilizer subsystem control processes section of Roy's Adaptation Model Practice Methodology.
- Data from evaluation of the Coping Processes–stabilizer subsystem control process section of Roy's Adaptation Model Practice Methodology are related to data from evaluation of the Adaptive Modes–role function mode section of Roy's Adaptation Model Practice Methodology.

Source: Roy and Zhan (2010).

BOX 8.5 Guidelines for Roy's Adaptation Model Quality Improvement Projects

The purpose of quality improvement (QI) projects is to test the association between nurses' use of Roy's Adaptation Model practice methodology (Roy's Adaptation Model Nursing Process) and nurse and/or patient adaptation to environmental stimuli.

The phenomenon of interest for QI projects is the extent of nurses' use of Roy's Adaptation Model Nursing Process.

Data for QI projects are to be collected from nurses and/or patients in various settings, such as patients' homes, nurses' private practice offices, ambulatory clinics, hospitals, and communities.

Any methodological theory of change or QI may be used to guide the design of the QI project and the times for data collection. Checklists, rating scales, and responses to open-ended questions may be used to determine the extent to which nurses actually implement one or more components of Roy's Adaptation Model Nursing Process—assessment of stimuli, assessment of behavior, nursing diagnosis, goal setting, intervention, evaluation.

Descriptive statistics may be used to analyze data obtained from checklists or rating scales, and content analysis may be used to identify categories or themes found in responses to open-ended questions.

The results of Roy's Adaptation Model Nursing Process–based QI projects enhance understanding of how using Roy's Adaptation Model Nursing Process affects nurse and/or patient adaptation to environmental stimuli.

Adaptation Model Nursing Process; the relevant dimensions are assessment of behaviors and assessment of stimuli. The other conceptual model concept is Adaptive Modes; the relevant dimension of this concept is role function mode. The theory concepts are Roy Adaptation Model Assessment Tool Educational Program and Roy Adaptation Model Assessment Tool Utilization.

Roy Adaptation Model Assessment Tool Educational Program represents the assessment of behavior and assessment of stimuli dimensions of Roy's Adaptation Model Nursing Process. Roy Adaptation Model Assessment Tool Utilization represents the role function mode of Adaptive Modes.

Roy Adaptation Model Assessment Tool Educational Program is operationalized by the Roy Adaptation Model Assessment Tool Educational Program protocol. Kaur and Mahal (2012) cited Ryan's (2009) Integrated Theory of Health Behavior Change (ITHBC), which may be considered the methodological theory for their quality improvement project (see Appendix A).

Roy Adaptation Model Assessment Tool Utilization is measured by the investigator-developed Acceptability Scale and by the investigator-developed Like–Dislike Scale. Descriptive statistics (numbers, percents, means, standard deviations; see Appendix B) were used to analyze nurses' responses to the Acceptability Scale items and the Like–Dislike Scale items.

The CTE structure that was constructed from an interpretation of the content of Kaur and Mahal's (2012) journal article is illustrated in Figure 8.4. The non-relational and relational propositions for each component of the CTE structure are listed in Box 8.6.

BOX 8.6   An Example of a Conceptual–Theoretical–Empirical Structure for Roy's Adaptation Model Quality Improvement Project

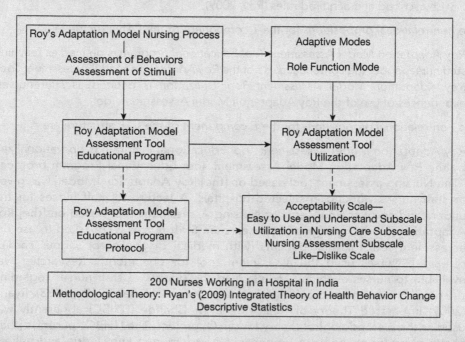

FIGURE 8.4 Conceptual–theoretical–empirical (CTE) structure for Roy's Adaptation Model quality improvement (QI) project—theory of effect of an educational program on utilization of Roy's Adaptation Model assessment tool.

The *non-relational propositions* for the *C component* of the conceptual–theoretical–empirical (CTE) structure are:

- *Roy's Adaptation Model Nursing Process* is defined as the nursing process.
- The relevant dimensions of Roy's Adaptation Model Nursing Process are assessment of behaviors and assessment of stimuli.
  o *Assessment of behaviors* is defined as systematic collection of data about the behavior of the human adaptive system and judgment about the current state of the coping proceess and of adaptation in each adaptive mode—physiological/physical mode, self-concept/group identity mode, role function mode, and interdependence mode.
  o *Assessment of stimuli* is defined as identification of the internal and external focal and contextual stimuli that are influencing the behaviors of particular interest, in the order of priority established at the end of the assessment of behavior dimension of Roy's Adaptation Model Nursing Process.

(continued)

BOX 8.6   An Example of a Conceptual–Theoretical–Empirical Structure for Roy's Adaptation Model Quality Improvement Project *(continued)*

- *Adaptive Modes* is defined as ways in which human adaptive systems respond to stimuli from the environment that are processed through the coping processes.
- The relevant dimension of Adaptive Modes is the role function mode.
  - o *Role function mode* is defined as behaviors—or activities—that are associated with ascribed and acquired roles (Roy, 2009).

The *non-relational propositions* for the *T component* of the CTE structure are:

- *Roy Adaptation Model Assessment Tool Educational Program* is defined as teaching staff nurses about the content and use of the Roy Adaptation Model Assessment Tool.
- *Roy Adaptation Model Assessment Tool Utilization* is defined as staff nurses' experiences of use of the Roy Adaptation Model Assessment Tool.

The *non-relational propositions* for the *E component* of the CTE structure are:

- Roy Adaptation Model Assessment Tool Educational Program is operationalized by the Roy Adaptation Model Assessment Tool Educational Program protocol. "The Nursing assessment tool based on [the] Roy Adaptation [Model] was given to staff nurses working in selected hospitals. A lecture to staff nurses for the understanding of the concepts of Nursing Assessment tool based on [the] Roy Adaptation [Model] was given by researcher. Staff nurses were asked to use the assessment tool for their patients [with medical diagnoses of various cardiac diseases]. Nurses used the assessment tool for one month. Researcher was available to nurses everyday and clarified the doubts of staff nurses regarding the nursing assessment tool if they had any" (Kaur & Mahal, 2012, p. 133). Ryan's (2009) Integrated Theory of Health Behavior Change (ITHBC) apparently was used as the methodological theory for the QI project. The ITHBC "purports [that] health behavior change can be enhanced by fostering knowledge and beliefs, increasing self-regulation skills and abilities, and enhancing social facilitation" (Ryan, 2009, p. 164). Kaur and Mahal (2012) fostered staff nurses' knowledge and beliefs by providing the lecture about the assessment tool. Their availability to clarify doubts about the assessment tool increased the staff nurses' self-regulation skills and abilities and social facilitation.
- Roy Adaptation Model Assessment Tool Utilization is measured by the investigator-developed Acceptability Scale (Kaur & Mahal, 2012). The Acceptability Scale is made up of 21 items, each of which is rated on a 5-point Likert scale (see Appendix B) of 1 = strongly disagree, 2 = disagree, 3 = neutral, 4 = agree, and 5 = strongly agree. The items are arranged in three subscales—easy to use and understand (9 items), usefulness in nursing care (6 items), and nursing assessment (6 items).
- Roy Adaptation Model Assessment Tool Utilization also is measured by the investigator-developed Like–Dislike Scale (Kaur & Mahal, 2012). The Like–Dislike Scale contains one item addressing overall impression of use of the Roy Adaptation Model Assessment Tool. The item is rated on a 5-point scale of "I disliked it very much," "I disliked it," "I liked it somewhat," "I liked it," and "I liked it very much."

Source: Kaur and Mahal (2012).

APPLICATION TO NURSING RESEARCH

The guidelines for Roy's Adaptation Model nursing research are listed in Box 8.7.

BOX 8.7   Guidelines for Roy's Adaptation Model Research

The purpose of Roy's Adaptation Model–based basic nursing research is to understand and explain people adapting within their life situations, including descriptions of individual and group coping processes and adaptation to environmental stimuli and explanations of the relation between adaptation and health. The purpose of Roy's Adaptation Model–based clinical nursing research is to develop and test interventions designed to enhance positive life processes and patterns.

The phenomena to be studied include basic life processes and how nursing maintains or enhances adaptive responses or changes ineffective responses to adaptive responses. The particular foci of inquiry are focal and contextual stimuli; adaptation level; regulator and cognator coping processes in individuals and stabilizer and innovator coping processes in groups; and responses in the physiological/physical, self-concept/group identity, role function, and interdependence adaptive modes.

Within the context of basic nursing research, phenomena of particular interest are the person or group as an adaptive system, including coping processes (cognator and regulator processes for individuals, stabilizer and innovator processes for groups); stability of adaptive patterns; dynamics of evolving adaptive patterns; cultural and other influences on the development and interrelatedness of the adaptive modes; and adaptation related to health, including person–environment interaction and integration of the adaptive modes. Within the context of clinical nursing research, the phenomena of particular interest are changes in the effectiveness of coping processes; changes within and among the adaptive modes; and nursing interventions that promote adaptive behavioral responses, in times of transition, during changes in the environment, and during acute and chronic illness, injury, treatment, and threats from use of health technology.

The problems to be studied are those stemming from the attempts made by the human adaptive system to meet needs for physiological integrity (individuals), resource adequacy (groups), psychic and spiritual integrity (individuals), identity integrity (groups), social integrity (individuals), role clarity (groups), and relational integrity (individuals and groups). Particular interest is in situations in which adaptive behavioral responses are threatened by health technologies and behaviorally induced health problems.

Research participants may be individuals or groups who are well or who have acute or chronic medical conditions.

Descriptive, correlational, experimental, and/or mixed-methods research designs are required to study the phenomena encompassed by Roy's Adaptation Model. Qualitative and/or quantitative methods of data collection are appropriate. Data can be gathered in any health care setting in which human adaptive systems are found. Research instruments should reflect the unique focus and intent of Roy's Adaptation Model and include the instruments that have been directly derived from Roy's Adaptation Model.

(continued)

BOX 8.7   Guidelines for Roy's Adaptation Model Research   *(continued)*

Data analysis techniques encompass qualitative content analysis and nonparametric and parametric statistical procedures, with an emphasis on statistical techniques that facilitate analysis of nonlinear and reciprocal relations.

Roy's Adaptation Model–based research enhances understanding of the human adaptive system and the role of nursing intervention in the promotion of adaptation.

Adapted from Fawcett and DeSanto-Madeya (2013).

A CTE Structure for a Systematic Literature Review

The journal article by Bowers and Wetsel (2014) is an example of a report of a systematic literature review. The purposes of their literature review were to "(1) describe the utilization of [music therapy] MT for symptom management, (2) discuss the efficacy of MT as an intervention, and (3) present the implications for [advanced practice nursing] APN education, practice, and research" (p. 232). Their special interest was people receiving palliative care or hospice care.

Bowers and Wetsel (2014) identifed several inclusion and exclusion criteria for the literature review:

> Inclusion criteria were that the articles were available in the English language, were peer reviewed, were limited to the adult population, related to those symptoms experienced by patients at end-of-life, and studied the use of music as an adjunct therapy. Exclusion criteria were that the articles were related to program development/ evaluation, pediatrics, and mechanical injury symptoms and/or were of a nonresearch nature. (p. 232)

The inclusion and exclusion criteria were applied to a search of several electronic databases, including the Cumulative Index to Nursing and Allied Health Literature (CINAHL), Academic Search Alumni Edition, Psychology and Behavioral Sciences Collection, Cochrane Database, Medline, Humanities, Health Source-Consumer Edition, and ProQuest and Allied Health. The search terms were "Music Therapy," "Symptom Management," and "Hospice." The search included publcations from 2006 to 2013, as well as "five articles published before 2006…as they were found to be frequently referenced in the literature reviewed" (Bowers & Wetsel, 2014, p. 232). A total of 17 reports of research published as journal articles were reviewed.

The theory is the effects of music therapy on anxiety, pain, depression, and quality of life. The two conceptual model concepts are Roy's Adaptation Model Nursing Process and Adaptive Modes. The relevant dimension of Roy's Adaptation Model Nursing Process is intervention. The relevant dimension of

Adaptive Modes is self-concept mode; the two subdimensions of self-concept mode are physical self and personal self. The four theory concepts are Music Therapy, Pain, Anxiety, Depression, and Quality of Life, which were extracted from the review of the 17 journal articles.

The CTE structure that was constructed from an interpretation of the content of Bowers and Wetsel's (2014) journal article is illustrated in Figure 8.5. The non-relational propositions for each component of the CTE structure, along with a relational proposition for the T component, that were extracted from the literature review are listed in Box 8.8.

BOX 8.8 An Example of a Conceptual–Theoretical–Empirical Structure for Roy's Adaptation Literature Review

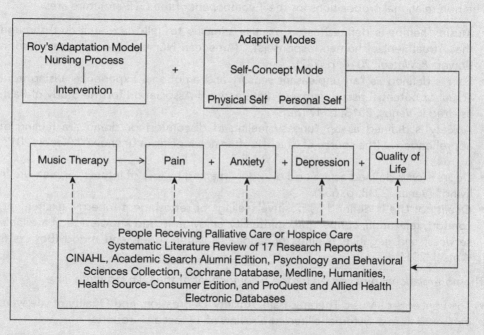

FIGURE 8.5 Conceptual–theoretical–empirical (CTE) structure for Roy's Adaptation Model literature review—theory of the effects of music therapy on anxiety, pain, depression, and quality of life.

CINAHL, Cumulative Index to Nursing and Allied Health Literature.

The *non-relational propositions* for the *C component* of the conceptual–theoretical–empirical (CTE) structure are:

- *Roy's Adaptation Model Nursing Process* is defined as the nursing process.
- The relevant dimension of Roy's Adaptation Model Nursing Process is intervention.
  o *Intervention* is defined as management of stimuli using nursing approaches that have a high probability of changing stimuli or strengthening adaptive processes. Stimuli may be altered, increased, decreased, removed, or maintained.

(continued)

BOX 8.8   An Example of a Conceptual–Theoretical–Empirical Structure for Roy's Adaptation Literature Review   *(continued)*

- *Adaptive Modes* is defined as ways in which human adaptive systems respond to stimuli from the environment that are processed through the coping processes.
- The relevant dimension of Adaptive Modes is self-concept mode.
  - o *Self-concept mode* is defined as behavior "pertaining to the personal aspect of human systems" (Roy, 2009, p. 95).
  - o The two subdimensions of self-concept mode are physical self and personal self.
    - ■ *Physical self* is defined as "appraisal of one's own physical being" (Roy, 2009, p. 323).
    - ■ *Personal self* is defined as "appraisal of one's own characteristics, expectations, values, and worth" (Roy, 2009, p. 323).

The *non-relational propositions* for the *T component* of the CTE structure are:

- *Music Therapy* is defined as "a positive stimulus to '[alleviate suffering] through the…treatment of human response[s]'" (American Nurses Assocation, as cited in Bowers & Wetsel, 2014, p. 232).
- *Pain* is defined as "an unpleasant sensory and emotional experience arising from actual or potential tissue damage" (International Association for the Study of Pain, as cited in Venes, 2013, p. 1716).
- *Anxiety* is defined as an "uneasy feeling of discomfort or dread…a feeling of apprehension…[the source of which] is often nonspecific or unknown" (Venes, 2013, p. 164).
- *Depression* is defined as a mood disorder "marked by loss of interest or pleasure in living" (Venes, 2013, p. 652).
- *Quality of Life* is defined as positive feelings of refreshment, energy, excitement, comfort, relaxation, connection, spirituality, enjoyment, and knowledge of available services, and negative feelings of fatigue, isolation, grief, and mood (Bowers & Wetsel, 2014).

The *non-relational proposition* for the *E component* of the CTE structure is:

- The concepts of Music Therapy, Pain, Anxiety, Depression, and Quality of Life were extracted from a systematic literature review of 17 research reports.

The *relational proposition* for the *T component* of the CTE structure is:

- Music Therapy has effects on Pain, Anxiety, Depression, and Quality of Life.

Source: Bowers and Wetsel (2014).

A CTE Structure for Instrument Development

Phillips's (2011) journal article is an example of a report of Roy's Adaptation Model instrument development. The purpose of his article was "to describe the development of an instrument to measure internalized stigma of HIV/AIDS that taps the dimensions of the self-concept as described in the Roy adaptation model" (p. 307).

The theory is internalized stigma beliefs. The conceptual model concept is Adaptive Modes. The relevant dimension of Adaptive Modes is self-concept, and the subdimensions of self-concept are physical self and personal self. The theory concept is Internalized Stigma Beliefs. The three dimensions of Internalized Stigma Beliefs are body image, self-ideal, and moral–ethical–spiritual self. Body image represents the self-concept subdimension of physical self. Self-ideal and moral–ethical–spiritual self represent the personal self subdimension. Internalized Stigma Beliefs and its three dimensions are measured by the Internalized Stigma of AIDS Tool (ISAT; Phillips, 2011; Phillips, Moneyham, &Tavakoli, 2011).

Phillips et al. (2011) reported that the ISAT items were generated by means of a literature review and interviews with persons living with HIV/AIDS. They explained that item analysis (see Appendix B) revealed that none of the 10 ISAT items should be deleted. They reported that the ISAT has adequate estimates of internal consistency reliability using Cronbach's alpha and construct validity using exploratory factor analysis. Inasmuch as the factor analysis revealed that the concept of Internalized Stigma Beliefs is unidimensional, the ISAT has no subscales. They also reported an adequate estimate of convergent validity, which they determined by calculating the correlation (r) between the ISAT and the Centers for Epidemiological Studies Depression Scale (Radloff, 1977; see Appendix B).

The CTE structure that was constructed from the content of Phillips's (2011) journal article is illustrated in Figure 8.6. The non-relational propositions for each component of the CTE structure are listed in Box 8.9.

A CTE Structure for Descriptive Qualitative Research

A journal article by de Queiroz Frazão, Bezerra, de Paiva, and de Carvalho Lira (2014) is an example of a report of Roy's Adaptation Model descriptive qualitative research. The purpose of their research was to "Identify the changes in the self-concept mode of Roy's [Adaptation] model in women undergoing hemodialysis" (p. 215).

The researchers used a simple descriptive research design (see Appendix A). They interviewed 178 patients who had a medical diagnosis of chronic kidney disease and were receiving hemodialysis at a clinic in Brazil. Their journal article is a report of the results of their analysis of interviews with 24 of the women patients.

The theory is feelings about self. The conceptual model concept is Adaptive Modes. The relevant dimension of the concept is self-concept mode and the subdimensions of self-concept mode are physical self and personal self. The theory concept is Feelings About Self. The two dimensions of Feeling About Self are low self-esteem and sexual dysfunction.

The theory concept and its two dimensions were discovered by means of content analysis (see Appendix B) of the women's responses to an interview. de Queiroz Frazão et al. (2014) did not provide any information about the content of the interview or the type of questions asked.

BOX 8.9 An Example of a Conceptual–Theoretical–Empirical Structure for Roy's Adaptation Model Instrument Development

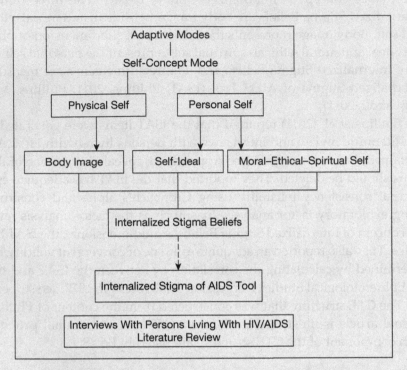

FIGURE 8.6 Conceptual–theoretical–empirical (CTE) (structure for Roy's Adaptation Model instrument development—theory of internalized stigma beliefs.

The *non-relational propositions* for the *C component* of the conceptual–theoretical–empirical (CTE) structure are:

- *Adaptive Modes* is defined as ways in which human adaptive systems respond to stimuli from the environment that are processed through the coping processes.
- The relevant dimension of Adaptive Modes is self-concept.
  - o *Self-concept* is defined as "psychological and spiritual characteristics of the person. One's self-concept consists of all the beliefs and feelings that one has formed about oneself" (Andrews & Roy, as cited in Phillips, 2011, pp. 307–308).
  - o The two subdimensions of self-concept mode are physical self and personal self.
    - *Physical self* is defined as "the person's appraisal of one's own characteristics, physical attributes, functioning, sexuality, health–illness states, and appearance" (Roy & Andrews, as cited in Phillips, 2011, p. 308).
    - *Personal self* is defined as "an individual's appraisal of one's own characteristics, expectations, values, and worth" (Roy & Andrews, as cited in Phillips, 2011, p. 308).

The *non-relational propositions* for the *T component* of the CTE structure are:

- *Internalized Stigma Beliefs* is defined as "Socially constructed views and negative stereotypes about HIV/AIDS and persons with HIV/AIDS that become incorporated into the self-concept" (Phillips et al., 2011, p. 360).

(continued)

> **BOX 8.9   An Example of a Conceptual–Theoretical–Empirical Structure for Roy's Adaptation Model Instrument Development (continued)**
>
> - The three dimensions of Internalized Stigma are body image, self-ideal, and moral–ethical–spiritual self.
>   - *Body image* is defined as "the level of satisfaction with appearance" (Roy & Andrews, as cited in Phillips, 2011, p. 308).
>   - *Self-ideal* is defined as "what one would like to be or do related to what one is capable of being of doing" (Roy & Andrews, as cited in Phillips, 2011, p. 308).
>   - *Moral–ethical–spiritual self* is defined as "that aspect of the personal self which includes a belief system and an evaluation of who one is in relation to the universe" (Roy, 2009, p. 323).
>
> The *non-relational proposition* for the E component of the CTE structure is:
>
> - Internalized Stigma Beliefs and its three dimensions are measured by the Internalized Stigma of AIDS Tool (ISAT; Phillips, 2011; Phillips et al., 2011). The ISAT is made up of 10 items that are rated on a 5-point scale of 1 = strongly disagree, 2 = disagee, 3 = neither agree nor disagree, 4 = agree, and 5 = strongly agree. Body image is measured by two items; self-ideal, by five items; and moral–ethical–spiritual self, by three items.
>
> *Source*: Phillips (2011).

The CTE structure that was constructed from the content of de Queiroz Frazão et al.'s journal article is illustrated in Figure 8.7. The non-relational propositions for each component of the CTE structure are listed in Box 8.10.

A CTE Structure for Correlational Research

Aktan's (2012) journal article is an example of a report of Roy's Adaptation Model correlational research. The purpose of her study was to examine the relations between social support and state and trait anxiety.

Aktan (2012) explained that she conducted a secondary analysis of data from a longitudinal study (see Appendix A) of 177 women during the third trimester of pregnancy and the sixth week postpartum. The study sample included

> Healthy pregnant and postpartum women with no known prenatal or postnatal complications attending childbirth preparation classes or prenatal visits or who are members of or were referred by a local community women's organization. Pregnant women in their third trimester of gestation meeting the criteria for study comprised the sample of convenience and the sample was delimited to pregnant women who can read and comprehend English. (Aktan, 2012, p. 187)

BOX 8.10 An Example of a Conceptual–Theoretical–Empirical Structure for Roy's Adaptation Model Descriptive Qualitative Research

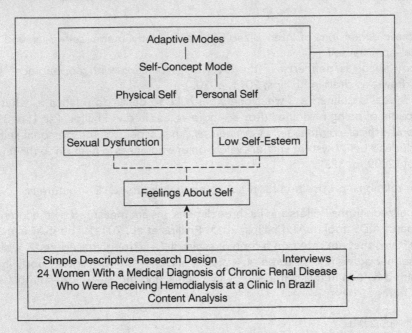

FIGURE 8.7 Conceptual–theoretical–empirical (CTE) structure for Roy's Adaptation Model descriptive qualitative research—theory of feelings about self.

The *non-relational propositions* for the *C component* of the conceptual–theoretical–empirical (CTE) structure are:

- *Adaptive Modes* is defined as ways in which human adaptive systems respond to stimuli from the environment that are processed through the coping processes (Roy, 2009).
- The relevant dimension of Adaptive Modes is self-concept mode.
  - o *Self-concept mode* is defined as behavior "pertaining to the personal aspect of human systems" (Roy, 2009, p. 95).
  - o The two subdimensions of self-concept mode are physical self and personal self.
    - ■ *Physical self* is defined as "appraisal of one's own physical being" (Roy, 2009, p. 323).
    - ■ *Personal self* is defined as "appraisal of one's own characteristics, expectations, values, and worth" (Roy, 2009, p. 323).

The *non-relational propositions* for the *T component* of the CTE structure are:

- *Feelings About Self* is defined as "thoughts of women undergoing hemodialysis" (de Queiroz Frazão et al., 2014, p. 217).
- The two dimensions of Feelings About Self are low self-esteem and sexual dysfunction.

(continued)

BOX 8.10   An Example of a Conceptual–Theoretical–Empirical Structure for Roy's Adaptation Model Descriptive Qualitative Research (continued)

- o *Low self-esteem* is defined as "the verbalization of negative feelings about the body; preoccupation with bodily changes; [and] thoughts about feelings of shame [and] feelings of sadness, fear, anxiety and insecurity" (de Queiroz Frazão et al., 2014, p. 218).
- o *Sexual dysfunction* is defined as "loss of libido" (de Queiroz Frazão et al., 2014, p. 218).

The *non-relational proposition* for the E component of the CTE structure is:

- Feelings About Self and its two dimensions—low self-esteem and sexual dysfunction—were generated from content analysis of interviews with 24 women who had a medical diagnosis of chronic kidney disease and were receiving hemodialysis at a clinic in Brazil.

Source: de Queiroz Frazão, Bezerra, de Paiva, and de Carvalho Lira (2014).

Aktan (2012) used a bivariate correlational research design (see Appendix A). Accordingly, she used the Pearson Product Moment Coefficient of Correlation (*r*; see Appendix B) to analyze the data.

The theory is the relation between social support and anxiety. The conceptual model concept is Adaptive Modes. The two relevant dimensions of Adaptive Modes are interdependence mode and self-concept mode. The theory concepts are Social Support and Anxiety. The two dimensions of Anxiety are state anxiety and trait anxiety.

The interdependence mode dimension of Adaptive Modes is represented by Social Support, and the self-concept mode dimension is represented by Anxiety and its two dimensions. Social Support is measured by the Personal Resource Questionnaire (PRQ 85-Part 2; Brandt & Weinert, 1981). Anxiety is measured by the State Trait Anxiety Inventory (STAI; Spielberger, 1983). The state anxiety dimension of Anxiety is measured by the STAI S-Anxiety Scale, and the trait anxiety dimension is measured by the STAI T-Anxiety Scale.

The CTE structure that was constructed from the content of Aktan's (2012) journal article is illustrated in Figure 8.8. The non-relational and relational propositions for each component of the CTE structure are listed in Box 8.11.

A CTE Structure for Experimental Research

Reis, Walsh, Young-McCaughan, and Jones's (2013) journal article is a report of Roy's Adaptation Model experimental research. The purpose of their

BOX 8.11 An Example of a Conceptual–Theoretical–Empirical Structure for Roy's Adaptation Model Correlational Research

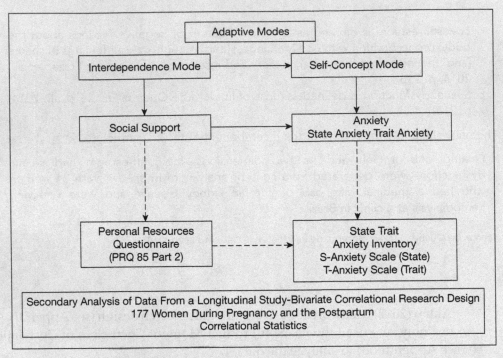

FIGURE 8.8 Conceptual–theoretical–empirical (CTE) structure for Roy's Adaptation Model correlational research—theory of relation between social support and anxiety.

The *non-relational propositions* for the C component of the conceptual–theoretical–empirical (CTE) structure are:

- *Adaptive Modes* is defined as ways in which human adaptive systems respond to stimuli from the environment that are processed through the coping processes (Roy, 2009).
- The relevant dimensions of Adaptive Modes are interdependence mode and self-concept mode.
  - o *Interdependence Mode* is defined as "interactions related to the giving and receiving of love, respect, and value" (Roy, 2009, p. 45).
  - o *Self-concept mode* is defined as behavior "pertaining to the personal aspect of human systems" (Roy, 2009, p. 95).

The *non-relational propositions* for the T component of the CTE structure are:

- *Social Support* is defined as "the six categories of relational provisions: attachment, social integration, the opportunity for nurturance, a reassurance of worth, a sense of reliable alliance, and the obtaining of guidance" (Weiss, as cited in Aktan, 2012, p. 184).

(continued)

BOX 8.11   An Example of a Conceptual–Theoretical–Empirical Structure for Roy's Adaptation Model Correlational Research (continued)

- *Anxiety* is defined as "both subjective feelings of apprehension and activation of the autonomic nervous system and...as a nonobservable subjective experience that is unpleasant, uncomfortable, and characterized by feelings of dread, apprehension, and tension" (Spielberger, as cited in Aktan, 2012, p. 184).
- The two dimensions of anxiety are state anxiety and trait anxiety.
  o *State anxiety* is defined as "a transitory emotional state or condition that is characterized by subjective, consciously perceived feelings of tension and apprehension and heightened autonomic system activity" (Gaudry & Speilberger, as cited in Aktan, 2012, p. 184).
  o *Trait anxiety* is defined as "relatively stable individual differences in anxiety proneness or differences between people in the tendency to respond to situations perceived as threatening" (Gaudry & Speilberger, as cited in Aktan, 2012, p. 184).

The *non-relational propositions* for the *E component* of the CTE structure are:

- Social Support is measured by the Personal Resource Questionnaire (PRQ 85-Part 2; Brandt & Weinert, 1981). The PRQ 85-Part 2 contains 25 items, each of which is rated on a 7-point scale of 1 = strongly disagree to 7 = strongly agree. Each of the five subscales—intimacy, social integration, nurturance, worth, and assistance—includes five items.
- The state anxiety dimension of Anxiety is measured by the State Trait Anxiety Inventory S-Anxiety Scale (STAI S-Anxiety Scale; Spielberger, 1983). The STAI S-Anxiety Scale contains 20 items that are rated on a 4-point scale of 1 = not at all, 2 = somewhat, 3 = moderately so, and 4 = very much so.
- The trait anxiety dimension of Anxiety is measured by the State Trait Anxiety Inventory T-Anxiety Scale (STAI T-Anxiety Scale; Spielberger, 1983) The STAI T-Anxiety Scale contains 20 items that are rated on a 4-point scale of 1 = almost never, 2 = sometimes, 3 = often, and 4 = almost always.

The *relational propositions* for the *C* and *T components* of the CTE structure are:

- Adaptive Modes are interrelated.
- Therefore, Social Suport is related to Anxiety.

The *relational proposition* for the *E component* of the CTE structure is:

- Scores for the PRQ are inversely related to scores for the STAI during pregnancy and the postpartum.

Source: Aktan (2012).

study was "to compare the effects of a 12-week Nia [exercise] program to usual care in women with breast cancer undergoing radiation therapy...[on] fatigue, [quality of life] QOL, aerobic capacity, and shoulder flexibility" (p. E375).

The study was conducted as a longitudinal experimental randomized controlled trial (see Appendix A). Reis et al. (2013) explained,

> Randomization was stratified by stage of disease (II, III) and age (59 years or younger, 60 years and older) in an attempt to ensure equal representation of these groups in both interventions. Participants were assessed for fatigue, QOL, aerobic capacity, and shoulder flexibility at baseline, 6 weeks, and 12 weeks. Because some women required more than six weeks of radiation therapy, the timing of the three assessments was altered slightly to correspond to the start of radiation therapy, the completion of radiation therapy, and six weeks after completion. (p. E376)

The sample included 41 women with a medical diagnosis of breast cancer who were receiving radiation therapy. The experimental Nia exercise treatment group included 22 women, and the usual care treatment group included 19 women.

The theory is effects of Nia exercise or usual care on fatigue, quality of life, aerobic capacity, and shoulder flexibility. The conceptual model concepts are Roy's Adaptation Model Nursing Process and Adaptive Modes. The relevant dimension of Roy's Adaptation Model Nursing Process is intervention. Reis et al. (2013) identified the relevant dimensions of Adaptive Modes as the physiological mode and the psychosocial modes (self-concept, role function, interdependence). One theory concept is Type of Interventions; the two dimensions of this concept are Nia exercise and usual care. The other theory concepts are Fatigue, Quality of Life, Aerobic Capacity, and Shoulder Flexibility.

The intervention dimension of Roy's Adaptation Model Nursing Process is represented by Type of Intervention. The physiological mode dimension of Adaptive Modes is represented by Aerobic Capacity and Shoulder Flexibility. The psychosocial modes dimension of Adaptive Modes is represented by Fatigue and Quality of Life. Fatigue may be regarded as a body sensation, which is an aspect of the physical self subdimension of the self-concept mode.

The Nia exercise dimension of Type of Intervention is operationalized by the Nia exercise protocol, and the usual care dimension is operationalized by the usual care protocol. Both dimensions of Type of Intervention are also operationalized by an Exercise Log maintained by the research participants. Fatigue is measured by the Functional Assessment of Chronic Illness Therapy-Fatigue, Version 4 (FACIT-F, version 4; Yellen, Cella, Webster, Blendowski, & Kaplan, 1997; www.facit.org/FACITOrg/Questionnaires). Quality of Life is measured by the Functional Assessment of Cancer Therapy-General, Version 4 (FACT-G, version 4; Yellen et al., 1997; www.facit.org/FACITOrg/Questionnaires). Aerobic Capacity is measured by the Six-Minute Walk Test (6MWT; ATS Committee on Proficiency Standards for Clinical Pulmonary Function Laboratories, 2002). A goniometer is used to measure Shoulder Flexibility. Reis et al. (2013) stated that they used "Repeated-measures analysis of variance (ANOVA) and repeated-measured analysis of covariance [ANCOVA]…to assess change over time between the groups" (pp. 377–378; see Appendix B).

The CTE structure that was constructed from an interpretation of the content of Reis et al.'s (2013) journal article is illustrated in Figure 8.9. The non-relational and relational propositions for each component of the CTE structure are listed in Box 8.12.

BOX 8.12   An Example of a Conceptual–Theoretical–Empirical Structure for Roy's Adaptation Model Experimental Research

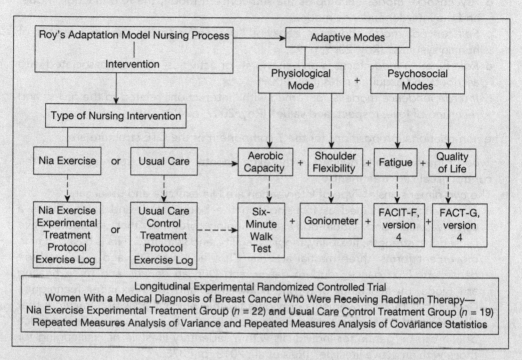

FIGURE 8.9 Conceptual–theoretical–empirical (CTE) structure for Roy's Adaptation Model experimental research—theory of effects of Nia exercise or usual care on fatigue, quality of life, aerobic capacity, and shoulder flexibility.

FACIT-F, Functional Assessment of Chronic Illness Therapy-Fatigue; FACT-G, Functional Assessment of Cancer Therapy-General.

The *non-relational propositions* for the *C* component of the conceptual–theoretical–empirical (CTE) structure are:

- *Roy's Adaptation Model Nursing Process* is defined as the nursing process.
- The relevant dimension is intervention.
  o *Intervention* is defined as management of stimuli using nursing approaches that have a high probability of changing stimuli or strengthening adaptive processes. Stimuli may be altered, increased, removed, or maintained.
- *Adaptive Modes* is defined as ways in which human adaptive systems respond to stimuli from the environment that are processed through the coping processes.
- The relevant dimensions are physiological mode and psychosocial modes (Reis et al., 2013).

(continued)

BOX 8.12   An Example of a Conceptual–Theoretical–Empirical Structure for Roy's Adaptation Model Experimental Research *(continued)*

- o *Physiological mode* is defined as "the manifestation of the physiologic activities of all the cells, tissues, organs, and systems comprising the human body" (Roy, 2009, p. 90).
- o *Psychosocial modes* encompass the self-concept mode, the role function mode, and the interdependence mode.
- o *Self-concept mode* addresses behavior "pertaining to the personal aspect of human systems" (Roy, 2009, p. 95).
- o *Role function mode* focuses on behaviors—or activities—that are associated with ascribed and acquired roles (Roy, 2009).
- o *Interdependence mode* is concerned with "interactions related to the giving and receiving of love, respect, and value" (Roy, 2009, p. 45).

The *non-relational propositions* for the *T component* of the CTE structure are:

- *Type of Intervention* is defined as the experimental Nia exercise treatment or the control usual care treatment.
- The two dimensions of Type of Intervention are Nia exercise and usual care.
  - o *Nia exercise* is defined as focusing "on the body, mind, and spirit. Nia is a cardiovascular and whole-body conditioning program that integrates five sensations: strength, flexibility, mobility, agility, and stability...Nia is based in nine movement forms: three martial arts (Tai Chi, Tae Kwon Do, and Aikido), three dance arts (jazz dance, modern dance, and Duncan dance), and three healing arts (yoga, the teachings of Moshe Feldenkrais, and the Alexander Technique). Collectively, those movements provide a flexible physical activity framework that allows individuals to direct movements according to their own needs. The practice of Nia can be gentle for individuals with a sedentary lifestyle or challenging for those with an active lifestyle" (Reis et al., 2013, p. E375).
  - o *Usual care* is defined as usual exercise engaged in by study participants (Reis et al., 2013).
- *Fatigue* is defined as "an overwhelming, debilitating, and sustained sense of exhaustion that decreases one's ability to carry out daily activities, including the ability to work effectively and to function at one's usual level in family or other social roles" (Smith, Lai, & Cella, 2010, p. 359).
- *Quality of Life* is defined as a composite of the person's perceptions of his or her physical, social or family, emotional, and functional well-being.
- *Aerobic Capacity* is defined as the functional capability of the cardiorespiratory system.
- *Shoulder Flexibility* is defined as extent of movement of the shoulder, including flexion and extension (Reis et al., 2013).

The *non-relational propositions* for the *E component* of the CTE structure are:

- The Nia exercise dimension of Type of Intervention is operationalized by the Nia exercise protocol. Reis et al. (2013) explained, "Participants received instructions and a demonstration about the Nia techniques and a Nia DVD for home use.

(continued)

BOX 8.12 An Example of a Conceptual–Theoretical–Empirical Structure for Roy's Adaptation Model Experimental Research (continued)

Participants were advised to practice Nia 20 to 60 minutes at least three times per week for 12 weeks and record their activities in an exercise log. At 6 weeks and 12 weeks, participants met individually with the principal investigator and discussed variations in movement to enhance Nia practice" (p. E376).

- The usual care dimension of Type of Intervention is operationalized by the usual care protocol. Reis et al. (2013) explained, "Control group participants also met individually with the principal investigator. Participants were instructed to maintain their current exercise regimen and record their activities in an exercise log. At 6 weeks and 12 weeks, participants met individually with the principal investigator and discussed topics such as physical, emotional, mental, and spiritual well-being. Following the 12-week assessment, participants in the control group were given the opportunity to participate in a group Nia class (offered outside of the study) and were given the Nia DVD" (p. E376).

- Fatigue is measured by the Functional Assessment of Chronic Illness Therapy-Fatigue, Version 4 (FACIT-F, version 4; Yellen et al., 1997; www.facit.org/FACITOrg/Questionnaires. The FACIT-F contains 13 items that are rated on a 5-point scale of 0 = not at all, 1 = a little bit, 2 = somewhat, 3 = quite a bit, and 4 = very much.

- Quality of Life is measured by the Functional Assessment of Cancer Therapy-General, Version 4 (FACT-G, version 4; www.facit.org/FACITOrg/Questionnaires). The FACT-G includes 27 items that address four domains of quality of life—physical well-being (seven items), social/family well-being (seven items), emotional well-being (six items), and functional well-being (seven items). Each item is rated on a 5-point scale of 0 = not at all, 1 = a little bit, 2 = somewhat, 3 = quite a bit, and 4 = very much.

- Aerobic Capacity is measured by the Six-Minute Walk Test (6MWT; ATS Committee on Proficiency Standards for Clinical Pulmonary Function Laboratories, 2002). "Participants in the current study walked on a 100-foot tiled corridor that was marked at 10-foot intervals (every 3 meters). The starting line and turnaround point were marked with brightly colored tape. The 6MWT was self-paced; study participants were permitted to stop during the 6 minutes. The total number of laps walked plus any additional distance was rounded up to the nearest foot. If a participant was unable to walk for six minutes, the test was stopped and the reason documented on the data collection form" (Reis et al., 2013, p. E377).

- Shoulder Flexibility was measured as shoulder flexion and shoulder extension by means of a goniometer. "In the current study, shoulder flexion was measured by having participants stand with the palms of their hands facing the body and placing the goniometer over the acromion process with the stationary and moving arm of the goniometer aligned at the midline of the humerus. Keeping the stationary arm in place, participants raised their arm. Shoulder extension was measured by placing the goniometer over the acromion process, with the stationary and moving arms of the goniometer aligned at the midline of the humerus. Participants turned their heads away

(continued)

BOX 8.12   An Example of a Conceptual–Theoretical–Empirical Structure for Roy's Adaptation Model Experimental Research (continued)

from the shoulder and kept their elbow slightly bent, lifting the arm as far as able. For both flexion and extension, the degree of movement was measured on the moving arm and recorded" (Reis et al., 2013, p. E377).

The *relational propositions* for the C and T components of the CTE structure are:

- Roy's Adaptation Model Nursing Process is related to Adaptive Modes.
- Therefore, Type of Intervention (Nia exercise or usual care) has effects on Fatigue, Quality of Life, Aerobic Capacity, and Shoulder Flexibility.

The *relational proposition* for the E component of the CTE structure is:

- Use of the Nia exercise protocol has more positive effects than use of the usual care protocol on scores for the FACIT-F, FACT-G, and the 6MWT, and for goniometer readings, such that the Nia exercise protocol group will have lower FACIT-F scores, higher FACT-G scores, better scores for the 6MWT, and better goniometer readings than the usual care protocol group after 12 weeks.

Source: Reis, Walsh, Young-McCaughan, and Jones (2013).

A CTE Structure for Mixed-Methods Research

Weiss, Fawcett, and Aber's (2009) journal article is an example of a report of Roy's Adaptation Model mixed-methods research (QUAL + QUAN). One purpose of their study was to examine the relations of type of cesarean birth, cultural identity, and parity to cesarean-delivered women's physical, emotional, functional, and social adaptation, and to their postpartum concerns and learning needs (henceforth referred to as P1). Another purpose of their study was to identify cesarean-delivered women's postpartum problems or needs and associated nursing interventions (henceforth referred to as P2).

The mixed-methods research design included collection of both qualitative data and quantitative data. All qualitative data were quantified. A descriptive comparative research design (see Appendix A) was used for the P1 portion of the study, and a simple descriptive research design (see Appendix A) was used for the P2 portion. The study is part of a research program that integrates faculty scholarship and undergraduate nursing student learning (Fawcett, Aber, & Weiss, 2003). Integration occurs as students gather clinical information from patients and, with the patients' consent, the faculty use the information as research data.

The sample included "233 English-speaking women at least 18 years old who gave birth by caesarean at urban hospitals in Midwestern and Northeastern regions of the United States. The sample was limited to women who had an uncomplicated hospital course and were discharged by the fourth postpartum day with their infants" (Weiss et al., 2009, p. 2941). The clinical information was gathered via home visit or telephone interview by nursing students within 1 month following each woman's delivery, with a target of during the second week postpartum.

The theory is women's adaptation to cesarean birth. The conceptual model concepts are Stimuli, Adaptive Modes, and Roy's Adaptation Model Nursing Process. The two relevant dimensions of Stimuli are focal stimulus and contextual stimuli. The four dimensions of Adaptive Modes are physiological mode, self-concept mode, role function mode, and interdependence mode. The two relevant dimensions of Roy's Adaptation Model Nursing Process are assessment of stimuli and intervention.

The theory concepts are Type of Cesarean Birth, Cultural Identity, Parity, Physical Adaptation, Emotional Adaptation, Functional Adaptation, Social Adaptation, Postpartum Concerns, Learning Needs, Problems or Needs, and Recommended Interventions. The two dimensions of Type of Cesarean Birth are planned and unplanned. The two dimensions of Cultural Identity are race and ethnicity. The two dimensions of Parity are primipara and multipara. The four dimensions of Problems or Needs are physiological mode, self-concept mode, role function mode, and interdependence mode. The four dimensions of Recommended Interventions are health teaching, treatments and procedures, case management, and surveillance.

Type of Cesarean Birth and its two dimensions represent the focal stimulus dimension of Stimuli, and Cultural Identity and Parity and their dimensions represent the contextual stimuli dimension of Stimuli. Physical Adaptation, Emotional Adaptation, Functional Adaptation, Social Adaptation represent the physiological mode, self-concept mode, role function mode, and interdependence mode dimensions of Adaptive Modes, respectively. Postpartum Concerns represents all four dimensions of Adaptive Modes. Learning Needs represents the role function dimension of Adaptive Modes. Problems and Needs and its dimensions represent the assessment dimension of Roy's Adaptation Model Nursing Process. Recommended Interventions and its dimensions represent the intervention dimension of Roy's Adaptation Model Nursing Process.

Type of Cesarean Birth, Cultural Identity, and Parity and their dimensions are measured items on the investigator-developed Background Data Sheet (BDS). Physical Adaptation, Emotional Adaptation, Functional Adaptation, and Social Adaptation are measured by the investigator-developed Post-Cesarean Adaptation Interview Schedule (PCAIS). Postpartum Concerns is measured by the Maternal Concerns Questionnaire (MCQ; Bull, 1979, 1981; Moxon, 1989). Learning Needs is measured by the investigator-developed Postpartum Self and Infant Knowledge and Behaviors Inventory (PKBI). Problems or Needs are recorded on the investigator-developed Roy's Adaptation Model (RAM) Post-Discharge Assessment Record. Recommended Interventions are categorized using the Omaha System Intervention Scheme (Martin & Scheet, 1992).

For the P1 portion of their study, Weiss et al. (2009) used content analysis for the qualitative data and quantified those data using descriptive statistics (numbers, percents, means, standard deviations), *t*-tests, and analysis of variance statistics (see Appendix B). For the P2 portion of their study, Weiss et al. (2009) used content analysis (see Appendix B) to extract Problems or Needs and Recommended Interventions from the data obtained from the RAM Post-Discharge Assessment Record and the Omaha System Intervention Scheme. They used descriptive statistics (numbers, percents; see Appendix B) to quantify the two concepts and their dimensions.

The CTE structure that was constructed from the content of Weiss et al.'s (2009) journal article is illustrated in Figure 8.10. The non-relational and relational propositions for each component of the CTE structure are listed in Box 8.13, along with the relational propositions for the P1 portion of the study.

BOX 8.13   An Example of a Conceptual–Theoretical–Empirical Structure for Roy's Adaptation Model Mixed-Methods Research

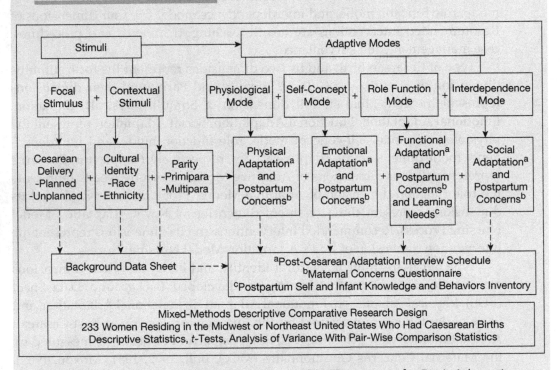

FIGURE 8.10 Conceptual–theoretical–empirical (CTE) structure for Roy's Adaptation Model mixed-methods research—theory of women's adaptation to cesarean birth—quantitative portion. *(continued)*

(continued)

BOX 8.13   An Example of a Conceptual–Theoretical–Empirical Structure for Roy's Adaptation Model Mixed-Methods Research *(continued)*

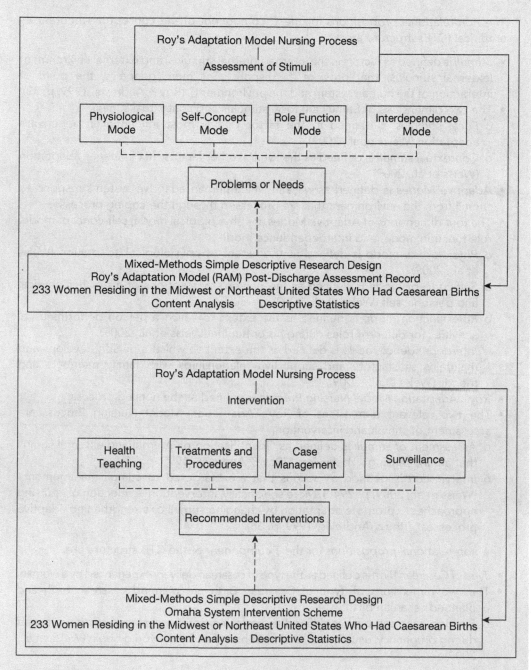

FIGURE 8.10 Qualitative portions.   *(continued)*

(continued)

BOX 8.13   An Example of a Conceptual–Theoretical–Empirical Structure for Roy's Adaptation Model Mixed-Methods Research (continued)

The *non-relational propositions* for the *C component* of the conceptual–theoretical–empirical (CTE) structure are:

- *Stimuli* is defined as factors in the internal (internal stimulus) and external environment (external stimulus) that provoke "a response, or more generally, the point of interaction of the human system and the environment" (Roy & Andrews, 1999, p. 32).
- The two dimensions of Stimuli are focal stimulus and contextual stimuli.
  o *Focal stimulus* is defined as the factor that is most influential in a person's adaptation (Weiss et al., 2009).
  o *Contextual stimuli* is defined as the total of other factors that influence adaptation (Weiss et al., 2009).
- *Adaptive Modes* is defined as ways in which human adaptive systems respond to stimuli from the environment that are processed through the coping processes.
- The four dimensions of Adaptive Modes are physiological mode, self-concept mode, role function mode, and interdependence mode.
  o *Physiological mode* is defined as the extent of physiological adaptation (Weiss et al., 2009).
  o *Self-concept mode* is defined as the person's perceptions of his or her physical and personal self (Weiss et al., 2009).
  o *Role function mode* is defined as the extent to which a person performs usual activities for different roles during his or her life (Weiss et al., 2009).
  o *Interdependence mode* is defined as the extent to which a person develops and maintains satisfactory and supportive relationships with family members and friends (Weiss et al., 2009).
- *Roy's Adaptation Model Nursing Process* is defined as the nursing process.
- The two relevant dimensions of Roy's Adaptation Model Nursing Process are assessment of stimuli and intervention.
  o *Assessment of stimuli* is defined as "identification of internal and external stimuli that are influencing...behaviors" (Roy & Andrews, 1999, p. 71).
  o *Intervention* is defined as actions that are "targeted to stimuli management" (Weiss et al., 2009, p. 2940). More specifically, intervention is selection of "nursing approaches...promote adaptation by changing stimuli or strengthening adaptive processes" (Roy & Andrews, 1999, p. 66).

The *non-relational propositions* for the *T component* of the CTE structure are:

- *Type of Cesarean Birth* is defined as the type of cesarean delivery experienced by a woman.
- The two dimensions of Type of Cesarean Birth are planned cesarean birth and unplanned cesarean birth.
  o *Planned cesarean birth* is defined as performance of a cesarean section planned during pregnancy, usually weeks or months before labor would begin (Weiss et al., 2009).

(continued)

BOX 8.13   An Example of a Conceptual–Theoretical–Empirical Structure for Roy's Adaptation Model Mixed-Methods Research (continued)

- o *Unplanned cesarean birth* is defined as performance of a cesarean section when labor was not going to result in a vaginal delivery (Weiss et al., 2009)
- *Cultural Identity* is defined as behavioral responses such as lifestyle, beliefs, and customs, acquired from and accepted by a community (Giger et al., as cited in Weiss et al., 2009).
- The two dimensions of Cultural Identity are race and ethnicity.
  - o *Race* is defined as biological characteristics such as skin color or "a social grouping based on arbitrarily selected physical characteristics" (Outlaw, 1997, p. 134).
  - o *Ethnicity* is defined as a person's awareness of belonging to a group that differs from other groups due to a shared past and continuing interests in symbolic markers such as culture, biology, or territory (Outlaw, 1997).
- *Parity* is defined as number of live children a woman has delivered.
- The two dimensions of Parity are primipara and multipara.
  - o *Primipara* is defined as a woman who has given birth to one live child.
  - o *Multipara* is defined as a woman who has given birth to two or more live children.
- *Physical Adaptation* is defined as women's reports of their physical feelings since hospital discharge following childbirth (Weiss et al., 2009).
- *Emotional Adaptation* is defined as women's reports of their emotional feelings since hospital discharge following childbirth (Weiss et al., 2009).
- *Functional Adaptation* is defined as women's reports of their adjustmet to being a new mother (primiparas) or to a new infant at home (multiparas) (Weiss et al., 2009).
- *Social Adaptation* is defined as women's reports of their husband's or partner's adjustment to the infant (Weiss et al., 2009).
- *Postpartum Concerns* is defined as the woman's questions and/or expressions of worries or problems during the early postpartum period (Weiss et al., 2009).
- *Learning Needs* is defined as the woman's need and desire for information in the early postpartum period (Weiss et al., 2009).
- *Problems or Needs* is defined as women's actual, potential, or health promotion problem or need during the early postpartum period (Weiss et al., 2009).
- *Recommended Interventions* is defined as actions needed to address women's problems and needs during the early postpartum period, categorized as health teaching, treatments and procedures, case management, or surveillance (Weiss et al., 2009).

The *non-relational propositions* for the *E component* of the CTE structure are:

- Type of Cesarean Birth is measured by an item on the investigator-developed Background Data Sheet (BDS) asking for self-report of when the woman found out that she would have a cesarean birth (Weiss et al., 2009).
- Cultural Identity is measured by two items on the investigator-developed BDS. One item is the woman's self-report of her ethnicity as Mexican, Puerto Rican, Cuban, South or Central American, or other Spanish culture or origin, regardless of race; the

(continued)

BOX 8.13   An Example of a Conceptual–Theoretical–Empirical Structure for Roy's Adaptation Model Mixed-Methods Research (continued)

other item is the woman's self-report of her race as American Indian or Alaska Native, Asian, Black, Native Hawaiian or Other Pacific Islander, White, or Other. Responses to the two items are combined and categorized as White, non-Hispanic; Black, non-Hispanic; Asian; and Hispanic (Weiss et al., 2009).

- Parity is measured by an item on the investigator-developed BDS asking for self-report of number of children; responses are categorized as primipara or multipara.
- Physical Adaptation, Emotional Adaptation, Functional Adaptation, and Social Adaptation are measured by content analysis and quantification of open-ended questions on the investigator-developed Post-Cesarean Adaptation Interview Schedule (PCAIS). Separate and combined PCAIS scores were calculated for Physical Adaptation, Emotional Adaptation, Functional Adaptation, and Social Adaptation by dividing adaptive responses by adaptive + ineffective responses and multiplying by 100, to yield an adaptive response proportion score, which can range from 0 to 100 (Weiss et al., 2009).
  o Physical Adaptation is measured by asking the woman how she has been feeling physically since hospital discharge (Weiss et al., 2009).
  o Emotional Adaptation is measured by asking the woman how she has been feeling emotionally since hospital discharge (Weiss et al., 2009).
  o Functional Adaptation is measured by asking the woman how she has been adjusting to motherhood (primipara) or how she has been adjusting to another baby (multipara) (Weiss et al., 2009).
  o Social Adaptation is measured by asking the woman how her husband/partner has been adjusting to the baby (Weiss et al., 2009).

Frequencies (n, %) were calculated for the results of the content analysis of women's responses to the questions.

- Postpartum Concerns is measured by the Maternal Concerns Questionnaire (MCQ; Bull, 1979, 1981; Moxon, 1989). The MCQ contains 50 items that are rated on a 4-point scale of 1 = "no concerns" to 4 = "much concern." Items were categorized according to the four Roy's Adaptation Model modes of adaptation, with 11 physiological mode items, 7 self-concept mode items, 17 role function mode items, and 15 interdependence mode items. Item wording was modified slightly for women who had a cesarean birth. (Weiss et al., 2009).
- Learning Needs is measured by the investigator-developed Postpartum Self and Infant Knowledge and Behaviors Inventory (PKBI). The PKBI includes 16 questions addressing the extent to which the woman acquired knowledge from a hospital discharge teaching program (Weiss et al., 2009). Responses to the questions are scored as 0 = "incorrect" or 1 = "correct."
- Problems or Needs is measured by each student nurse's identification of problems or needs in three priority areas according to the student's assessment of a woman while she was in a hospital as well as the student's post-discharge interview with the woman (Weiss et al., 2009). Each student recorded the identified problems or needs on the investigator-developed Roy's Adaptation Model (RAM) Post-Discharge

(continued)

BOX 8.13 An Example of a Conceptual–Theoretical–Empirical Structure for Roy's Adaptation Model Mixed-Methods Research (continued)

Assessment Record. Problems and Needs are categorized as actual, potential, or health promotion for each adaptive mode—physiological, self-concept, role function, and interdependence. Each category is quantified as a tally using frequency statistics (Weiss et al., 2009).

- Recommended Interventions are measured by each student nurse's identification of an action for each of the three priority problems or needs he or she had identified for a woman. The recommended interventions are categorized as health teaching, treatments and procedures, case management, or surveillance using the Omaha System Intervention Scheme (Martin & Scheet, 1992). Each category is quantified as a tally using frequency statistics (Weiss et al., 2009).

For the P1 portion of the study, the *relational propositions* for the *C and T components* of the CTE structure are:

- Stimuli are related to Adaptive Modes.
- Therefore, Type of Cesarean Birth, Cultural Identity, and Parity influence Physical Adaptation, Emotional Adaptation, Functional Adaptation, Social Adaptation, Postpartum Concerns, and Learning Needs.

For the postpartum concerns and learning needs (P1) portion of the study, the *relational proposition* for the *E component* of the CTE structure is:

- Women's self-reports for items on the BDS for Type of Cesarean Birth (categorized as planned or unplanned), Cultural Identity (categorized as White, non-Hispanic; Black, non-Hispanic; Asian; or Hispanic, and Parity (categorized as primipara or multipara) influence scores for the PCAIS, MCQ, and the PKBI.

Source: Weiss, Fawcett, and Aber (2009).

CONCLUSION

Roy's Adaptation Model is a distinctive, holistic perspective of individuals and groups as they adapt to the environment. Roy expressed her confidence that Roy's Adaptation Model "is compatible with futurists' views of the universe as progressing in structure, organization, and complexity" (Roy & Andrews, 1999, p. 34).

Roy's Adaptation Model has been applied extensively in nursing practice, research, education, and administration. The wide acceptance and application of the model is evident in the examples of its use as a guide for practice, quality improvement projects, and research given in this chapter. Especially noteworthy are the compendia of research guided by the model (Boston-Based Adaptation

Research Nursing Society, 1999) and middle-range theories derived from the model (Roy, 2014).

NOTE

1. Portions of this chapter are adapted from Fawcett, J., & DeSanto-Madeya, S. (2013). *Contemporary nursing knowledge: Analysis and evaluation of nursing models and theories* (3rd ed., Chapter 10). Philadelphia, PA: F. A. Davis, with permission.

REFERENCES

Aktan, N. M. (2012). Social support and anxiety in pregnant and postpartum women: A secondary analysis. *Clinical Nursing Research, 21,* 183–194.

ATS Committee on Proficiency Standards for Clinical Pulmonary Function Laboratories. (2002). ATS statement: Guidelines for the six-minute walk test. *American Journal of Respiratory and Critical Care Medicine, 166,* 111–117.

Boston-Based Adaptation Research in Nursing Society (1999). *Roy Adaptation Model-based research: 25 years of contributions to nursing science.* Indianapolis, IN: Sigma Theta Tau International Center Nursing Press.

Bowers, T. A., & Wetsel, M. A. (2014). Utilization of music therapy in palliative and hospice care. *Journal of Hospice and Palliative Nursing, 16,* 231–239.

Brandt, P. A., & Weinert, C. (1981). The PRQ: A social support system. *Nursing Research, 30,* 277–280.

Bull, M. (1979). *A study of the change in concerns of first time mothers after one week at home.* (Unpublished master's thesis). University of Wisconsin-Milwaukee, Milwaukee.

Bull, M. (1981). Change in concerns of first time mothers after one week home. *Journal of Obstetric, Gynecologic and Neonatal Nursing, 10,* 391–394.

de Queiroz Frazão, C. F., Bezerra, C. B., de Paiva, M. N., & de Carvalho Lira, A. B. (2014). Changes in the self-concept mode of women undergoing hemodialysis: A descriptive study. *Online Brazilian Journal of Nursing, 13,* 215–222. Available from http://www.objnursing.uff.br/index.php/nursing/article/view/4209

Fawcett, J., Aber, C., & Weiss, M. (2003). Teaching, practice and research: an integrative approach benefiting students and faculty. *Journal of Professional Nursing, 19,* 17–21.

Fawcett, J., & DeSanto-Madeya, S. (2013). *Contemporary nursing knowledge: Analysis and evaluation of nursing models and theories* (3rd ed.). Philadelphia, PA: F. A. Davis.

Kaur, H., & Mahal, R. (2012). A study on nurses' acceptability for utilization of theory based nursing assessment tool. *International Journal of Nursing Education, 4,* 132–136.

Martin, K. S., & Scheet, N. J. (1992). *The Omaha system: Applications for community health nursing.* Philadelphia, PA: Saunders.

Moxon, B. E. (1989). *A study of the intensity of concerns of postpartum mothers who live in the northwest perinatal region of Wisconsin prior to discharge.* Unpublished master's thesis, University of Wisconsin-Milwaukee, Milwaukee.

Outlaw, F. H. (1997). Culture, ethnicity and race in mental health and illness. In A. W. Burgess (Ed.), *Psychiatric nursing: Promoting mental health* (pp. 131–140). Stamford, CT: Appleton and Lange.

Phillips, K. D. (2011). Conceptual development of an instrument to measure the internalized stigma of AIDS based on the Roy Adaptation Model. *Nursing Science Quarterly, 24,* 306–310.

Phillips, K. D., Moneyham, L., & Tavakoli, A. (2011). Development of an instrument to measure internalized stigma of HIV/AIDS. *Issues in Mental Health Nursing, 32,* 359–366.

Radloff, L. S. (1977). The CES-D Scale: A self-report depression scale for research in the general population. *Applied Psychological Measurement, 1*, 385–401.

Reis, D., Walsh, M. E., Young-McCaughan, S., & Jones, T. (2013). Effects of Nia exercise in women receiving radiation therapy for breast cancer. *Oncology Nursing Forum, 40*, E374–E381.

Roy, C. (2009). *The Roy Adaptation Model* (3rd ed.). Upper Saddle River, NJ: Pearson.

Roy, C. (2014). *Generating middle range theory: From evidence to practice.* New York, NY: Springer Publishing.

Roy, C., & Andrews, H. A. (1999). *The Roy Adaptation Model* (2nd ed.). Stamford, CT: Appleton & Lange.

Roy, C., & Zhan, L. (2010). Sister Callista Roy's Adaptation Model. In M. E. Parker & M. C. Smith (Eds.), *Nursing theories and nursing practice* (3rd ed., pp. 167–181). Philadelphia, PA: F. A. Davis.

Ryan, P. (2009). Integrated theory of health behavior change: Background and intervention development. *Clinical Nurse Specialist: The Journal of Advanced Nursing Practice, 23*, 161–170.

Smith, E., Lai, J-S., & Cella, D. (2010). Building a measure of fatigue: The functional assessment of Chronic Illness Therapy Fatigue Scale. *PM&R: The Journal of Injury, Function and Rehabilitation, 2*, 359–363.

Spielberger, C. D. (1983). *Manual for the state-trait anxiety inventory: STAI (Form Y).* Palo Alto, CA: Consulting Psychologists.

Venes, D. (Ed.). (2013). *Taber's cyclopedic medical dictionary* (22nd ed.). Philadelphia, PA: F. A. Davis.

Weiss, M. A., Fawcett, J., & Aber, C. (2009). Adaptation, postpartum concerns, and learning needs in the first two weeks after cesarean birth. *Journal of Clinical Nursing, 18*, 2938–2948.

Yellen, S. B., Celia, D. F., Webster, K., Blendowski, C, & Kaplan, E. (1997). Measuring fatigue and other anemia-related symptoms with the Functional Assessment of Cancer Therapy (FACT) measurement system. *Journal of Pain and Symptom Management, 13*, 63–74.

CHAPTER 9

THE SYNERGY MODEL

The Synergy Model focuses on the extent to which nurses' competencies match the patients' characteristics. The goal of Synergy Model nursing is to "restore a patient to an optimal level of wellness as defined by the patient. Death can be an acceptable outcome, in which the goal of nursing care is to move a patient toward a peaceful death" (American Association of Critical Care Nurses [AACN], 2014, p. 9).

SYNERGY MODEL: CONCEPTS AND NON-RELATIONAL PROPOSITIONS

This section of the chapter includes the concepts of the Synergy Model and the definitions (non-relational propositions) of the concepts and the dimensions of the multidimensional concepts (AACN, 2014; Curley, 2007a; Hardin & Kaplow, 2005).

Synergy is defined as the result of the match of the needs and characteristics of a patient with a nurse's competencies (AACN, 2014).

Patient Characteristics is defined as the unique health-related characteristics and needs of each person who is a patient and his or her family members. The eight dimensions of Patient Characteristics are resiliency, vulnerability, stability, complexity, resource availability, participation in care, participation in decision making, and predictability.

Resiliency is defined as "The capacity to return to a restorative level of functioning using compensatory/coping mechanisms; the ability to bounce back quickly after an insult" (AACN, 2014, p. 1).

Vulnerability is defined as "Susceptibility to actual or potential stressors that may adversely affect patient outcomes" (AACN, 2014, p. 1).

Stability is defined as "The ability to maintain steady-state equilibrium" (AACN, 2014, p. 2).

Complexity is defined as "The intricate entanglement of two or more systems" (AACN, 2014, p. 2).

Resource availability is defined as the "Extent of resources... the patient/family/community bring to the situation" (AACN, 2014, p. 2).

Participation in care is defined as the "Extent to which patient/family engages in aspects of care" (AACN, 2014, p. 3).

Participation in decision making is defined as the "Extent to which patient/family engages in decision making" (AACN, 2014, p. 3).

Predictability is defined as "A characteristic that allows one to expect a certain course of events or course of illness" (AACN, 2014, p. 3).

Nurse Competencies is defined as the nurse's integration of his or her "knowledge, skills, experience, and attitudes needed to meet the needs of patients and families" (AACN, 2014, p. 4) and to optimize patient and family member outcomes (Curley, 2007a). Nurse Competencies "are essential for... providing care" (Hardin & Kaplow, 2005, p. 5). The eight dimensions of Nurse Competencies for nursing practice are clinical judgment, advocacy and moral agency, caring practices, collaboration, systems thinking, response to diversity, facilitation of learning, and clinical inquiry.

Clinical judgment is defined as "Clinical reasoning, which includes clinical decision-making, critical thinking, and a global grasp of the situation, coupled with nursing skills acquired through a process of integrating formal and informal experiential knowledge and evidence based guidelines" (AACN, 2014, p. 4).

Advocacy and moral agency is defined as "Working on another's behalf and representing the concerns of the patient/family and nursing staff; serving as a moral agent in identifying and helping to resolve ethical and clinical concerns within and outside the clinical setting" (AACN, 2014, p. 4).

Caring practices is defined as "Nursing activities that create a compassionate, supportive, and therapeutic environment for patients and staff, with the aim of promoting comfort and healing and preventing unnecessary suffering. Includes, but is not limited to, vigilance, engagement, and responsiveness of caregivers, including family and healthcare personnel" (AACN, 2014, p. 5).

Collaboration is defined as "Working with others... in a way that promotes/encourages each person's contributions toward achieving optimal/realistic patient/family goals" (AACN, 2014, p. 6).

Systems thinking is defined as the "Body of knowledge and tools that allow the nurse to manage whatever environmental and system resources exist for the patient/family and staff, within or across healthcare and nonhealthcare systems" (AACN, 2014, p. 6).

Response to diversity is defined as "The sensitivity to recognize, appreciate and incorporate differences into the provision of care" (AACN, 2014, p. 7).

Facilitation of learning is defined as "The ability to [formally and informally] facilitate learning for patients/families, nursing staff, other members of the healthcare team, and community" (AACN, 2014, p. 7).

Clinical inquiry is defined as "The ongoing process of questioning and evaluating practice and providing informed practice. Creating practice changes through research utilization and experiential learning" (AACN, 2014, p. 8).

Patient and Family Outcomes is defined as results derived from patients and their family members and from the synergy of the characteristics of a patient and his or her family members with the competencies of a nurse. The seven dimensions of Patient and Family Outcomes[1] are symptom and disease management, resolution of ethical problems, achievement of appropriate self-care, demonstration of health-promoting behavior, health-related quality of life, rescue phenomena, and patient/family perception of being well cared for (Curley, 2007a).

Symptom and disease management is defined as results such as improvements in symptoms and disease processes.

Resolution of ethical problems is defined as results such as improved decision making about ethical issues.

Achievement of appropriate self-care is defined as a result such as learning to competently care for self.

Demonstration of health-promoting behavior is defined as a result such as achievement of goals that are mutually acceptable to the patient and the nurse.

Health-related quality of life is defined as a result such as improvements in all aspects of function.

Rescue phenomena is defined as results such as occurrence of fewer adverse events, decreased effects of expected complications, early identification of unexpected complications, and reduction of risk of mortality.

Patient/family perception of being well cared for is defined as results such as improved patient and family trust in nurses, patient and family identification of these nurses, and enhanced patient and family satisfaction with nursing care (Curley, 2007a).

Unit Outcomes is defined as results occurring at the level of the nursing unit (Curley, 2007a). The two dimensions of Unit Outcomes[2] are shared accountability and authority for unit operations and performance, and more experienced nurses catalyzing the advancement of less experienced nurses (Curley, 2007a).

Shared accountability and authority for unit operations and performance is defined as results such as an increased number of occurrences of level decisions, as well as an increased number of nurses who participate actively in shared governance (Curley, 2007a).

More experienced nurses catalyzing the advancement of less experienced nurses is defined as activities such as additional mentoring and coaching, championing interest in graduate education and certification, and developing creative educational programs that support nursing practice (Curley, 2007a).

System Outcomes is defined as results "derived from the health care system" (Hadin & Kaplow, 2005, p. 9). The five dimensions of System Outcomes[3] are nurse satisfaction, staffing costs, resource utilization and patient charges, multidisciplinary teamwork and satisfaction, and cross-system innovation (Curley, 2007a).

Nurse satisfaction is defined as results such as nurses' increased autonomy, and their perception of high-quality care, sufficient support, enough time to complete work, and positive relationships with health care team members (Curley, 2007a).

Staffing costs is defined as results such as increased retention and desire to continue in the health care system, which decreases turnover, unfilled positions, absenteeism, and per diem staff needs (Curley, 2007a).

Resource utilization and patient charges is defined as a result such as fewer supplies wasted (Curley, 2007a).

Multidisciplinary teamwork and satisfaction is defined as a result such as increased collaboration (Curley, 2007a).

Cross-system innovation is defined as a result such as enhanced learning within the health care system (Curley, 2007a).

SYNERGY MODEL: RELATIONAL PROPOSITIONS

The statements of associations between concepts of the Synergy Model were extracted from AACN (2014), Curley (1998, 2007a), and Fontaine and Prevost (2005). These relational propositions are listed here.

- The dimensions of Patient Characteristics are interrelated.
- The dimensions of Nurse Competencies are interrelated.
- Patient Characteristics and Nurse Competencies are related.
- Patient and Family Outcomes are interrelated.
- Unit Outcomes are interrelated.
- System Outcomes are interrelated.
- Patient and Family Outcomes, Unit Outcomes, and System Outcomes are interrelated.
- Patient Characteristics are related to Synergy.
- Nurse Competencies are related to Synergy.
- Patient Characteristics have a positive effect on Patient and Family Outcomes, Unit Outcomes, and System Outcomes.

- Nurse Competencies have a positive effect on Patient and Family Outcomes, Unit Outcomes, and System Outcomes.
- Synergy (the match between Patient Characteristics and Nurse Competencies) results in optimal Patient and Family Outcomes, Unit Outcomes, and System Outcomes.

SYNERGY MODEL: APPLICATION TO NURSING PRACTICE

The guidelines for Synergy Model nursing practice are listed in Box 9.1. These guidelines were extracted from publications about the application of the Synergy Model to nursing practice, especially book chapters by Curley (2007b) and Reed, Cline, and Kerfoot (2007). A diagram of the practice methodology for the Synergy Model is illustrated in Figure 9.1. The diagram is based on content primarily from Curley's journal article (1998) and book chapter (2007a). The components of the Synergy Model practice methodology are assessment of patient characteristics; assessment of nurse competencies; determination of synergy, that is, the match between patient characteristics

---

BOX 9.1 Guidelines for Synergy Model Practice

The purpose of Synergy Model nursing practice is to foster a match between patient characteristics and nurse competencies (Curley, 2007b).

Practice problems encompass eight patient characteristics (resiliency, vulnerability, stability, complexity, resource availability, participation in care, participation in decision making, and predictability) and eight nurse competencies (clinical judgment, advocacy and moral agency, caring practices, collaboration, systems thinking, response to diversity, facilitation of learning, and clinical inquiry).

The Synergy Model can be used in all practice settings, ranging from hospital critical care units to ambulatory settings, such as outpatient clinics and the community.

Legitimate participants in Synergy Model nursing practice are all persons who are in actual or potential crisis and who seek nursing services.

The components of the Synergy Model Nursing Process are assessment of patient characteristics, assessment of nurse competencies, determination of synergy, intervention by use of the nurse competencies, and evaluation of patient-level, unit-level, and system-level outcomes.

Synergy Model–based nursing practice contributes to "organization of . . . data about patients so that their needs are consistently identified and continuity of care is maintained" (Reed et al., 2007, p. 7). Furthermore, Synergy Model–based nursing practice contributes to identification of the "important role that professional nursing plays in the healthcare system and, when facilitated by the organization, defines the impact professional nursing can have not only on patient outcomes but also on organization transformation and success" (Reed et al., 2007, p. 10).

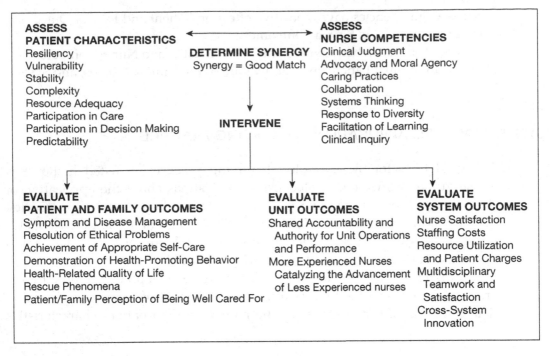

ASSESS
PATIENT CHARACTERISTICS ←————————→ **ASSESS**
NURSE COMPETENCIES

DETERMINE SYNERGY
Synergy = Good Match

Resiliency
Vulnerability
Stability
Complexity
Resource Adequacy
Participation in Care
Participation in Decision Making
Predictability

Clinical Judgment
Advocacy and Moral Agency
Caring Practices
Collaboration
Systems Thinking
Response to Diversity
Facilitation of Learning
Clinical Inquiry

INTERVENE

EVALUATE
PATIENT AND FAMILY OUTCOMES
Symptom and Disease Management
Resolution of Ethical Problems
Achievement of Appropriate Self-Care
Demonstration of Health-Promoting Behavior
Health-Related Quality of Life
Rescue Phenomena
Patient/Family Perception of Being Well Cared For

EVALUATE
UNIT OUTCOMES
Shared Accountability and
Authority for Unit Operations
and Performance
More Experienced Nurses
Catalyzing the Advancement
of Less Experienced nurses

EVALUATE
SYSTEM OUTCOMES
Nurse Satisfaction
Staffing Costs
Resource Utilization
and Patient Charges
Multidisciplinary
Teamwork and
Satisfaction
Cross-System
Innovation

FIGURE 9.1 The Synergy Model practice methodology.

and nurse competencies; intervention using one or more of the nurse competencies; and evaluation of patient and family outcomes, unit outcomes, and system outcomes.

An example of a practice tool that includes all aspects of the Synergy Model practice methodology is given in Box 9.2. The content of the tool was extracted primarily from publications by AACN (2014), Curley (2007a), and Reed et al. (2007).

A Conceptual–Theoretical–Empirical Structure for Assessment

One section of Arashin's (2010) journal article serves as an example of Synergy Model–guided assessment. The purpose of the article was to describe Synergy Model–based nursing care of a 60-year-old man with a medical diagnosis of cardiac disease who had been:

> Admitted in stable condition to the acute care unit with telemetry monitoring for a right lower lobe infiltrate and fever. . . . Approximately 1 hour into the night shift [the day after admission], the nurse finds him pale, diaphoretic, and more dyspneic than he was on admission. He appears anxious and states that his "chest feels funny" and that "he cannot catch his breath." . . . The nurse . . . calls the operator to page the Rapid Response Team (RRT) to the patient's bedside. Within 5 minutes, the response team's critical care nurse has arrived and began to assess [the patient's] condition. (p. 120)

BOX 9.2   The Synergy Model Practice Methodology Tool

ASSESS PATIENT CHARACTERISTICS

The nurse determines the patient's needs by assessing and rating each of the eight patient characteristics using subjective data from the patient and/or his or her family members and objective data from holistic examination of the patient and laboratory and other test results.

Resiliency is rated as 1 = minimally resilient, 3 = moderately resilient, or 5 = highly resilient.

Vulnerability is rated as 1 = highly vulnerable, 3 = moderately vulnerable, or 5 = minimally vulnerable.

Stability is rated as 1 = minimally stable, 3 = moderately stable, or 5 = highly stable.

Complexity is rated as 1 = highly complex, 3 = moderately complex, or 5 = minimally complex.

Resource availability is rated as 1 = few resources, 3 = moderate resources, or 5 = many resources.

Participation in care is rated as 1 = no participation, 3 = moderate level of participation, or 5 = full participation.

Participation in decision making is rated as 1 = no participation, 3 = moderate level of participation, or 5 = full participation.

Predictability is rated as 1 = not predictable, 3 = moderately predictable, or 5 = highly predictable.

   The nurse uses an acuity system based on the ratings of patient characteristics to classify the patient in a holistic manner (Curley, 2007b; Reed et al., 2007).

ASSESS NURSE COMPETENCIES

The nurse determines his or her level of expertise for eight competencies, or the charge nurse determines the level of expertise of each nurse working in the practice setting.

   The eight nurse competencies are *clinical judgment, advocacy and moral agency, caring practices, collaboration, systems thinking, response to diversity, facilitation of learning,* and *clinical inquiry.*

   Each of the eight nurse competencies is rated as 1 = competent, 3 = proficient, or 5 = expert (Reed et al., 2007).

DETERMINE SYNERGY

The nurse identifies the extent of the match between the patient characteristics and the nurse competencies. Based on the match, the charge nurse assigns the nurse or nurses with the most relevant expertise to meet the patient's needs.

INTERVENE

The nurse implements evidence-based nursing interventions within the context of the eight nurse competencies.

(continued)

BOX 9.2   The Synergy Model Practice Methodology Tool   *(continued)*

EVALUATE OUTCOMES

The nurse evaluates patient and family, unit, and system outcomes (Curley, 2007a).

Patient and family outcomes are symptom and disease management, resolution of ethical problems, achievement of appropriate self-care, demonstration of health-promoting behavior, health-related quality of life, rescue phenomena, and patient/family perception of being well cared for.

Unit outcomes are shared accountability and authority for unit operations and performance, and more experienced nurses catalyzing the advancement of less experienced nurses.

System outcomes are nurse satisfaction, staffing costs, resource utilization and patient charges, multidisciplinary teamwork and satisfaction, and cross-system innovation.

The theory used to guide practice is rapid response team assessment. The conceptual model concept is Patient Characteristics. The four relevant dimensions are vulnerability, stability, complexity, and predictability. The theory concept is rapid response team assessment.

Rapid response team assessment represents the four dimensions of Patient Characteristics. The assessment is operationalized by nurse interactions with the patient, physical assessment, and review of laboratory test results and the cardiac rhythm strip.

The conceptual–theoretical–empirical (CTE) structure that was constructed from the assessment content of Arashin's (2010) journal article is illustrated in Figure 9.2. The non-relational propositions for each component of the CTE structure are listed in Box 9.3.

A CTE Structure for Intervention

Another section of Arashin's (2010) journal article serves as an example of Synergy Model–guided intervention. Arashin explained that the assessment of the vulnerability, stability, complexity, and predictability dimensions of Patient Characteristics provided the information needed to quickly intervene to prevent further deterioration of the 60-year-old man's condition (see Assessment section of this chapter).

The theory is an effect of rapid response team nursing interventions on transfer to the intensive care unit (ICU). The conceptual model concepts are Nurse

BOX 9.3   An Example of a Conceptual–Theoretical–Empirical Structure for Synergy Model Nursing Practice: Assessment

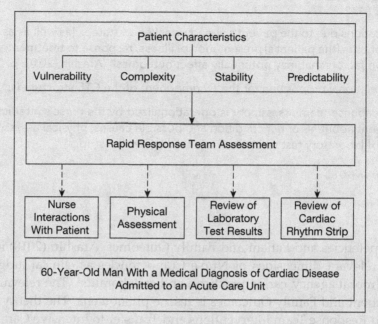

FIGURE 9.2 Conceptual–theoretical–empirical (CTE) structure for Synergy Model practice: Assessment—theory of rapid response team assessment.

The *non-relational propositions* for the *C component* of the conceptual–theoretical–empirical (CTE) structure are:

- *Patient Characteristics* is defined as "common characteristics demonstrated by patients when faced with an insult to their health.... These characteristics help nurses to anticipate the patient's path and provide the most optimal care based on the patient's unique needs" (Arashin, 2010, p. 121).
- The four relevant dimensions of Patient Characteristics are vulnerability, stability, complexity, and predictability.
  - *Vulnerability* is defined as "susceptibility to actual or potential stressors that may adversely affect patient outcomes" (Arashin, 2010, p. 121).
  - *Stability* is defined as "the patient's ability to maintain a steady state equilibrium" (Arashin, 2010, p. 122).
  - *Complexity* is defined as "the intricate entanglement of 2 or more systems" (Arashin, 2010, p. 122)
  - *Predictability* is defined as "a summative characteristic that allows one to expect a certain trajectory" (Arashin, 2010, p. 122).

The *non-relational propositions* for the *T component* of the CTE structure are:

- *Rapid response team assessment* is defined as assessment of "the patient's circumstances and [anticipation of] the potential for negative outcomes or

(continued)

> **BOX 9.3 An Example of a Conceptual–Theoretical–Empirical Structure for Synergy Model Nursing Practice: Assessment (continued)**
>
> complications due to the patient's already weakened state...[as well as assessment] of subleties in [the patient's] presentation of illness, response to treatment, and other unknown factors that may potentially affect outcomes" (Arashin, 2010, p. 122).
>
> The *non-relational proposition* for the *E component* of the CTE structure is:
>
> • Rapid response team assessment is operationalized by the nurse's interactions with the patient about his or her condition and possible causes, physical assessment, and review of laboratory test results and the cardiac rhythm strip.
>
> *Source*: Arashin (2010).

Competencies and Patient and Family Outcomes. Arashin (2010) identified the four relevant dimensions of Nurse Competencies as clinical judgment, advocate/moral agency, caring practices, and collaboration. The relevant dimension of Patient and Family Outcomes is rescue phenomena. The theory concepts are Rapid Response Team Interventions and Transfer to Intensive Care Unit.

The four dimensions of Nurse Competencies are represented by Rapid Response Team Interventions. The rescue phenomena dimension of Patient and Family Outcomes is represented by Transfer to Intensive Care Unit. Rapid Response Team Interventions is operationalized by the Rapid Response Team Interventions protocol. Transfer to Intensive Care Unit is operationalized by the Transfer to Intensive Care Unit protocol.

The CTE structure that was constructed from an interpretation of the intervention content of Arashin's (2010) journal article is illustrated in Figure 9.3. The non-relational and relational propositions for each component of the CTE structure are listed in Box 9.4.

SYNERGY MODEL: APPLICATION TO QUALITY IMPROVEMENT PROJECTS

The guidelines for Synergy Model quality improvement (QI) projects are listed in Box 9.5. These guidelines were extracted from the content and intent of the Synergy Model as described primarily by Curley (1998, 2007a, 2007b), Hardin and Kaplow (2005), and Kaplow and Hardin (2007).

A CTE Structure for a QI Project

Sanderson's (2014) report of an evidence-based staffing project is an example of a Synergy Model–guided QI project. Although Sanderson's (2014) report

BOX 9.4 An Example of a Conceptual–Theoretical–Empirical Structure for Synergy Model Nursing Practice: Intervention

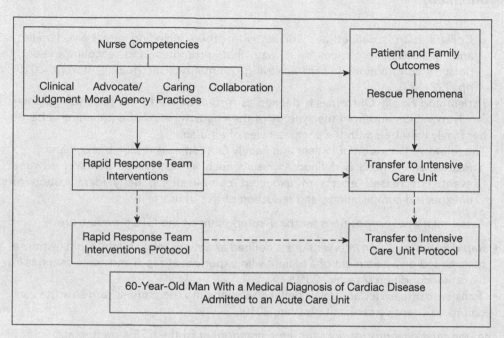

FIGURE 9.3 Conceptual–theoretical–empirical (CTE) structure for Synergy Model practice: Intervention—theory of effects of Rapid Response Team Interventions on transfer to intensive care unit.

The *non-relational propositions* for the *C component* of the conceptual–theoretical–empirical (CTE) structure are:

- *Nurse Competencies* is defined as the nurse's integration of "knowledge, skill, and experience into actions that guide nursing practice for promoting the best patient outcomes" (Arashin, 2010, p. 121).
- The four relevant dimensions of Nurse Competencies are clinical judgment, advocate/ moral agency, caring practices, and collaboration (Arashin, 2010).
  - o *Clinical judgment* is defined as "the use of clinical reasoning including decision-making, critical thinking, and a global grasp of a situation, coupled with nursing skills acquired through a process of integrating education, experiential knowledge and evidence-based guidelines" (Arashin, 2010, p. 122).
  - o *Advocate/moral agency* is defined as "working on another's behalf and representing the concerns of the patient...[and ensuring] that the patient's wishes, rights, and dignity are preserved during a crisis" (Arashin, 2010, p. 122).
  - o *Caring practices* is defined as "the constellation of nursing activities that are responsive to the uniqueness of the patient's needs" (Arashin, 2010, p. 122).

(continued)

BOX 9.4   An Example of a Conceptual–Theoretical–Empirical Structure for Synergy Model Nursing Practice: Intervention (*continued*)

- o *Collaboration* is defined as "working with others including physicians, families, and healthcare providers in a way that promotes and encourages each person's contributions toward achieving optimal realistic goals" (Arashin, 2010, pp. 122–123).
- *Patient and Family Outcomes* is defined as results derived from patients and their family members and from the synergy of the characteristics of a patient and his or her family members with the competencies of a nurse.
- The relevant dimension of Patient and Family Outcomes is rescue phenomena.
- o *Rescue phenomena* is defined as results such as occurrence of fewer adverse events, decreased effects of expected complications, early identification of unexpected complications, and reduction of risk of mortality.

The *non-relational propositions* for the *T component* of the CTE structure are:

- *Rapid Response Team Interventions* is defined as actions taken by the rapid response team based on assessment of a patient who experiences rapid and acute changes in his or her condition (Arashin, 2010).
- *Transfer to Intensive Care Unit* is defined as relocating the patient from an acute care unit to an intensive care unit (Arashin, 2010).

The *non-relational propositions* for the *E component* of the CTE structure are:

- Rapid Response Team Interventions is operationalized by the Rapid Response Team Interventions protocol, which specifies that immediate actions are directed toward providing "potentially lifesaving care and treatment by ensuring that the patient's needs are met" (Arashin, 2010, p. 123).
- Transfer to Intensive Care Unit is operationalized by the Transfer to Intensive Care Unit protocol, which specifies that the rapid response team "prepares [the patient] for further testing including a chest computed tomography angiogram to confirm the suspected diagnosis of pulmonary embolism and transfer to the intensive care unit" (Arashin, 2010, p. 124).

The *relational propositions* for the *C* and *T components* of the CTE structure are:

- Nurse Competencies have a positive effect on Patient and Family Outcomes.
- Therefore, Rapid Response Team Interventions have a positive effect on Transfer to Intensive Care Unit.

The *relational proposition* for the *E component* of the CTE structure is:

- Implementation of the Rapid Response Team Interventions protocol results in implementation of the Transfer to Intensive Care Unit protocol.

Source: Arashin (2010).

BOX 9.5 Guidelines for Synergy Model Quality Improvement Projects

The purpose of Synergy Model quality improvement (QI) projects is to determine the extent to which nurses assess patient characteristics and nurse competencies, determine synergy, and evaluate patient and family-, unit-, and system-level outcomes.

Phenomena of interest for Synergy Model QI projects include assessment of patient characteristics and of nurse competencies, determination of synergy, and evaluation of patient and family-, unit-, and system-level outcomes.

Data for QI projects are to be collected from nurses caring for patients in various acute care and ambulatory settings.

Any methodological theory of change or QI may be used to guide the design of the QI project and the times for data collection. Checklists, rating scales, and responses to open-ended questions may be used to determine the extent to which nurses actually implement one or more components of the Synergy Model practice methodology—assessment of patient characteristics, assessment of nurse competencies, determination of synergy, intervention using one or more of the nurse competencies, and evaluation of patient and family-level, unit-level, and system-level outcomes.

Descriptive statistics may be used to analyze data obtained from checklists or rating scales, and content analysis may be used to identify categories or themes found in responses to open-ended questions.

The results of Synergy Model–based QI projects enhance understanding of how using the Synergy Model practice methodology affects patient and family-level, unit-level, and system-level outcomes.

---

is available only as an abstract, sufficient detail is given for construction of a CTE structure. The purpose of the QI project was to develop and implement an evidence-based approach that would decrease or eliminate poor outcomes experienced by patients hospitalized on a medical ICU.

The theory is the effects of a workload assignment tool educational program on adverse events. The conceptual model concepts are Synergy and Patient and Family Outcomes. The relevant dimension of Patient and Family Outcomes is rescue phenomena. The theory concepts are Workload Assignment Tool Education Program and Adverse Events. The five dimensions of Adverse Events are catheter-associated urinary tract infection, central catheter–associated bloodstream infection, ventilator-associated pneumonia, pressure ulcers, and falls.

Synergy is represented by Workload Assignment Tool Education Program, and the rescue phenomenon of Patient and Family Outcomes is represented by Adverse Events and its five dimensions. Workload Assignment Tool Education Program is operationalized by the Workload Assignment Tool Education Program protocol. Sanderson (2014) did not identify the methodological theory that guided the QI project. However, the content of the Methods section of her report is consistent with the Plan-Do-Study-Act methodological theory for

QI (Gillam & Siriwardena, 2013; see Appendix A). The five dimensions of Adverse Events are measured by medical ICU record reviews before and after implementation of the protocol. Descriptive statistics (numbers; see Appendix B) are used to determine changes in rates of the dimensions of Adverse Events before and after implementaion of the protocol.

The CTE structure that was constructed from an interpretation of the content of Sanderson's (2014) report is illustrated in Figure 9.4. The non-relational and relational propositions for each component of the CTE structure are listed in Box 9.6.

BOX 9.6   An Example of a Conceptual–Theoretical–Empirical Structure for a Synergy Model Quality Improvement Project

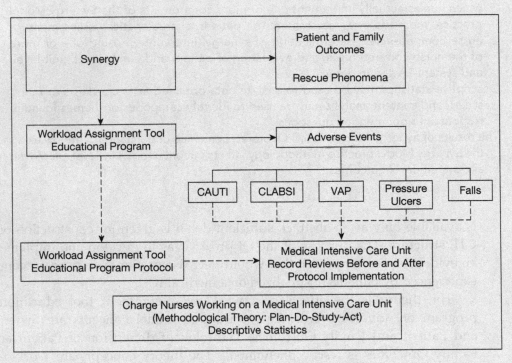

FIGURE 9.4 Conceptual–theoretical–empirical (CTE) structure for a Synergy Model quality improvement project—theory of effects of a workload assignment tool educational program on adverse events.

CAUTI, catheter-associated urinary tract infections; CLABSI, central catheter–associated bloodstream infections; VAP, ventilator-associated pneumonia.

The *non-relational propositions* for the *C component* of the conceptual–theoretical–empirical (CTE) structure are:

- *Synergy* is defined as "an evolving phenomenon that occurs when individuals work together in mutually enhancing ways toward a common goal" (Curley, 1998, p. 64),

---

(continued)

BOX 9.6 An Example of a Conceptual–Theoretical–Empirical Structure for a Synergy Model Quality Improvement Project (continued)

the result of the match of the needs and characteristics of a patient with a nurse's competencies (American Association of Critical Care Nurses [AACN], 2014).

- *Patient and Family Outcomes* is defined as results derived from patients and their family members and from the synergy of the characteristics of a patient and his or her family members with the competencies of a nurse.
- The relevant dimension of Patient and Family Outcomes is rescue phenomena.
  o *Rescue phenomena* is defined as results such as occurrence of fewer adverse events, decreased effects of expected complications, early identification of unexpected complications, and reduction of risk of mortality.

The *non-relational propositions* for the *T component* of the CTE structure are:

- *Workload Assignment Tool Education Program* is defined as teaching charge nurses to use a new workload assignment tool based on a Synergy Model–guided staffing model (Sanderson, 2014).
- *Adverse Events* is defined as "poor outcomes experienced by hospitalized patients" (Sanderson, 2014, p. E10).
- The five dimensions of Adverse Events are catheter-associated urinary tract infection, central catheter–associated bloodstream infection, ventilator-associated pneumonia, pressure ulcers, and falls.
  o *Catheter–associated urinary tract infection* is defined as urinary tract infections associated with indwelling urinary catheters.
  o *Central catheter–associated bloodstream infection* is defined as infections manifested in the bloodstream associated with indwelling central catheters.
  o *Ventilator-associated pneumonia* is defined as lung inflammation associated with invasive mechanical ventilation (Venes, 2013).
  o *Pressure ulcers* is defined as "Localized areas of tissue necrosis that tend to develop when soft tissue is compressed between a bony prominence and an external surface for a prolonged period" (National Pressure Ulcer Advisory Panel, as cited in Burd et al., 1992, p. 31).
  o *Falls* is defined as accidental drops to the floor, ground, or a lower level, such as a chair (Venes, 2013).

The *non-relational propositions* for the *E component* of the CTE structure are:

- Workload Assignment Tool Education Program is operationalized by the Workload Assignment Tool Education Program protocol, which stipulates that "All of the charge nurses were trained to use the tool, and we also provided training to the relief charge staff nurses to promote a consistent approach to staffing decisions" (Sanderson, 2014, p. E10). Although the methodological theory is not explicit, development of the protocol could be guided by the Plan-Do-Study-Act methodological theory. The three steps of this methodological theory are (1) "develop a plan and define the

(continued)

BOX 9.6   An Example of a Conceptual–Theoretical–Empirical Structure for a Synergy Model Quality Improvement Project *(continued)*

objective (plan)," (2) "carry out the plan and collect data (do), then analyze the data and summarize what was learned (study)," and (3) "plan the next cycle with necessary modifications (act)" (Gillam & Siriwardena, 2013, p. 125). Sanderson (2014) reported that she and her colleagues used the Synergy Model to develop a staffing model and workload assignment tool to reduce or eliminate adverse events experienced by patients hospitalized on a medical intensive care unit (plan). They then collected data for rates of adverse events (study), implemented the Workload Assignment Tool Education Program protocol (do), and collected adverse events data again (study). Sanderson (2014) indicated that adverse event rates decreased substantially after implementation of the protocol. Thus, it is likely that the Workload Assessment Tool will continue to be used (act).

- All five dimensions of Adverse Events are measured by medical intensive care record reviews before and after implementation of the Workload Assignment Tool Education Program protocol (Sanderson, 2014).

The *relational propositions* for the *C* and *T components* of the CTE structure are:

- Synergy (the match between Patient Characteristics and Nurse Competencies) results in optimal Patient and Family Outcomes.
- Therefore, the Workload Assignment Tool Education Program has a negative effect on Adverse Events.

The *relational proposition* for the *E component* of the CTE structure is:

- Medical record reviews of catheter-associated urinary tract infection, central catheter-associated bloodstream infection, ventilator-associated pneumonia, pressure ulcers, and falls after implementation of the Workload Assignment Tool Education Program protocol will reveal decreased rates when compared with rates prior to implementation of the protocol.

Source: Sanderson (2014).

SYNERGY MODEL: APPLICATION TO NURSING RESEARCH

The guidelines for Synergy Model nursing research are listed in Box 9.7. These guidelines were constructed primarily from content in Curley's (1998) journal article and Brewer's (2007) book chapter.

A CTE Structure for a Systematic Literature Review

No publications that are explicit reports of Synergy Model–guided literature reviews could be located. However, Wysong and Driver's (2009) journal article includes a section that can serve as an example of a review of literature that is

BOX 9.7 Guidelines for Synergy Model Nursing Research

The ultimate purpose of Synergy Model research is to determine the effect of synergy (the match between patient characteristics and nurse competencies) on patient and family outcomes, unit outcomes, and system outcomes.

The phenomena to be studied are patient characteristics, nurse competencies, and patient and family outcomes, unit outcomes, and system outcomes.

The primary problem to be studied is how synergy is achieved.

Data may be collected from nurses and patients, as well as from nursing clinical units and clinical agencies.

Synergy Model–based research encompasses clinically focused qualitative, quantitative, and/or mixed-methods designs. Longitudinal designs are especially relevant, as these designs allow tracking of changes in patient characteristics, nurse competencies, patient and family outcomes, unit outcomes, and system outcomes. Instruments directly derived from the Synergy Model are most appropriate although other instruments that can be clearly linked to concepts of the Synergy Model may be used. Data are collected primarily by nurses, although patient self-report is appropriate.

Data analysis techniques include those that are appropriate for analysis of qualitative and quantitative data. Regression techniques, especially canonical correlation, should be used to test the match between patient characteristics and nurse competencies, as well as the effect of synergy on outcomes. Structural equation modeling may be used to test the interrelations of patient characteristics, of nurse competencies, and of outcomes at each level—patient and family, unit, and system.

Synergy Model–based research contributes to understanding the "epistemological links and outcomes posited within the Synergy Model…[and] to the quality of patients' care, containment of costs, and patients' outcomes" (Curley, 1998, p. 71).

relevant for the Synergy Model. The purpose of their article was to report the results of a study designed "to explore patients' perceptions of nurses' skill in a progressive care unit (PCU)" (p. 24). They included a detailed report of the results of their review of 15 studies of patients' thoughts about nurses' and physicians' skills. The review included studies published between 1994 and 2007. The studies were conducted in the United States ($n = 7$), Canada ($n = 2$), Iceland ($n = 2$), Australia ($n = 1$), Denmark ($n = 1$), the United Kingdom ($n = 1$), and a multisite study in Sweden, the United Kingdom, and the United States ($n = 1$). Eight studies focused only on perceptions of nurses; six, only on perceptions of physicians; and one, on perceptions of the staff of a neonatal intensive care unit (NICU), including nurses.

Although Wysong and Driver (2009) did not mention the databases they searched, all 15 publications are in the Medline electronic database. Ten of the publications, including all nine publications about nurses, also are in the Cumulative Index to Nursing and Allied Health Literature (CINAHL Complete) electronic database.

Wysong and Driver (2009) included the parents' perceptions of NICU staff publication with their discussion of the nurses-only studies. Therefore, discussion of the results of their literature review for this chapter includes the eight studies of nurses only and the one study of NICU staff.

The theory is patient satisfaction with and perceptions of nurses' skillful care. The conceptual model concept is Patient and Family Outcomes; the relevant dimension is patient/family perception of being well cared for. The theory concepts are Patient Satisfaction with Nursing Care and Patient Perceptions of Quality of Nursing Care, which were extracted from Wysong and Driver's (2009) analysis of the literature they reviewed.

The CTE structure that was constructed from an interpretation of the literature review section of Wysong and Driver's (2009) journal article is illustrated in Figure 9.5. The non-relational propositions for each component of the CTE structure are listed in Box 9.8.

A CTE Structure for Instrument Development

Kohr, Hickey, and Curley's (2012) journal article is an example of a report of Synergy Model instrument development. The purpose of their study was to explore the feasibility of using the AACN Synergy Model for Patient Care "as a conceptual framework for a nursing productivity system that describes nursing work on the basis of the needs of patient[s] and their family members. Specifically, we wanted to know (a) what charge nurses considered when assigning nurses to patients/families and (b) what experienced nurses linked to 3 levels of nursing workload" (p. 421).

The theory is nurse productivity. The conceptual model concept is Patient Characteristics; all seven dimensions are relevant—stability, predictability, vulnerability, complexity, resiliency, patient and/or family participation in care and in decision making, and available resources; Kohr et al. (2012) combined the two patient and/or family participation characteristics in their report.

The theory concept is Nurse Productivity, which represents the seven dimensions of Patient Characteristics identified by Kohr et al. (2012). Nurse Productivity is measured by the Nurse Productivity System Visual Analog Scale (NPS-VAS).

In Phase 1 of their study, Kohr et al. (2012) generated items for the NPS-VAS from content analysis (see Appendix B) of transcripts from focus groups with 30 charge nurses who worked in the medical–surgical, cardiac, or neonatal ICU of a large pediatric hospital. The charge nurses were asked to respond to open-ended questions for each dimension of Patient Characteristics by identifying "patient and family indicators that [they] considered when making nurse-patient assignments" (Kohr et al., 2012, p. 422). An estimate of face validity (see Appendix B) for the items was obtained from the nurse managers from the three ICUs in which the charge nurses worked.

In Phase 2 of the study, the items were used to develop the NPS-VAS, which was administered as three different surveys to 33 level II and level III staff nurses working in pediatric ICUs. Each of the three surveys reflects one of three levels of work—light, typical, or heavy—required for the care of one patient on

Box 9.8   An Example of a Conceptual–Theoretical–Empirical Structure for a Synergy Model Literature Review

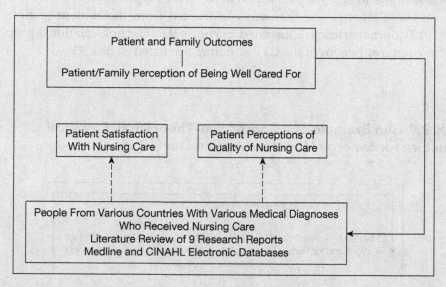

FIGURE 9.5 Conceptual–theoretical–empirical (CTE) structure for a Synergy Model literature review—theory of patient satisfaction with and perceptions of nurses' skillful nursing care.

CINAHL, Cumulative Index to Nursing and Allied Health Literature.

The *non-relational propositions* for the *C component* of the conceptual–theoretical–empirical (CTE) structure are:

- *Patient and Family Outcomes* is defined as results derived from patients and their family members and from the synergy of the characteristics of a patient and his or her family members with the competencies of a nurse.
- The relevant dimension of Patient and Family Outcomes is patient/family perception of being well cared for.
  - o *Patient/family perception of being well cared for* is defined as results such as improved patient and family trust in nurses, patient and family identification of these nurses, and enhanced patient and family satisfaction with nursing care (Curley, 2007a).

The *non-relational propositions* for the *T component* of the CTE structure are:

- *Patient Satisfaction with Nursing Care* is defined as patients' expressed satisfaction with the skillful care they received from nurses.
- *Patient Perceptions of Quality of Nursing Care* is defined as patients' expressions of the quality of skillful care they received from nurses.

The *non-relational proposition* for the *E component* of the CTE structure is:

- The concepts of Patient Satisfaction with Care and Patient Perceptions of Quality of Care were discovered in a review of nine research reports.

Source: Wysong and Driver (2009).

any day. Each survey includes all dimensions of Patient Characteristics, and each dimension is rated on the VAS from best-case scenario to worst-case scenario. Kohr et al. (2012) used descriptive statistics (numbers, percents) and cluster analysis to analyze the NPS-VAS data (see Appendix B).

The CTE structure that was constructed from the content of Kohr et al.'s (2012) journal article is illustrated in Figure 9.6. The non-relational propositions for each component of the CTE structure are listed in Box 9.9.

BOX 9.9 An Example of a Conceptual–Theoretical–Empirical Structure for Synergy Model Instrument Development

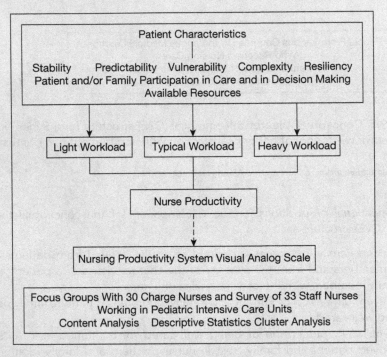

FIGURE 9.6 Conceptual–theoretical–empirical (CTE) structure for Synergy Model instrument development—theory of nurse productivity.

The *non-relational propositions* for the *C component* of t]he conceptual–theoretical–empirical (CTE) structure are:

- *Patient Characteristics* is defined as the unique health-related characteristics and needs of each person who is a patient and his or her family members.

(continued)

BOX 9.9 An Example of a Conceptual–Theoretical–Empirical Structure for Synergy Model Instrument Development *(continued)*

- The eight dimensions of Patient Characteristics are resiliency, vulnerability, stability, complexity, resource availability, participation in care, participation in decision making, and predictability.
  - *Resiliency* is defined as "The capacity to return to a restorative level of functioning using compensatory/coping mechanisms; the ability to bounce back quickly after an insult" (AACN, 2014, p. 1).
  - *Vulnerability* is defined as "Susceptibility to actual or potential stressors that may adversely affect patient outcomes" (AACN, 2014, p. 1).
  - *Stability* is defined as "The ability to maintain steady-state equilibrium" (AACN, 2014, p. 2).
  - *Complexity* is defined as "The intricate entanglement of two or more systems" (AACN, 2014, p. 2).
  - *Resource availability* is defined as the "Extent of resources...the patient/family/community bring to the situation" (AACN, 2014, p. 2).
  - *Participation in care* is defined as the "Extent to which patient/family engages in aspects of care" (AACN, 2014, p. 3).
  - *Participation in decision making* is defined as the "Extent to which patient/family engages in decision making" (AACN, 2014, p. 3).
  - *Predictability* is defined as "A characteristic that allows one to expect a certain course of events or course of illness" (AACN, 2014, p. 3).

The *non-relational propositions* for the *T component* of the CTE structure are:

- *Nurse Productivity* is defined as the level of nursing work based on pediatric patient and family needs (Kohr et al., 2012).
- The three dimensions of Nurse Productivity are light workload, typical workload, and heavy workload.
  - *Light workload* is defined as an "easy" pediatric patient for a particular intensive care unit, "specifically, a patient with stable vital signs, receiving routine care, whose trajectory of illness is on target, and who is tolerating procedures. The diagnosis may be new for the family and the home environment is stable with extended family resources" (Kohr et al., 2012, pp. 422, 426).
  - *Typical workload* is defined as a "usual" pediatric patient for a particular intensive care unit, "specifically, a patient who is similar to the patients in the [light workload] category but whose direction of illness is in question, with a number of more severe problems. The developmental level of the patient and the knowledge base and/or educational level of the parents are important" (Kohr et al., 2012, pp. 422, 426).
  - *Heavy workload* is defined as a "hard" pediatric patient for a particular intensive care unit (ICU), "specifically, a patient without physiological reserve, with a number of invasive catheters, interventions, and ICU therapies or complex technologies" (Kohr et al., 2012, pp. 422, 426).

(continued)

> **BOX 9.9   An Example of a Conceptual–Theoretical–Empirical Structure for Synergy Model Instrument Development** *(continued)*
>
> The *non-relational proposition* for the *E component* of the CTE structure is:
>
> • Nurse Productivity is measured by three different Nurse Productivity System Visual Analog Scales (NPS-VAS), one each for light workload, typical workload, and heavy workload. Each NPS-VAS includes a definition of and indicators for all eight dimensions of Patient Characteristics. Each dimension is rated on a VAS that is "5 inches (12.7 cm) in length. . . . Anchors on the left [end of the VAS] reflected the best-case scenario, and anchors on the right [end of the VAS] reflected the worst-case scenario, for example, stability on the left and instability on the right. Mid VAS anchors were also identified as 'moderate' or 'somewhat'" (Kohr et al., 2012, p. 422).
>
> *Source:* Kohr, Hickey, and Curley (2012).

A CTE Structure for Descriptive Qualitative Research

Cypress's (2013) journal article is an example of a Synergy Model–guided report of descriptive qualitative research. The purpose of her study was "to understand the lived experiences of patients, their family members, and nurses during critical illness in the [emergency department] ED" (Cypress, 2013, p. 312).

Cypress (2013) used a hermeneutic phenomenological research design for conduct of the study (van Manen, 1990; see Appendix A). The 23 research participants included 10 persons who were "acutely, crucially ill patients in the ED prior to their transfer to either the regular, medical floor, or the intensive care unit;" five family members who were "the patient's immediate family, primary support system, and caregivers;" and eight registered nurses who "held a bachelor of science in nursing . . . and had at least 2 years of critical care experience in the ED" (p. 313).

The theory is the lived experience of critical illness during emergency department care. The conceptual model concept is Nurse Competencies. Cypress (2013) identified seven relevant dimensions of Nurse Competencies as clinical judgment, advocacy and moral agency, caring practices, collaboration, response to diversity, systems thinking, and facilitator of learning. She explained that "Clinical inquiry, the ongoing process of questioning and evaluating practice through research utilization and experiential learning, was the only [dimension] not identified from the themes that were illuminated from the study" (p. 314).

The theory concept is Lived Experience of Critical Illness During Emergency Department Care. The dimensions of the concept are patients and family members on nurses and nurses on patients and family members. The subdimensions of patients and family members on nurses are critical thinking, communication, and sensitivity and caring. The subdimensions of nurses on patients and family members are response to physiological deficit and patients and families as co-participants in the human care processes.

The Lived Experience of Critical Illness During Emergency Department Care and its dimensions and subdimensions were discovered in the data provided by patients, family members, and nurses. Cypress (2103) used van Manen's (1990) method of analysis of qualitative data (see Appendix B) to discover the theory concept and its dimensions and subdimensions in the participants' answers to open-ended questions on an unstructured interview guide.

The CTE structure that was constructed from the content of Cypress's (2013) journal article is illustrated in Figure 9.7. The non-relational propositions for each component of the CTE structure are listed in Box 9.10.

A CTE Structure for Correlational Research

Tejero's (2012) journal article is an example of a report of Synergy Model–guided correlational research. The purpose of her study was "to test the direct and indirect relations of nurse-characteristics and patient characteristics to patient satisfaction, as mediated by nurse–patient dyad bonding" (Tejero, 2012, p. 996).

Tejero (2102) used a correlational path model research design (see Appendix A). The research participants included 210 nurses and the 210 patients for whom the nurses provided nursing care during the day or evening shift. The sample inclusion criteria were "nurses and patients...from the medical-surgical, obstetrics–gynaecological, otorhinolaryngological, ophthalmological units and the trauma ward and medical [intensive care units] ICUs, of two government and two private hospitals in the Philippines" (Tejero, 2012, p. 996). The exclusion criteria were "Patients with psychiatric illness or speech impediment and those on immediate post-anaesthesia" (Tejero, 2102, p. 996).

Explaining the creation of the nurse–patient dyads, Tejero (2102) stated,

> Although a nurse had several patients, only one patient was paired with a particular nurse for the observation of nurse–patient interaction. For each pair or dyad, only one episode of interaction was observed. The choice of episode was determined by chance, that is, whichever novel dyad-in-interaction was chanced upon by the observer was observed as data. (p. 996)

The theory is the relations of patient characteristics and nurse-characteristics to patient satisfaction, mediated by nurse–patient dyad bonding. The conceptual model concepts are Patient Characteristics, Nurse Competencies, Synergy, and Patient and Family Outcomes. The three relevant dimensions of Patient Characteristics are complexity, vulnerability, and predictability. The two relevant dimensions of Nurse Competencies are clinical judgment and facilitation

BOX 9.10 An Example of a Conceptual–Theoretical–Empirical Structure for Synergy Model Descriptive Qualitative Research

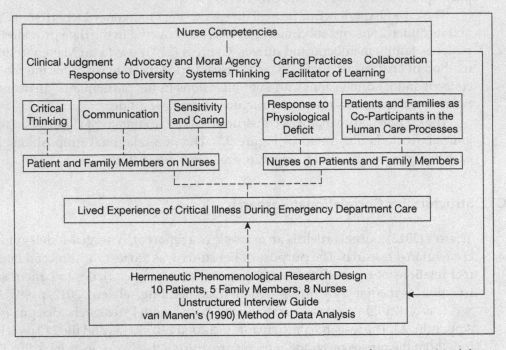

FIGURE 9.7 Conceptual–theoretical–empirical (CTE) structure for Synergy Model descriptive qualitative research—theory of the lived experience of critical illness during emergency department care.

The *non-relational propositions* for the *C component* of the conceptual–theoretical– empirical (CTE) structure are:

- *Nurse Competencies* is defined as the nurse's integration of his or her "knowledge, skills, experience, and attitudes needed to meet the needs of patients and families" (AACN, 2014, p. 4) and to optimize patient and family member outcomes (Curley, 2007a). Nurse competencies "are essential for … providing care" (Hardin & Kaplow, 2005, p. 5).
- The seven relevant dimensions of Nurse Competencies are clinical judgment, advocacy and moral agency, caring practices, collaboration, response to diversity, systems thinking, and facilitator of learning (Cypress, 2013).
  o *Clinical judgment* is defined as "clinical reasoning that includes clinical decision making, critical thinking, and a global grasp of the situation, coupled with nursing skills acquired through a process of integrating formal and informal experiential knowledge and evidence based guidelines" (AACN, as cited in Cypress, 2013, p. 314).
  o *Advocacy and moral agency* is defined as "working on another's behalf and representing the concerns of the patient, family, and nursing staff; serving as a moral agent in identifying and helping to resolve ethical and clinical concerns within and outside the clinical setting" (AACN, as cited in Cypress, 2013, p. 316).

(continued)

BOX 9.10 An Example of a Conceptual–Theoretical–Empirical Structure for Synergy Model Descriptive Qualitative Research (continued)

- o *Caring practices* is defined as "nursing activities that create a compassionate, supportive, and therapeutic environment for patients and staff, with the aim of promoting comfort and healing and preventing unnecessary suffering. It includes, but is not limited to, vigilance, engagement, and responsiveness of caregivers, including family and healthcare personnel" (AACN, as cited in Cypress, 2013, p. 316).
- o *Collaboration* is defined as "working with others such as the patients, families, and healthcare providers in a way that promotes each person's contributions toward achieving optimal and realistic patient and family goals" (AACN, as cited in Cypress, 2103, p. 317).
- o *Response to diversity* is defined as "the sensitivity to recognize, appreciate, and incorporate differences into the provision of care. Differences may include, but are not limited to, cultural differences, spiritual beliefs, sex, race, ethnicity, lifestyle, socioeconomic status, age, and values" (AACN, as cited in Cypress, 2013, p. 318).
- o *Systems thinking* is defined as the "body of knowledge and tools that allow the nurse to manage whatever environmental and system resources [that] exist for the patients, families, and staff, within or across healthcare. This also includes anticipating the needs of patients" (AACN, as cited in Cypress, 2013, p. 318).
- o *Facilitator of learning* is defined as "the ability to facilitate learning for patients and families by integrating education in the plan of care" (AACN, as cited in Cypress, 2013, p. 318).

The *non-relational propositions* for the *T component* of the CTE structure are:

- *Lived Experience of Critical Illness During Emergency Department Care* is defined as perceptions of critically ill patients, their family members, and their nurses about their experiences in the emergency department.
- The two dimensions of Lived Experience of Critical Illness During Emergency Department Care are patients and family members on nurses and nurses on patients and family members.
  - o *Patients and family members on nurses* is defined as perceptions of critically ill patients and their family members about the work done by nurses in the emergency department.
  - o The three subdimensions of patients and family members on nurses are critical thinking, communication, and sensitivity and caring.
    - ■ *Critical thinking* is defined as "ability in decision making; expertise in flexible, individualized, situation-specific problem solving; and clinical judgment... [including] quick triage and decision making, tests that are done promptly, and frequent assessment and monitoring" (Cypress, 2013, pp. 314, 315).
    - ■ *Communication* is defined as "identifying self as a nurse, greeting and listening...interacting with patients and family members, [and] giving information...about procedures, treatments including medications, test results, [and] transfer" (Cypress, 2013, pp. 314, 315, 317).

(continued)

BOX 9.10   An Example of a Conceptual–Theoretical–Empirical Structure for Synergy Model Descriptive Qualitative Research *(continued)*

- ■ *Sensitivity and caring* is defined as "avoiding ill remarks, complaining, and gossiping; empathizing for the nurses; and advocating for patients and families that includes privacy and confidentiality, culture, and socioeconomic status" (Cypress, 2013, p. 316).
- o *Nurses on patients and family members* is defined as nurses' perceptions of the work they do with critically ill patients and their family members during their time in the emergency department.
- o The two subdimensions of nurses on patients and family members are response to physiological deficit and patients and families as co-participants in the human care processes.
  - ■ *Response to physiological deficit* is defined as "expediting care and anticipating care as well as interventions, changes in signs and symptoms, and status and concern for outcomes" (Cypress, 2013, p. 318).
  - ■ *Patients and families as co-participants in the human care processes* is defined as nurses "Interacting, working with the family, and involving [patients and their family members] in the plan of care are the ways that patients and family members can coparticipate in the care processes" (Cypress, 2013, p. 317).

The *non-relational propositions* for the *E component* of the CTE structure are:

- • Lived Experience of Critical Illness During Emergency Department Care and its dimensions and subdimensions were discovered in patients', family members', and nurses' answers to open-ended questions on an unstructured interview guide constructed by Cypress (2103), who did not indicate what questions were asked. Participants were interviewed twice. After transcription of the first interview, "the participants were given the opportunity to review and modify the transcripts as needed" (Cypress, 2013, p. 313). In keeping with hermeneutic phenomenology, as the researcher Cypress "was the sole instrument of the study who worked closely with participants to collect data as a participant observer, interviewer, and analyzer of data....van Manen's [1990] holistic, selective, and detailed line-by-line approach was used to analyze the data" (Cypress, 2013, p. 313).

Source: Cypress (2013).

---

of learning. The relevant dimension of Patient and Family Outcomes is patient/family perception of being well cared for.

The theory concepts are Patient Characteristics, Nurse-Characteristics, Nurse–Patient Dyad Bonding, and Patient Satisfaction. The five dimensions of the theory concept of Patient Characteristics are comorbidities, weight, nosocomial infection, medication intake, and response to treatment. The two dimensions of Nurse-Characteristics are clinical judgment and facilitation of learning, which are the same dimensions of the conceptual model concept of Nurse Competencies.

The conceptual model concept Patient Characteristics complexity dimension is represented by the theory concept Patient Characteristics comorbidities dimension; the vulnerability dimension, by the weight and nosocomial infection dimensions; and the predictability dimension, by the medication intake and response to treatment dimensions. Nurse Competencies and its dimensions are represented by the dimensions of Nurse-Characteristics. Synergy is represented by Nurse–Patient Dyad Bonding. The patient/family perception of being well cared for dimension of Patient and Family Outcomes is represented by Patient Satisfaction.

The theory concept Patient Characteristics is measured by the investigator-developed Patient Characteristics Checklist of the contents of patients' charts and results from patient interviews. Nurse-Characteristics was measured by the investigator-developed Nurse-Characteristics Checklist of the contents of patients' chart reviews, observations of the nurses, and information obtained from the nurses and from the patients and their companions. Nurse–Patient Dyad Bonding is measured by the Nurse–Patient Bonding Instrument (Tejero 2010). Patient Satisfaction is measured by the Patient Satisfaction with Nursing Care instrument (Villarruz-Sulit, Dans, & Javeloza, 2009).

Path analysis with multiple regression statistics (see Appendix B) was used to examine the direct relations of the dimensions of Patient Characteristics and the dimensions of Nurse-Characteristics with Nurse–Patient Dyad Bonding and with Patient Satisfaction, as well as the direct relation between Nurse–Patient Dyad Bonding and Patient Satisfaction. Multiple regression statistics following Baron and Kenny's (1986) mediation technique (see Appendix B) were used to examine the indirect relations of the dimensions of Patient Characteristics and the dimensions of Nurse-Characteristics with Patient Satisfaction through Nurse–Patient Dyad Bonding.

The CTE structure that was constructed from an interpretation of the content of Tejero's (2012) journal article is illustrated in Figure 9.8. The non-relational and relational propositions for each component of the CTE structure are listed in Box 9.11.

A CTE Structure for Experimental Research

No reports of Synergy Model–guided experimental research could be located, which was confirmed by M. A. Q. Curley (personal communication, November 23, 2014). Consequently, a hypothetical experimental study is proposed, based on the contents of journal articles by Smith (2006, 2011) and by Smith and her colleagues (Pérez et al., 2011).

The purpose of the hypothetical study is to examine the differential effect of two types of spiritual care—experimental auditory bibliotherapy treatment or

BOX 9.11   An Example of a Conceptual–Theoretical–Empirical Structure for Synergy Model Correlational Research

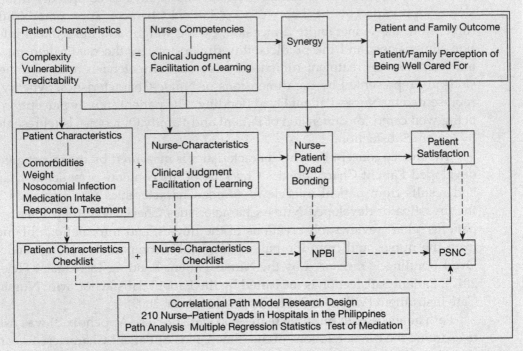

FIGURE 9.8 Conceptual–theoretical–empirical (CTE) structure for Synergy Model correlational research—theory of relations of patient characteristics and nurse-characteristics to patient satisfaction, mediated by nurse–patient dyad bonding.

NPBI, Nurse–Patient Bonding Instrument; PSNC, Patient Satisfaction With Nursing Care Instrument.

The *non-relational propositions* for the C component of the conceptual–theoretical–empirical (CTE) structure are:

- *Patient Characteristics* is defined as the unique health-related characteristics and needs of each person who is a patient and his or her family members.
- The three relevant dimensions of Patient Characteristics are complexity, vulnerability, and predictability.
    - o *Complexity* is defined as "the intricate entanglement of two or more systems" (AACN, 2014, p. 2).
    - o *Vulnerability* is defined as "susceptibility to stressors that may adversely affect patient outcomes" (AACN, 2014, p. 2).
    - o *Predictability* is defined as the expectation of "a certain trajectory of illness" (Curley, 2007a, p. 27).
- *Nurse Competencies* is defined as the nurse's integration of his or her "knowledge, skills, experiences, and attitudes needed to meet the needs of patients and families" (AACN, 2014, p. 4) and to optimize patient outcomes (Curley, 2007a).

(continued)

BOX 9.11   An Example of a Conceptual–Theoretical–Empirical Structure for Synergy Model Correlational Research   *(continued)*

- The two relevant dimensions of Nurse Competencies are clinical judgment and facilitation of learning.
  - o *Clinical judgment* is defined as "clinical reasoning, which includes clinical decision-making, critical thinking, and a global grasp of the situation, coupled with nursing skills acquired through a process of integrating formal and informal experiential knowledge and evidence based guidelines" (AACN, 2014, p. 4).
  - o *Facilitation of learning* is defined as "the ability to [formally and informally] facilitate learning for patient/families, nursing staff, other members of the healthcare team, and community" (AACN, 2014, p. 7).
- *Synergy* is defined as the meeting of the nurse and the patient "in the process [of] achieving [an] optimum outcome for the patient" (Tejero, 2012, p. 995), the result of the match of the needs and characteristics of a patient with a nurse's competencies (AACN, 2014).
- *Patient and Family Outcomes* is defined as results derived from patients and their family members and from the synergy of the characteristics of a patient and his or her family members with the competencies of a nurse.
- The relevant dimension of Patient and Family Outcomes is patient/family perception of being well cared for.
  - o *Patient/family perception of being well cared for* is defined as results such as improved patient and family trust in nurses, patient and family identification of these nurses, and enhanced patient and family satisfaction with nursing care (Curley, 2007a).

The *non-relational propositions* for the *T component* of the CTE structure are:

- *Patient Characteristics* is defined as the unique health-related characteristics and needs of each person who is a patient and his or her family members.
- The five dimensions of Patient Characteristics are comorbidities, weight, nosocomial infection, medication intake, and response to treatment.
  - o *Comorbidities* is defined as presence of medical diagnoses of diseases that exist "simultaneously with and worsens or affects of primary disease" (Venes, 2013, p. 533).
  - o *Weight* is defined as the patient's body weight.
  - o *Nosocomial infection* is defined as presence of a hospital-acquired infection (Venes, 2013).
  - o *Medication intake* is defined as medications taken by the patient during hospitalization.
  - o *Response to treatment* is defined as the patient's reaction to interventions.
- *Nurse-Characteristics* is defined as the nurse's integration of his or her "knowledge, skills, experiences, and attitudes needed to meet the needs of patients and families" (AACN, 2014, p. 4) and to optimize patient outcomes (Curley, 2007a).
- The dimensions of Nurse-Characteristics are clinical judgment and facilitation of learning.

(continued)

BOX 9.11 An Example of a Conceptual–Theoretical–Empirical Structure for Synergy Model Correlational Research *(continued)*

- o *Clinical judgment* is defined as "clinical reasoning, which includes clinical decision-making, critical thinking, and a global grasp of the situation, coupled with nursing skills acquired through a process of integrating formal and informal experiential knowledge and evidence based guidelines" (AACN, 2014, p. 4).
- o *Facilitation of learning* is defined as "the ability to [formally and informally] facilitate learning for patients/families, nursing staff, other members of the healthcare team, and community (AACN, 2014, p. 7).
- *Nurse–Patient Dyad Bonding* is defined as "the respective openness and engagement of nurse and patient during interaction. Patient-openness refers to the patient's readiness to manifest [his or her own self] to the nurse, whereas nurse-openness refers to the nurse's gathering of as much information [as possible] pertinent to the treatment and care of the patient. Nurse engagement refers to the effective provision of care by the nurse to the patient, whereas patient-engagement refers to the patient's involvement in this care" (Tejero, 2012, p. 996).
- *Patient Satisfaction* is defined as the patient's level of satisfaction with the nurse "as a caring person, as an information provider and as a competent and skilled healthcare provider" (Tejero, 2012, p. 997).

The *non-relational propositions* for the *E component* of the CTE structure are:

- The five dimensions of Patient Characteristics—comorbidities, weight, nosocomial infection, medication intake, and response to treatment—are measured by the investigator-developed Patient Characteristics (PC) Checklist. The PC Checklist is used to document the contents of patients' charts and results from patient interviews regarding comorbidities, weight, nosocomial infection, medication intake, and response to treatment.
- The two dimensions of Nurse-Characteristics are measured by the investigator-developed Nurse-Characteristics (N-C) Checklist. The N-C Checklist is used to document results from patients' chart reviews, nonparticipant observations of the nurses, and information obtained from the nurses and from the patients and their companions. Scoring for both clinical judgment and facilitation of learning is "based on the levels set by AACN [Brewer, 2007], that is, nurse activities pertaining to levels 1, 3, 5 were given scores of 1, 3, 5, respectively" (Tejero, 2012, p. 997).
- Nurse–Patient Dyad Bonding is measured by the Nurse–Patient Bonding Instrument (NPBI; Tejero, 2010). The NPBI is "an observation checklist with 52 behavioural indicators of the dimensions of openness and engagement of both nurse and patient...trained observers checked each of the 52 behaviours [as] present, absent or not applicable. Behaviours that are present are scored 1 or 2 points, whereas absent behaviours are given −1, −2 or −3 points. The weight depends on how strongly or directly the behaviour measures [openness or engagement]. The weighted scores were then summed algebraically, yielding [a] patient–nurse openness score...and [a] patient–nurse engagement score" (Tejero, 2012, p. 996).

(continued)

BOX 9.11   An Example of a Conceptual–Theoretical–Empirical Structure for Synergy Model Correlational Research   *(continued)*

- Patient Satisfaction is measured by the Patient Satisfaction with Nursing Care instrument (PSNC; Villarruz-Sulit et al., 2009). The PSNC is made up of 19 items that are rated on a 5-point Likert-type scale of 1 = totally disagree, 2 = disagree, 3 = uncertain, 4 = agree, and 5 = totally agree for positively worded items; reverse scoring is used for negatively worded items.

The *relational propositions* for the *C* and *T components* of the CTE structure are:

- Patient Chacteristics have a positive effect on Patient and Family Outcomes.
- Nurse Competencies have a positive effect on Patient and Family Outcomes.
- Therefore, Patient Characteristics and Nurse-Characteristics are positively related to Patient Satisfaction.
- Patient Characteristics are related to Synergy.
- Nurse Competencies are related to Synergy.
- Therefore, Patient Characteristics and Nurse-Characteristics are positively related to Nurse–Patient Dyad Bonding.
- Synergy (the match between Patient Characteristics and Nurse Competencies) results in optimal Patient and Family Outcomes.
- Therefore, Nurse–Patient Dyad Bonding is positively related to Patient Satisfaction.
- And, Nurse–Patient Dyad Bonding mediates the relations of Patient Characteristics and Nurse-Characteristics with Patient Satisfaction (Tejero, 2012).

The *relational propositions* for the *E component* of the CTE structure are:

- Scores for the PC Checklist and scores for the N-C Checklist are related to scores for the NPBI.
- Scores for the PC Checklist and scores for the N-C Checklist are related to scores for the PSNC instrument.
- Scores for the NPBI are related to scores for the PSNC instrument.
- Scores for the NPBI mediate the relations of scores for the PC Checklist and for the N-C Checklist with scores for the PSNC instrument.

Source: Tejero (2012).

control presence treatment—on depression. An experimental pretest–posttest research design would be used (see Appendix A). The hypothetical research participants are 30 women and 30 men who are patients hospitalized on a medical intermediate care unit. Random assignment using the sealed opaque envelope technique (see Appendix B) would be used to assign 15 women and 15 men to one group and 15 women and 15 men to another group. Random assignment of the groups to experimental auditory bibliotherapy or control presence also would be done. Following the completion of the study, auditory bibliotherapy would be offered to the control presence group participants.

The theory is the effect of spiritual care on depression. The conceptual model concepts are Nurse Competencies and Patient and Family Outcomes. The relevant dimensions of Nurse Competencies are caring practices and response to diversity, and the relevant dimension of Patient and Family Outcomes is health-related quality of life. The theory concepts are Type of Spiritual Care and Depression. The two dimensions of Type of Spiritual Care are auditory bibliotherapy and presence.

Type of Spiritual Care represents the caring practices and response to diversity dimensions of Nurse Competencies. Depression represents the health-related quality of life dimension of Patient and Family Outcomes. The two dimensions of Type of Spiritual Care are operationalized by the experimental auditory bibliotherapy protocol and the control presence protocol. Depression is measured by the Center for Epidemiological Studies-Depression Scale (CES-D; Radloff, 1977). The theory would be tested using analysis of covariance statistics (see Appendix B) with pretest CES-D scores and gender (women, men) as the covariates.

The CTE structure that was constructed from the hypothetical experimental study is illustrated in Figure 9.9. The non-relational and relational propositions for each component of the CTE structure are listed in Box 9.12.

A CTE Structure for Mixed-Methods Research

No reports of Synergy Model–guided mixed-methods research could be located, which was confirmed by M. A. Q. Curley (personal communication, November 23, 2014). Consequently, a hypothetical mixed-methods study was proposed, based on the contents of an abstract by Smith (2007) and a journal article by Belcher and Griffiths (2005).

The purpose of the hypothetical mixed methods study is to describe nurses' spiritual care perspectives. The QUAN + QUAL mixed-methods study would use a simple descriptive design (see Appendix A). The QUAN portion of the study comes directly from research conducted by Smith (2007) with a sample of 35 nurses from two medical intermediate care units. The QUAL portion is extracted from the findings of Belcher and Griffiths's (2005) study of the spiritual perspectives of 204 hospice nurses, which were applied to the hypothetical mixed-methods study supposing the same sample used for the QUAN portion.

The theory is spiritual care perspectives. The conceptual model concept is Nurse Competences, and the relevant dimension is caring practices. The theory concept is Spiritual Care Perspectives. Eight dimensions of the concept are extracted from the data for the QUAL portion of the study—expression of spirituality in personal life, expression of spirituality in professional life, role conflict in spiritual expression, knowledge base of spiritual care needs and professional responsibilities, assessment of spiritual needs, interdisciplinary relationships, role comfort, and informational needs.

BOX 9.12   An Example of a Conceptual–Theoretical–Empirical Structure for Synergy Model Experimental Research

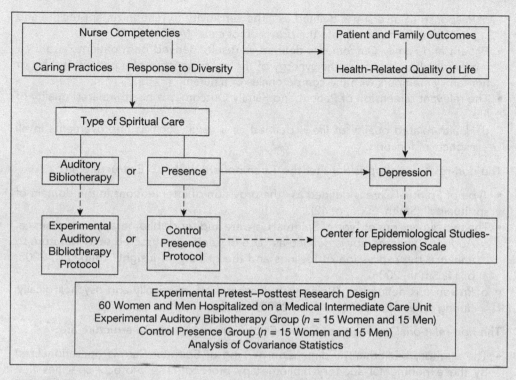

FIGURE 9.9 Conceptual–theoretical–empirical (CTE) structure for Synergy Model experimental research—theory of effect of spiritual care on depression.

The *non-relational propositions* for the *C component* of the conceptual–theoretical–empirical (CTE) structure are:

- *Nurse Competencies* is defined as the nurse's integration of his or her "knowledge, skills, experience, and attitudes needed to meet the needs of patients and families" (AACN, 2014, p. 4) and to optimize patient and family member outcomes (Curley, 2007a).
- The two relevant dimensions of Nurse Competencies are caring practices and response to diversity.
  - o *Caring practices* is defined as "Nursing activities that create a compassionate, supportive, and therapeutic environment for patients and staff, with the aim of promoting comfort and healing and preventing unnecessary suffering. Includes, but is not limited to, vigilance, engagement, and responsiveness of caregivers, including family and healthcare personnel" (AACN, 2014, p. 5).

(continued)

BOX 9.12   An Example of a Conceptual–Theoretical–Empirical Structure for Synergy Model Experimental Research   (continued)

- o *Response to diversity* is defined as "The sensitivity to recognize, appreciate and incorporate differences into the provision of care" (AACN, 2014, p. 7).
- *Patient and Family Outcomes* is defined as results derived from patients and their family members and from the synergy of the characteristics of a patient and his or her family members with the competencies of a nurse.
- The relevant dimension of Patient and Family Outcomes is health-related quality of life.
  - o *Health-related quality of life* is defined as a result such as improvements in all aspects of function.

The *non-relational propositions* for the *T component* of the CTE structure are:

- *Type of Spiritual Care* is defined as "the provision of interventions in the domain of spirituality" (Smith, 2006, p. 42).
- The two dimensions of Type of Spiritual Care are auditory bibliotherapy and presence.
  - o *Auditory bibliotherapy* is defined as "Use of [readings of sacred text] literature to enhance the expression of feelings and the gaining of insight" (Burkhart, 2005, p. 11, Smith, 2006).
  - o *Presence* is defined as "Being with another, both physically and psychologically, during times of need" (Burkhart, 2005, p. 11).

The *non-relational propositions* for the *E component* of the CTE structure are:

- The auditory bibliotherapy dimension of Type of Spiritual Care is operationalized by the experimental auditory bibliotherapy protocol. The protocol specifies that the nurse first asks the patient which sacred text is preferred (e.g., Old Testament portion of the Christian Bible, the Tanakh [Hebrew Bible], New Testament portion of the Christian Bible, the Book of Mormon, the Koran, the Gospel of Buddha, the Rig Veda, the Confucian Canon, the Tao Te Ching). The selected sacred text is then retrieved from the Internet via a smart phone or tablet app. The patient and the nurse listen to the reading of selected passages of the sacred text and discuss the text (Cress-Ingebo & Chrisagis, 1998; A. R. Smith, personal communication, December 2, 2014). The nurse applies the protocol three times each day, once during each 8-hour shift.
- The presence dimension of Type of Spiritual Care is operationalized by the control presence protocol. The protocol specifies that the nurse is physically and psychologically available to the patient and is at the patient's bedside with no expectation of responses from the patient whenever the nurse enters the patient's room. The nurse physically helps the patient with activities of daily living, demonstrates an accepting attitude, orally communicates empathy and understanding of the patient's experience, establishes trust with the patient, conveys positive regard of the patient, listens to the patient's concerns, and touches the patient with his or her permission to express concern (Cavendish et al., 2003). The nurse applies the protocol three times each day, once during each 8-hour shift.

(continued)

> **BOX 9.12   An Example of a Conceptual–Theoretical–Empirical Structure for Synergy Model Experimental Research** *(continued)*
>
> - Depression is measured by the Center for Epidemiological Studies-Depression Scale (CES-D; Radloff, 1977). The CES-D is made up of 20 items that address cognitive, affective, and somatic symptoms. Each item is rated on a 4-point scale of 0 = rarely or none of the time, 1 = some or a little of the time, 2 = occasionally or a moderate amount of time, to 3 = most or all of the time.
>
> The *relational propositions* for the *C* and *T components* of the CTE structure are:
>
> - Nurse Competencies have a positive effect on Patient and Family Outcomes.
> - Therefore, Type of Spiritual Care has a positive effect on Depression.
>
> The *relational proposition* for the *E component* of the CTE structure is:
>
> - Research participants who receive the experimental auditory bibliotherapy protocol will have lower scores on the CES-D Scale than research participants who receive the control presence protocol.
>
> *Sources:* Constructed for this chapter from Pérez et al. (2011) and Smith (2006, 2011).

The caring practices dimension of Nurse Competencies is represented by Spiritual Care Perspectives. For the QUAN portion of the study, Spiritual Care Perspectives is measured by the Spiritual Care Perspectives Scale (Chism & Magnan, 2009; Taylor, 2006). Descriptive statistics (mean, range) are used to analyze the data (see Appendix B). For the QUAL portion of the study, the eight dimensions of Spiritual Care Perspectives were discovered in the participants' responses to questions on an investigator-developed survey (Belcher & Griffiths, 2005). Miles and Huberman's (1994) method of data analysis was used to extract and code the responses (see Appendix B).

The CTE structure that was constructed from the contents of Smith's (2007) and Belcher and Griffiths's (2005) research reports is illustrated in Figure 9.10. The non-relational propositions for each component of the CTE structure are listed in Box 9.13.

CONCLUSION

The Synergy Model began as a conceptual framework for acute and critical care nursing practice. The relative simplicity of the model has been so attractive to many nurses that its use has extended to virtually every practice setting and many nursing clinical specialties. Arashin (2010) commented that nursing

BOX 9.13   An Example of a Conceptual–Theoretical–Empirical Structure for Synergy Model Mixed-Methods Research

This example of a hypothetical mixed-methods study was constructed for this chapter based on studies by Belcher and Griffiths (2005) and Smith (2007).

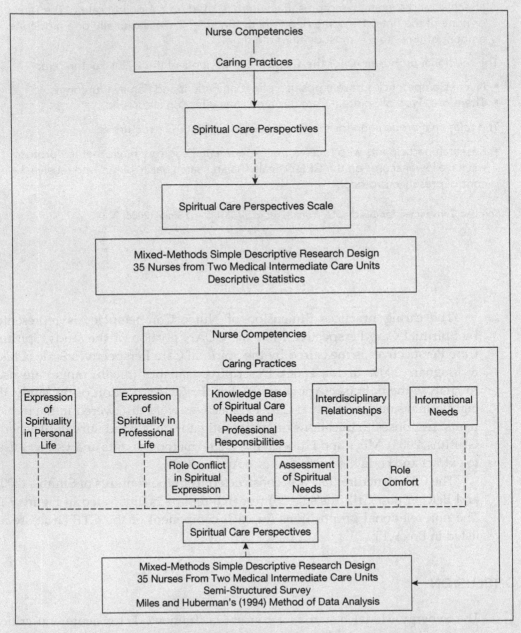

FIGURE 9.10 Conceptual–theoretical–empirical (CTE) structure for Synergy Model mixed-methods research: Quantitative portion—theory of spiritual care perspectives—quantitative and qualitative portions.

(continued)

BOX 9.13   An Example of a Conceptual–Theoretical–Empirical Structure for Synergy Model Mixed-Methods Research   *(continued)*

The *non-relational propositions* for the *C component* of the conceptual–theoretical–empirical (CTE) structure are:

- *Nurse Competencies* is defined as the nurse's integration of his or her "knowledge, skills, experience, and attitudes needed to meet the needs of patients and families" (AACN, 2014, p. 4) and to optimize patient and family member outcomes (Curley, 2007a).
- The two relevant dimensions of Nurse Competencies are caring practices and response to diversity.
    o *Caring practices* is defined as "Nursing activities that create a compassionate, supportive, and therapeutic environment for patients and staff, with the aim of promoting comfort and healing and preventing unnecessary suffering. Includes, but is not limited to, vigilance, engagement, and responsiveness of caregivers, including family and healthcare personnel" (AACN, 2014, p. 5).
    o *Response to diversity* is defined as "The sensitivity to recognize, appreciate and incorporate differences into the provision of care" (AACN, 2014, p. 7).

The *non-relational propositions* for the *T component* of the CTE structure are:

- *Spiritual Care Perspectives* is defined as "the attitudes and beliefs nurses have regarding spiritual care in nursing" (Chism & Magnan, 2009, p. 599).
- The eight dimensions of Spiritual Care Perspectives for the qualitative portion of the study are expression of spirituality in personal life, expression of spirituality in professional life, role conflict in spiritual expression, knowledge base of spiritual care needs and professional responsibilities, assessment of spiritual needs, interdisciplinary relationships, role comfort, and informational needs (Belcher & Griffiths, 2005).
    o *Expression of spirituality in personal life* is defined as attending and participating in church rituals, participating in activities of community ministries and fellowships, praying each day, studying scripture or spiritual readings, reflecting through meditation and journaling, and engaging with nature or music (Belcher & Griffiths, 2005).
    o *Expression of spirituality in professional life* is defined as the extent of openness about and comfort with provision of spiritual care, such as encouragement, attentive listening, and comfort for patients, as well as for coworkers and peers, especially in the form of support and encouragement (Belcher & Griffiths, 2005).
    o *Role conflict in spiritual expression* is defined as lack of congruence between personal and professional expressions of spirituality, the extent of openness about and comfort with provision of spiritual care for patients (Belcher & Griffiths, 2005).
    o *Knowledge base of spiritual care needs and professional responsibilities* is defined as how nurses learn about spiritual care and their professional responsibility for providing spiritual care (Belcher & Griffiths, 2005).
    o *Assessment of spiritual needs* is defined as recognition of the importance of and professional responsibility for assessing patients' needs for spiritual care (Belcher & Griffiths, 2005).

(continued)

BOX 9.13   An Example of a Conceptual–Theoretical–Empirical Structure for Synergy Model Mixed-Methods Research   (continued)

   o *Interdisciplinary relationships* is defined as having productive interactions with pastoral care personnel (Belcher & Griffiths, 2005).
   o *Role comfort* is defined as situations that elicit feelings of discomfort or comfort while caring for patients (Belcher & Griffiths, 2005).
   o *Informational needs* is defined as desire for more information about the beliefs and practices of various religions (Belcher & Griffiths, 2005).

The *non-relational propositions* for the *E component* of the CTE structure are:

- Spiritual Care Perspectives is measured for the quantitative portion of the study by the Spiritual Care Perspectives Scale (SCPS; Chism & Magnan, 2009; Taylor, 2006). The SCPS contains 12 items that address "nurses' attitudes, beliefs, comfort, and confidence related to the provision of spiritual care in nursing practice." Each item is rated on a 5-point scale of 1 = strongly agree to 5 = strongly disagree (Chism & Magnan, 2009, p. 600).
- The eight dimensions of Spiritual Care Perspectives for the qualitative portion of the study were discovered in the data from an investigator-developed semi-structured survey and analyzed using Miles and Huberman's (1994) method. The survey is made up of "15 open-ended questions that were designed to elicit the participants' thoughts about the issues and questions related to personal and professional expressions of spirituality, as well as their spiritual practices and self-determined ability to apply their spiritual values to patient care" (Belcher & Griffiths, 2005, p. 273). Only 1 of the 15 questions was included in Belcher and Griffiths's (2005) research report: "How did you learn about the spiritual needs of patients?" (p. 275).

Sources: Constructed for this chapter from Belcher and Griffiths (2005) and Smith (2007).

practice guided by the Synergy Model "ensures that needs are identified, the right resources are used, and the best outcomes for the patient can be realized" (p. 124).

Although the Synergy Model has been used extensively in nursing practice, to date relatively little Synergy Model nursing research has been conducted. Brewer (2007) discussed the need for development of instruments to measure the Synergy Model concepts and the subsequent need to test theory concepts and propositions derived from the Synergy Model. Generation and testing of theories derived from the Synergy Model is evident, although to a limited extent. Perhaps most important is the need to test theories of the effect of synergy—the match between patient characteristics and nurse competencies—on outcomes.

The several examples of actual applications of the Synergy Model discussed in this chapter clearly point to the utility of this conceptual model of nursing, which was introduced to the world of nursing in the late 1990s, a much more recent time than all other conceptual models included in this book, with the exception of the Transitions Framework, which is another recent addition to the discipline of nursing (see Chapter 10).

NOTES

1. In one previous version of the Synergy Model, seven dimensions of Patient and Family Outcomes were identified—functional changes, behavioral changes, trust, subjective and objective ratings, satisfaction, comfort, and quality of life (Curley, 1998). In another previous version, six dimensions were identified—functional changes, behavioral changes, trust, satisfaction, comfort, and quality of life (Hardin & Kaplow, 2005).

2. In previous versions of the Synergy Model, Nurse Outcomes were identified as one of three types of outcomes (Patient Outcomes, Nurse Outcomes, and System Outcomes). Three dimensions of Nurse Outcomes were identified as management of physiological changes, presence or absence of complications, and extent to which care or treatment objectives were attained (Curley, 1998; Hardin & Kaplow, 2005; Reed et al., 2007).

3. In one previous version of the Synergy Model, two dimensions of System Outcomes were identified—recidivism and costs/resource utilization (Curley, 1998). In another previous version, three dimensions were identified—readmission rate, length of stay, and cost utilization per case (Hardin & Kaplow, 2005).

REFERENCES

American Association of Critical Care Nurses. (2014). *The AACN Synergy Model for Patient Care*. Retrieved from http://www.aacn.org/wd/certifications/docs/synergymodelfor patientcare.pdf

Arashin, K. A. (2010). Using the Synergy Model to guide the practice of rapid response teams. *Dimensions of Critical Care Nursing, 29*, 120–124.

Baron, R. M., & Kenny, D. A. (1986). The moderator-mediator variable distinction in social psychological research: Conceptual, strategic, and statistical considerations. *Journal of Personality and Social Psychology 51*, 1173–1182.

Belcher, A., & Griffiths, M. (2005). The spiritual care perspectives and practices of hospice nurses. *Journal of Hospice and Palliative Nursing, 7*, 271–279.

Brewer, B. B. (2007). Measurement of the Synergy Model. In M. A. Q. Curley (Ed.), *Synergy: The unique relationship between nurses and patients. The AACN synergy model for patient care* (pp. 239–253). Indianapolis, IN: Sigma Theta Tau International.

Burd, C., Langemo, D. K., Olson, B., Hanson, D., Hunter, S., & Sauvage, T. (1992). Skin problems: Epidemiology of pressure ulcers in a skilled care facility. *Journal of Gerontological Nursing, 18*(9), 29–39.

Burkhart, L. (2005). A click away. Documenting spiritual care. *Journal of Christian Nursing, 22*(1), 6–12.

Cavendish, R., Konecny, L., Mitzeliotis, C., Russo, D., Luise, B. K., Lanza, M., . . . Bajo, M. A. M. (2003). Spiritual care activities of nurses using nursing interventions classification (NIC) labels. *International Journal of Nursing Terminologies and Classifications, 14*, 113–124.

Chism, L. A., & Magnan, M. A. (2009). The relationship of nursing students' spiritual care perspectives to their expressions of spiritual empathy. *Journal of Nursing Education, 48*, 597–605.

Cress-Ingebo, R., & Chrisagis, X. (1998). Try a good book: Bibliotherapy as spiritual care. *Journal of Christian Nursing, 15*(2), 14–17.

Curley, M. A. (1998). Patient-nurse synergy: Optimizing patient outcomes. *American Journal of Critical Care, 7*, 64–72.

Curley, M. A. Q. (2007a). The AACN Synergy Model for patient care revisited. In M. A. Q. Curley (Ed.), *Synergy: The unique relationship between nurses and patients. The AACN synergy model for patient care* (pp. 25–35). Indianapolis, IN: Sigma Theta Tau International.

Curley, M. A. Q. (2007b). The Synergy Model: From theory to practice. In M. A. Q. Curley (Ed.), *Synergy: The unique relationship between nurses and patients. The AACN synergy model for patient care* (pp. 1–23). Indianapolis, IN: Sigma Theta Tau International.

Cypress, B. S. (2013). Using the Synergy Model of Patient Care in understanding the lived emergency department experiences of patients, family members, and their nurses during critical illness: A phenomenological study. *Dimensions of Critical Care Nursing, 32,* 310–321.

Fontaine, D. K., & Prevost, S. S. (2005). Foreword. In S. R. Hardin & R. Kaplow (Eds.), *Synergy for clinical excellence: The AACN synergy model for patient care* (p. xi). Burlington, MA: Jones & Bartlett.

Gillam, S., & Siriwardena, A. N. (2013). Frameworks for improvement: Clinical audit, the plan–do–study–act cycle and significant event audit. *Quality in Primary Care, 21,* 123–130.

Hardin, S. R., & Kaplow, R. (2005). *Synergy for clinical excellence: The AACN synergy model for patient care.* Burlington, MA: Jones & Bartlett.

Kaplow, R., & Hardin, S. R. (Eds.). (2007). *Critical care nursing: Synergy for optimal outcomes.* Burlington, MA: Jones & Bartlett.

Kohr, L. M., Hickey, P. A., & Curley, M. A. Q. (2012). Building a nursing productivity measure based on the Synergy Model: First steps. *American Journal of Critical Care, 21,* 420–431.

Miles, M., & Huberman, A. (1994). *Qualitative data analysis: An expanded sourcebook.* Thousand Oaks, CA: Sage.

Pérez, J., Rex Smith, A., Norris, R., Canenguez, K., Tracey, E., & DeCristofaro, S. (2011). Types of prayer and depressive symptoms among cancer patients: The mediating role of rumination and social support. *Journal of Behavioral Medicine, 34,* 519–530.

Radloff, L. S. (1977). The CES-D scale: A self-report depression scale for research in the general population. *Applied Psychological Measurement, 1,* 385–401.

Reed, K., Cline, M., & Kerfoot, K. (2007). Implementation of the Synergy Model in critical care. In R. Kaplow & S. R. Hardin (Eds.), *Critical care nursing: Synergy for optimal outcomes* (pp. 3–12). Burlington, MA: Jones & Bartlett.

Sanderson, S. (2014). Evidence-based staffing: Using the Synergy Model to improve patient and nurse outcomes in the intensive care unit. *Critical Care Nurse, 34*(2), E9–E10.

Smith, A. R. (2006). Using the synergy model to provide spiritual nursing care in critical care settings. *Critical Care Nurse, 26,* 41–47.

Smith, A. R. (2007). Using the Synergy Model to study spirituality in intermediate care: Report of a pilot study. *American Journal of Critical Care, 16,* 314–315. [Abstract].

Smith, A. R. (2011). FAQs in spiritual care: What if a patient doesn't want prayer? *Journal of Christian Nursing, 28,* 235.

Taylor, E. (2006). *Spiritual Care Perspectives Scale (SCPS)-Revised. (Description and development of SCPS)* (Unpublished manuscript). Loma Linda University, Loma Linda, CA.

Tejero, L. M. S. (2010). Development and validation of an instrument to measure nurse-patient bonding. *International Journal of Nursing Studies 47,* 608–615.

Tejero, L. M. S. (2012). The mediating role of the nurse–patient dyad bonding in bringing about patient satisfaction. *Journal of Advanced Nursing, 68,* 994–1002.

van Manen, M. (1990). *Researching lived experience: Human science for an action sensitive pedagogy.* Albany, NY: State University Press.

Venes, D. (Ed.). (2013). *Taber's cyclopedic medical dictionary* (22nd ed.). Philadelphia, PA: F. A. Davis.

Villarruz-Sulit, M. V., Dans, A., & Javeloza, M. A. (2009). Measuring satisfaction with nursing care of patients admitted in the medical wards of the Philippine General Hospital. *Acta Medica Philippina, 43*(4), 52–56.

Wysong, P. R., & Driver, E. (2009). Patients' perceptions of nurses' skill. *Critical Care Nurse, 29*(4), 24–37.

CHAPTER 10

THE TRANSITIONS FRAMEWORK[1]

The Transitions Framework focuses on "the human experiences, the responses, [and] the consequences of transitions on the well-being of people" (Meleis, 2010c, p. 2). The goal of Transitions Framework nursing is "to help people go through healthy transitions, [including mastery of behaviors, sentiments, cues, and symbols associated with new roles and identities] and non-problematic processes, to enhance healthy outcomes" (Im, 2010, p. 417; Meleis, 2010c, p. 5).[2]

TRANSITIONS FRAMEWORK: CONCEPTS AND NON-RELATIONAL PROPOSITIONS

This section of the chapter includes the concepts of the Transitions Framework and the definitions (non-relational propositions) of the concepts and the dimensions of the multidimensional concepts.

Transition is defined as a process of "change in health status, or in role relationships, expectations, or abilities. It denotes changes in needs of all human systems. Transition requires the person to incorporate new knowledge, to alter behavior, and therefore to change the definition of self in social context" (Meleis, 2012, p. 100); "a passage from one fairly stable state to another fairly stable state" (Meleis, 2010b, p. 11); and "the experience of losses and gains, changes and transformations" (Meleis, 2010a, p. 619). "Transitions are both a result of and result in change in lives, health, relationships, and environments" (Meleis, Sawyer, Im, Hilfinger Messias, & Schumacher, 2000). The process of a transition includes anticipating, defined as expecting that a transition will occur; experiencing, defined as the actual experience of a transition; and completing, defined as finishing the process of a transition.

Transition Type is defined as various circumstances that require a process of change. The five dimensions of Transitions Type are developmental transition, situational transition, wellness/illness transition, organizational transition, and cultural transition.

Developmental transition is defined as a normative and dynamic process of biophysical, psychosocial, and spiritual change associated with the stages and phases of maturation throughout the lifespan (Clayton State University School of Nursing, 2012; Hanna, 2012).

Situational transition is defined as a process of change associated with circumstances that represent losses and gains occuring throughout the life span (Im, 2014).

Wellness/illness transition is defined as a process of biopsychosocial and spiritual change associated with development, diagnosis, and treatment of disease and full recovery from disease or development of chronic illness.

Organizational transition is defined as a process of change within an organization, specifically, "changing environmental conditions that affect the lives of clients and workers" (Im, 2014, p. 257).

Cultural transition is defined as "the process of moving from one culture to another and usually accompanies a geographic relocation. A cultural transition includes all of the variables within a culture such as language, food, social mores and behaviors, rules and laws, attitudes, and values" (Baird, 2012, p. 255). The subdimensions of a cultural transition are separation, liminality, and integration.[3]

Separation is defined as the first phase of a cultural transition, which involves "separation and displacement from [the] culture of origin and culture of identity" (Baird, 2012, p. 257). The separation may extend over time and involve many separations.

Liminality is defined as the second phase of a cultural transition, which involves feeling "being in an in-between or liminal space…[This subdimension] is central in the process of cultural transition. A liminal state is associated with a profound paradox. In one sense, being in a liminal state is negative as all past form and structure are lost. At the same time, the liminal state includes great potential…for change and positive transformation" (Baird, 2012, p. 258).

Integration is defined as the third phase of a cultural transition, which involves adjustment and adaptation to the new culture; " 'the simultaneous ethnic retention and adaptation to the new society'" (Phinney, Horenczyk, Liebkind, & Vedder, as cited in Baird, 2012, p. 258).

Transition Patterns is defined as aspects of transitions that may or may not overlap (Meleis et al., 2000, p. 18). The six dimensions of Transitions Patterns are single transition, multiple transitions, sequential transitions, simultaneous transitions, related transitions, and unrelated transitions.

Single transition is defined as one transition occuring at a particular time.

Multiple transitions is defined as more than one transition occuring at the same time.

Sequential transitions is defined as one transition leading directly to another transition that may or may not be related (Coffey, 2014).

Simultaneous transitions is defined as clusters of two or more transitions occuring at the same time that may or may not be related (Coffey, 2014).

Related transitions is defined as two or more transitions that are associated with each other.

Unrelated transitions is defined as two or more transitions that are not associated with each other.

Transition Properties is defined as complex interrelated processes that occur during the overall transition process (Meleis et al., 2000). The five dimensions of Transition Properties are awareness, engagement, change and difference, transition time span, and critical points and events.

Awareness is defined as "perception, knowledge, and recognition of a transition experience... [including] physical, emotional, social, or environmental changes" (Im, 2010, pp. 420–421). More specifically, awareness is the "degree of congruency between what is known about processes and responses and what constitutes an expected set of responses and perceptions of individuals undergoing similar transitions" (Meleis et al., 2000, pp. 18–19).

Engagement is defined as "the degree to which a person demonstrates involvement in the processes inherent in the transition" (Meleis et al., 2000, p. 19).

Change and difference. Change is defined as "Changes in a person's identities, roles, relationships, abilities, and behaviors" (Im, 2014, p. 358). Difference is defined as "unmet or divergent expectations, feeling different, being perceived as different, or seeing the world and others in different ways" (Meleis et al., 2000, p. 20).

Transition time span is defined as "a span of time with an identifiable starting point, extending from the first signs of anticipation, perception, or demonstration of change; moving through a period of instability, confusion, and distress; and on to an eventual ending with a new beginning or period of stability" (Im, 2014, p. 259), which may be difficult or impossible to document (Meleis et al., 2000).

Critical points and events is defined as "Final critical points are identified by a sense of comfort in new schedules, competence, lifestyles, and self-care behaviors" (Im, 2014, p. 259). These "identifiable marker event[s]... [are] often associated with increasing awareness of change or difference or more active engagement in dealing with the transition experience" (Meleis et al., 2000, p. 21).

Transition Conditions is defined as "those circumstances that influence the way a person moves through a transition, and that facilitate or hinder progress toward achieving a healthy transition" (Im, 2010, p. 421). The two dimensions of Transition Conditions are personal characteristics and environmental characteristics (Hanna, 2012).

Personal characteristics is defined as individual factors that can facilitate or inhibit the process of transition. The five subdimensions of personal characteristics are perceptions of and meanings attached to health, cultural beliefs, socioeconomic status, preparation, and knowledge.

Perceptions of and meanings attached to health is defined as "subjective appraisal of an anticipated event [i.e., a transition] and the evaluation of its likely effect on one's life" (Coffey 2014, p. 53), which "may facilitate or hinder healthy transitions" (Meleis et al., 2000, pp. 21–22).

Cultural beliefs is defined as hindrance to a transition if the transition is stigmatized in a culture (Meleis et al., 2000).

Socioeconomic status is defined as facilitator of or hindrance to a transition depending on level of education and category of occupation.

Preparation is defined as being informed about and having access to resources for the transition (J. B. Foust, personal communication, January 6, 2015). "Anticipatory preparation facilitates the transition experience, whereas lack of preparation is an inhibitor" (Meleis et al., 2000, p. 22).

Knowledge is defined as acquisition of information "about what to expect during a transition and what strategies may be helpful in managing it" (Meleis et al., 2000, p. 23).

Environmental Characteristics is defined as factors external to the individual that can facilitate or inhibit the process of transition. The two subdimensions of environmental characteristics are community resources and societal conditions.

Community resources is defined as extent of "availability of support from family, friends, and services; relevant information; role models; and advice" (Coffey, 2014, p. 53), which may facilitate or inhibit a transition (Meleis et al., 2000).

Societal conditions is defined as the views of society at large, which may facilitate or inhibit a transition. Societal stigmatization, stereotyping, and marginalization are inhibitors of a transition (Coffey, 2014; Meleis et al., 2000).

Nursing Therapeutics is defined as "all nursing activities and actions deliberately designed to care for nursing clients" (Barnard, as cited in Meleis, 2012, p. 105); especially "those interventions or actions that can modify or influence the outcomes of a transition" (Baird, 2012, p. 259). The dimensions of Nursing Therapeutics are assessment of readiness, risk assessment, transition preparation, role supplementation, creation of a healthy environment, and monitoring.

Assessment of readiness is defined as the determination of the person's readiness for the transition experience, which "requires multidisciplinary efforts and should be based on a comprehensive understanding of the client" (Im, 2014, p. 261).

Risk assessment is defined as determination of the actual or potential risk that the transition experience may pose (J. B. Foust, personal communication, September 23, 2013).

Transition preparation is defined as an intervention made by a nurse in collaboration with or referral to other members of the health care team directed toward the client's being informed about and having access to resources for the transition (J. B. Foust, personal communication, January 6, 2015) and toward promotion of "well-being and mastery of the changes that result from the transition" (Meleis, 2010a, p. 619).

Role supplementation is defined as a nursing intervention used to overcome client role insufficiency, which refers to difficulty with performance of role activities and occurs when the client is "not properly prepared for a transitional experience" (Meleis, 2010b, p. 11); Role supplementation is "the process of bringing into awareness the behaviors, sentiments, sensations, and goals involved in a given role...[which] involves facilitating new knowledge through role-modeling, support, and revision of skills and capabilities" (Coffey, 2014, p. 54).

Creation of a healthy environment is defined as a nursing intervention that involves the nurse working in collaboration with other members of the health care team and "with patient and family to create...healthy...physical, social, political and cultural surroundings...to meet their needs and to promote dignity and personal integrity...[by means of] mobilization of...personal, family, and community...resources" (Coffey, 2014, p. 55).

Monitoring is defined as determining the results of nursing interventions (J. B. Foust, personal communication, September 23, 2013), with emphasis on response patterns process indicators and outcome indicators.

Response Patterns is defined as "those factors that indicate movement toward enhanced or diminished well-being" (Baird, 2012, p. 259). The two dimensions of Response Patterns are process indicators and outcome indicators.

Process indicators is defined as responses manifested during and after the process of transition. The four subdimensions of process indicators are feeling connected, interacting, location and being situated, and developing confidence and coping.

Feeling connected is defined as "the need to feel and stay connected" to family members, friends, and health care team members (Meleis et al., 2000, p. 24), as well as to social networks and community services (Coffey, 2014).

Interacting is defined as "intra-dyadic interaction" (Meleis et al., 2000, p. 24).

Location and being situated is defined as living conditions and situating self "in terms of time, space, and relationships" (Coffey, 2014, p. 54).

Developing confidence and coping is defined as "experiencing an increase in...the level of understanding of the different processes inherent" in all aspects of the transition and developing strategies to manage the transition (Meleis et al., 2000, p. 25).

Outcome Indicators is defined as results of nursing intervention as the person is going through a transition. The five subdimensions of outcome indicators are mastery, fluid integrative identities, health outcomes, developmental outcomes, and behavioral outcomes (Hanna, 2012).

Mastery is defined as "the extent to which individuals demonstrate [competence and comfort with performance] of the skills needed to manage their new situations or environments" (Meleis et al., 2000, p. 26).

Fluid integrative identities is defined as "identity reformulation...[that is] fluid rather than static,...dynamic rather than stable" (Meleis et al., 2000, p. 26).

Health outcomes is defined as transition-specific wellness- or illness-related results of the transition and quality of life following the transition (Hanna, 2012).

Developmental outcomes is defined as the extent of "autonomy or independence in behaviors and decision-making related to [the transition] with a goal of ownership for [self-]care" (Hanna, 2012, p. 403).

Behavioral outcomes is defined as "how well [self-management] tasks are performed" (Hanna, 2012, p. 403). The goal of self-management is maintenance of wellness.

TRANSITIONS FRAMEWORK: RELATIONAL PROPOSITIONS

The statements of associations (relational propositions) among concepts of the Transitions Framework are listed here.

- Transition Properties are interrelated (Meleis et al., 2000)
- Transition Type, Transition Patterns, and Transition Properties are interrelated (Meleis et al., 2000).
- The personal characteristics and environmental characteristics dimensions of Transition Conditions are interrelated (Meleis et al., 2000).
- Transition Type, Transition Patterns, and Transition Properties are related to Transition Conditions (Meleis et al., 2000).
- The process indicators' and outcome indicators' dimensions of Response Patterns are interrelated (Meleis et al., 2000).
- Transitions Conditions are related to Response Patterns (Hanna, 2012; Meleis et al., 2000).
- The relations of Transition Type, Transition Patterns, and Transition Properties with Response Patterns are mediated by Transition Conditions (Meleis, 2010a).
- Nursing Therapeutics affects Transition Properties, Transition Conditions, and Response Patterns (Meleis et al., 2000).

TRANSITIONS FRAMEWORK: APPLICATION TO NURSING PRACTICE

The guidelines for Transitions Framework nursing practice are listed in Box 10.1. A diagram of the practice methodology for the Transitions Framework, which is called Nursing Therapeutics, is illustrated in Figure 10.1.

BOX 10.1 Guidelines for Transitions Framework Nursing Practice

The purpose of Transitions Framework–based nursing practice is to promote movement through transitions toward enhanced wellness by collaborating and cooperating with the person who is anticipating, experiencing, or completing a transition and other members of the health care team to address the person's "critical needs...during admission, discharge, recovery, and transfer" (Schumacher & Meleis, 1994, p. 125).

Practice problems of interest encompass consideration of the way in which people move through transitions, including developmental, situational, wellness/illness, organizational, and cultural transitions, recognizing that "Negotiating successful transitions depends on the development of an effective relationship between the nurse and client. This relationship is a highly reciprocal process that affects both the client and nurse" (Clayton State University School of Nursing, 2012).

Nursing may be practiced wherever people are experiencing transitions such as in their homes, in the community, and in clinical agencies.

Legitimate participants in nursing practice are all people who are anticipating or currently experiencing transitions and their family members.

The practice methodology is Nursing Therapeutics. The components of Nursing Therapeutics are assessment of readiness; risk assessment; intervention, including transition preparation, role supplementation, and creation of a healthy environment; and monitoring.

Transitions Framework–based nursing practice contributes to the well-being of people by facilitating their passage "from one fairly stable state to another fairly stable state" (Meleis, 2010b, p. 11).

Constructed from Baird (2012); Clayton State University School of Nursing (2012); Coffey (2014); Im (2014); and Meleis (2010b).

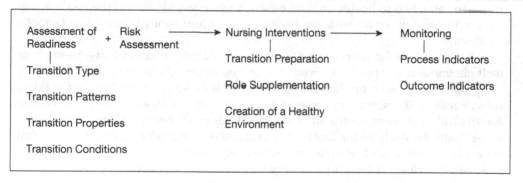

FIGURE 10.1 The Transitions Framework practice methodology: Nursing Therapeutics.

A practice tool that includes all aspects of the Transitions Framework practice methodology is given in Box 10.2.

A Conceptual–Theoretical–Empirical Structure for Assessment

Rossen's (2007/2010) reprinted journal article is an example of a report of explicit Transitions Framework–based practice focused on assessment. The purpose of

BOX 10.2 The Transitions Framework Practice Methodology Tool

Transitional care nursing practice is a comprehensive and holistic approach to caring for people who are anticipating, experiencing, or completing transitions.

The nurse first develops an effective relationship with the person who is anticipating, experiencing, or completing a transition and with his or her significant others, using effective communication techniques and a culturally sensitive approach. The nurse may mentor the person throughout the transition.

The nurse continuously collaborates and cooperates in interactive planning with other members of the health care team, with the person who is anticipating, experiencing, or completing a transition, and with his or her significant others.

The nurse ensures continuity of health care through consistency of health care providers throughout the transition. The nurse may accompany the person who is anticipating, experiencing, or completing a transition during visits to other providers.

ASSESSMENT OF READINESS

Together, the nurse and the person who is anticipating, experiencing, or completing a transition identify the transition type—developmental, wellness/illness, situational, organizational, or cultural.

The nurse then determines whether the person is aware of changes that occur with the transition, including the nature, time span, importance or severity of the changes, as well as expectations stemming from the changes and the person's level of comfort with and mastery of the changes.

The nurse also determines the extent of the person's engagement with the transition.

Next, the nurse develops a profile of the person's readiness for the transition by assessing each transition condition—the personal characteristics of perceptions of and meanings attached to health, cultural beliefs, socioeconomic status, preparation, and knowledge; and the environmental characteristics of community resources and societal conditions.

The nurse and the person together then identify the transition pattern—single or multiple transitions; if multiple, sequential or simultaneous, related or unrelated.

Finally, the nurse then determines whether the person is ready for the transition, using a scale of 0 = not ready, 1 = starting to be ready, 2 = almost ready, or 3 = ready. Alternatively, readiness for transition practice tools could be developed. An example is the Readiness Assessment Tool (Porter et al., 2014). Alternatively, practice tools that were initially developed as research instruments could be used. An example is the Readiness for Hospital Discharge Scale (Weiss & Piacentine, 2006).

RISK ASSESSMENT

Based on the results of the assessment of readiness, the nurse and the person who is anticipating, experiencing, or completing a transition together determine the extent of actual or potential risk that the transition may pose for the person, using a scale of 0 = no risk, 1 = some risk, or 2 = a great deal of risk.

(continued)

BOX 10.2 The Transitions Framework Practice Methodology Tool (continued)

INTERVENTION: TRANSITION PREPARATION

In collaboration with the person who is anticipating, experiencing, or completing a transition, his or her significant others, and other members of the health care team, the nurse designs and implements educational and supportive interventions that are age, gender, and culturally appropriate to create conditions that are optimal for movement through the processes of the transition.

INTERVENTION: ROLE SUPPLEMENTATION

In collaboration with the person who is anticipating, experiencing, or completing a transition, his or her significant others, and other members of the health care team, the nurse designs and implements interventions targeted to people who do not yet have mastery of the behaviors, sentiments, sensations, and goals required for the performance of activities associated with performance of new roles required by the transition. Interventions may include role modeling, provision of physical and psychological support, and teaching new skills.

INTERVENTION: CREATION OF A HEALTHY ENVIRONMENT

In collaboration with the person who is anticipating, experiencing, or completing a transition, his or her significant others, and other members of the health care team, the nurse designs and implements interventions that draw on available resources from the person, his or her family members, and the community to meet the person's needs and create physical, social, political, and cultural surroundings that are conducive to well-being.

MONITORING

The nurse determines the results of nursing interventions by evaluating response patterns, including the process indicators of feeling connected, interacting, location and being situated, and developing confidence and coping; and the outcome indicators of mastery, fluid integrative identities, health outcomes, developmental outcomes, and behavioral outcomes. The nurse asks the person to identify the extent of his or her overall subjective feeling of well-being, on a scale of 0 = not at all well to 10 = extreme well-being.

Constructed from J. B. Foust (personal communication, September 23, 2013) and from interpretations of Foust (1994); Im (2010); Meleis et al. (2000); Naylor et al. (2009); and Schumacher and Meleis (1994).

her journal article was to describe two assessment tools "for determining the readiness of an older person to move to independent congregate living and proposed areas for the older person to think about to promote readiness for the move" (p. 182).

The theory is assessment of readiness for later-life relocation. The conceptual model concept is Transition Type; the relevant dimension of the concept is situational transition. The theory concept is Later-Life Relocation, which represents the situational transition dimension of Transition Type. Later-Life Relocation is assessed by two investigator developed tools—the Readiness to Move Assessment Tool (RMAT) and the Self-Efficacy Relocation Scale (SERS; Rossen & Gruber, 2007).

The conceptual–theoretical–empirical (CTE) structure that was constructed from Rossen's (2007/2010) journal article is illustrated in Figure 10.2. The non-relational propositions for each component of the CTE structure are listed in Box 10.3.

A CTE Structure for Intervention

Kelley and Lakin's (1988/2010) reprinted journal article is an example of a report of explicit Transitions Framework–based practice focused on intervention. The purpose of their journal article was to describe "the use of role supplementation as a nursing intervention to promote effective adaptation, functioning, and growth in one family in which a member had Alzheimer's disease" (p. 572).

Kelley and Lakin (2010) described a case study of a married couple who received 17 home visits by a nurse during a period of 11 months. The husband was an 83-year-old "retired professional man, [who] was previously very active with community service, many hobbies, and travelling. . . . He was diagnosed with Alzheimer's disease (confusional phase) after an extensive medical work-up for the symptoms of agitation, extreme forgetfulness, and mild ataxia ataxia" (Kelley & Laking, 2010, p. 573). The wife was a 75-year-old woman who was the home manager, mother to one adult child and since her husband's diagnosis of Alzheimer's disease, his caregiver. During the past year, she had experienced frequent epigastric burning, decreased appetite, dizziness, headaches, interrupted sleep due to her husband's nighttime wandering, and a moderate level of anxiety. The wife told the visiting nurse that "her relationship with [her husband] had altered drastically during the past year. Problems with their interaction were clearly evident during early home visits" (Kelley & Lakin, 2010, p. 574). The wife also had decreased her contacts with friends.

The theory is the effect of role supplementation nursing intervention on role sufficiency. One conceptual model concept is Nursing Therapeutics. The relevant dimension of the concept is role supplementation. The other conceptual model concept is Response Patterns. The relevant dimension of the concept is outcome indicators, and the relevant subdimension of outcomes indicators is mastery.

One theory concept is Role Supplementation Nursing Interventions. The five dimensions of the concept are role clarification, role modeling, role rehearsal, reference group interactions, and role taking. The other theory concept is Role Sufficiency.

The role supplementation dimension of Nursing Therapeutics is represented by Role Supplementation Nursing Interventions and its dimensions.

BOX 10.3 An Example of a Conceptual–Theoretical–Empirical Structure for Transitions Framework Nursing Practice: Assessment

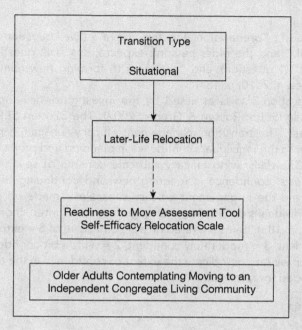

FIGURE 10.2 Conceptual–theoretical–empirical (CTE) structure for Transitions Framework practice: Assessment—theory of assessment of readiness for later-life relocation.

The *non-relational propositions* for the *C component* of the conceptual–theoretical–empirical (CTE) structure are:

- *Transition Type* is defined as various circumstances that require a process of change.
- The relevant dimension of Transition Type is situational transition.
  - o *Situational transition* is defined as "complex person-environment interactions embedded in the context and the situation that consist of both the disruption of the person's life and the person's responses to the disruption" (Rossen, 2010, p. 183).

The *non-relational propositions* for the *T component* of the CTE structure are:

- *Later-Life Relocation* is defined as "a situational transition . . . [that] comprises initiation of the move . . . to independent congregate living communities, . . . the actual move, and subsequent adjustment to the new setting" (Rossen, 2010, p. 182).

The *non-relational propositions* for the *E component* of the CTE structure are:

- Later-Life Relocation is assessed by the investigator-developed Readiness to Move Assessment Tool (RMAT), which may be administered as an interview. The RMAT includes 18 open-ended questions that assess older people's readiness to move to an independent living congregate community (ILC), including "choice in relocation"

(continued)

BOX 10.3 An Example of a Conceptual–Theoretical–Empirical
Structure for Transitions Framework Nursing Practice: Assessment
(continued)

(three questions), "preparation for the move" (five questions), "congruence
between the ILC and the older person's expectations" (six questions), "existence
of a confidant" (1 question), and "openness to forming new relationships" (three
questions) (Rossen, 2010, p. 184).
- Later-Life Relocation also is assessed by the investigator-developed Self-Efficacy
Relocation Scale (SERS; Rossen & Gruber, 2007). The 32-item SERS encompasses
three subscales: "The transition management efficacy subscale is made up of nine
items that refer to the individual's confidence in planning and preparing the activities
of moving.... The daily living efficacy subscale consists of seven items that refer
to the individuals' confidence in meeting new and continuing demands of living
at the ILC,... and the engagement efficacy subscale is made up of 16 items that
refer to the individual's confidence in engaging in social interactions and activities"
(Rossen, 2010, p. 185). Items are rated on a 5-point scale of 5 = extremely confident,
4 = very confident, 3 = moderately confident, 2 = a little bit confident, to 1 = not at
all confident; these ratings indicate the extent of confidence in the ability to perform
behaviors needed for relocation.

Source: Rossen (2010).

The mastery subdimension of outcomes indicators, which is a dimension of
Response Patterns, is represented by Role Sufficiency.

Role Supplementation Nursing Interventions is operationalized by the Role
Supplementation Nursing Intervention protocol. Role Sufficiency is evaluated
by indicators of physiological stress response (blood pressure, physical activity,
time to fall asleep, feeling relaxed, weight, appetite, headaches, and epigastric
burns) and by patterns of interacting with spouse and friends.

The CTE structure that was constructed from an interpretation of Kelley
and Lakin's (1988/2010) journal article is illustrated in Figure 10.3. The non-
relational and relational propositions for each component of the CTE structure
are listed in Box 10.4.

TRANSITIONS FRAMEWORK: APPLICATION
TO QUALITY IMPROVEMENT PROJECTS

The guidelines for Transitions Framework quality improvement (QI) projects
are listed in Box 10.5.

A CTE Structure for a QI Project

Porter et al.'s (2014) journal article is an example of a report of a QI project that
is consistent with the Transitions Framework. The purpose of their project was

BOX 10.4 An Example of a Conceptual–Theoretical–Empirical Structure for Transitions Framework Nursing Practice: Intervention

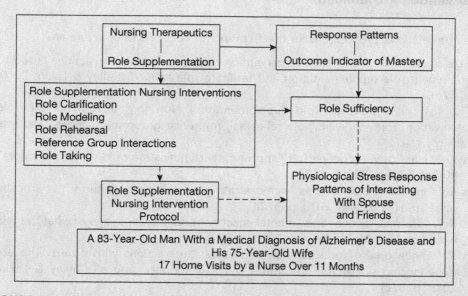

FIGURE 10.3 Conceptual–theoretical–empirical (CTE) structure for Transitions Framework practice: Intervention—theory of effect of role supplementation nursing intervention on role sufficiency.

The *non-relational propositions* for the *C* component of the conceptual–theoretical–empirical (CTE) structure are:

- *Nursing Therapeutics* is defined as "all nursing activities and actions deliberately designed to care for nursing clients" (Barnard, as cited in Meleis, 2012, p. 105); especially "those interventions or actions that can modify or influence the outcomes of a transition" (Baird, 2012, p. 259)
- The relevant dimension of Nursing Therapeutics is role supplementation.
  - o *Role supplementation* is defined as "the conveying of information or experience necessary to bring the role incumbent and significant others to full awareness of the anticipated behavior patterns, units, sentiments, sensations, and goals involved in each role and its complement. It includes necessary knowledge and experience that emphasizes heightened awareness of one's own roles and other's roles and the dynamics of the interrelationships" (Kelley & Lakin, 2010, p. 572)
- *Response Patterns* is defined as "those factors that indicate movement toward enhanced or diminished well-being" (Baird, 2012, p. 259).
- The relevant dimension of Response Patterns is outcome indicators.
  - o *Outcome indicators* is defined as results of nursing intervention as the person is going through a transition.
  - o The relevant subdimension of outcome indicators is mastery.

    - *Mastery* is defined as "the extent to which individuals demonstrate [competence and comfort with performance] of the skills needed to manage their new situations or environments" (Meleis et al., 2000, p. 26).

(continued)

BOX 10.4 An Example of a Conceptual–Theoretical–Empirical Structure for Transitions Framework Nursing Practice: Intervention *(continued)*

The *non-relational propositions* for the *T component* of the CTE structure are:

- *Role Supplementation Nursing Interventions* is defined as nursing actions "used to implement role supplementation and facilitate role taking" (Kelley & Lakin, 2010, p. 576).
- The five dimensions of Role Supplementation Nursing Interventions are role clarification, role modeling, role rehearsal, reference group interactions, and role taking.
  - o *Role clarification* is defined as "appropriate identification of new role behaviors" (Kelley & Lakin, 2010, p. 572).
  - o *Role modeling* is defined as "demonstrating behaviors associated with particular roles" (Kelley & Lakin, 2010, p. 572).
  - o *Role rehearsal* is defined as "mental enactment, fantasy, or image of what the role would be like" (Kelley & Lakin, 2010, p. 572).
  - o *Reference group interactions* is defined as "interactions with others who are experiencing similar role transitions, such as support groups" (Kelley & Lakin, 2010, p. 572).
  - o *Role taking* is defined as "effective demonstration of appropriate role behaviors" (Kelley & Lakin, 2010, pp. 572–573).
- *Role Sufficiency* is defined as an individual's "[clear] expectations of the knowledge, attitudes, values, and skills essential to performing a new role" (Kelley & Lakin, 2010, p. 572). Role insufficiency is unclear expectations.

The *non-relational propositions* for the *E component* of the CTE structure are:

- Role Supplementation Nursing Interventions is operationalized by the Role Supplementation Nursing Interventions protocol. The protocol includes 17 home visits made to an 83-year-old man who had a medical diagnosis of Alzheimer's disease and his 75-year-old wife over a period of 11 months. Early visits occurred every week and were "gradually decreased to every other week, and eventually, every third week" (Kelley & Lakin, 2010, p. 573). The protocol operationalizes the five dimensions of Role Supplementation Nursing Interventions. "To clarify her role, past and present family roles were discussed, and knowledge of the process and problems associated with Alzheimer's disease were provided at [the wife's] readiness....Role modeling was provided by [the visiting nurse] during interactions with [the husband and wife]....Role rehearsal was implemented by using mental imagery and role play, so that [the wife] could experience new behaviors during simulations of previous experiences....After about eight months,...[the wife] began to establish a modified reference group by sharing concerns with a neighbor whose husband had had an irreversible dementia and recently died....Some of the specific roles that [the wife]

(continued)

BOX 10.4 An Example of a Conceptual–Theoretical–Empirical Structure for Transitions Framework Nursing Practice: Intervention *(continued)*

was eventually able to change include improving her interactions with [her husband], managing yard maintenance (by hiring a volunteer from a local aging agency), and accepting budgetary assistance from her son and emotional support from friends" (Kelley & Lakin, 2010, p. 576).

- Role Sufficiency is measured by physiological stress response and patterns of interacting with spouse and friends (Kelley & Lakin, 2010). Physiological stress response is monitored by changes over the 11 months of home visits in several indicators, including the wife's blood pressure, physical activity, time to fall asleep, feeling relaxed, weight, appetite, headaches, and epigastric burning. Patterns of interacting are monitored by feedback from the wife about changes in the nature and content of her interactions with her husband and friends over the 11 months of home visits.

The *relational propositions* for the C and T *components* of the CTE structure are:

- Nursing Therapeutics affects Response Patterns.
- Therefore, the Role Supplementation Nursing Intervention affects Role Sufficiency. "Role supplementation is an intervention that can be used to reduce role stress and decrease, ameliorate, or prevent role insufficiency" (Kelley & Lakin, 2010, p. 572).

The *relational proposition* for the E *component* of the CTE structure is:

- Implementation of the Role Supplementation Nursing Intervention protocol affects changes in physiological stress response and changes in patterns of interacting with spouse and friends, such that Indicators of physiological stress response (blood pressure, physical activity, time to fall asleep, feeling relaxed, weight, appetite, headaches, and epigastric burning) become more positive, and feedback about patterns of interacting with spouse and friends becomes more positive.

Source: Kelley and Lakin (2010).

to describe "use of quality improvement methodology to evaluate the utility and impact of the newly created [sickle cell disease] SCD transition readiness assessment tool" (p. 264).

The theory is SCD care transition readiness. The conceptual model concept is Nursing Therapeutics; the relevant dimension is transition preparation. The theory concept, which represents the Nursing Therapeutics dimension of transition preparation, is SCD Care Transition Readiness Program.

SCD Care Transition Readiness Program is operationalized by the SCD Care Transition Readiness Program protocol and the investigator-developed Readiness Assessment Practice Tool (RAPT). Porter et al. (2104) used the Plan-Do-Study Act (PDSA) methodology (Walley & Gowland, 2004; see Appendix A) as the methodological theory for their quality improvement project. They

BOX 10.5 Guidelines for Transitions Framework Quality Improvement Projects

The purpose of Transitions Framework–based quality improvement (QI) projects is to test the extent to which nurses use one or more components of Nursing Therapeutics to enhance patient well-being during and after transitions.

The phenomenon of interest for a QI project is the extent of nurses' use of Nursing Therapeutics to enhance patient well-being during and after transitions.

Data for QI projects are to be collected from nurses and/or patients in various settings, including patients' homes, communities, nurses' private practice offices, ambulatory clinics, hospitals, and other clinical agencies.

Any methodological theory of change or QI may be used to guide the design of the QI project and the times for data collection. Checklists, rating scales, and responses to open-ended questions may be used to determine the extent to which nurses actually implement one or more components of Nursing Therapeutics—assessment of readiness, risk assessment, transition preparation, role supplementation, creation of a healthy environment, and monitoring. Descriptive statistics may be used to analyze data obtained from checklists or rating scales, and content analysis may be used to identify categories or themes found in responses to open-ended questions.

The results of Transitions Framework–based QI projects enhance the understanding of how using one or more components of Nursing Therapeutics affects the experience of transitions.

explained that three cycles of "PDSA...methodology [were] utilized to develop and evaluate the assessment tool" (Porter et al., 2014, p. 265). Descriptive statistics (numbers, percents, medians; see Appendix B) were used to document the number and percentage of adolescents who were assessed and their RAPT scores.

The CTE structure that was constructed from an interpretation of the content of Porter et al.'s (2014) journal article is illustrated in Figure 10.4. The non-relational propositions for each component of the CTE structure are listed in Box 10.6.

TRANSITIONS FRAMEWORK: APPLICATION TO NURSING RESEARCH

The guidelines for Transitions Framework nursing research are listed in Box 10.7.

A CTE Structure for a Systematic Literature Review

Kralik, Visentin, and van Loon's (2006) journal article is an example of a report of a literature review that is consistent with the Transitions Framework. The

BOX 10.6 An Example of a Conceptual–Theoretical–Empirical Structure for a Transitions Framework Quality Improvement Project

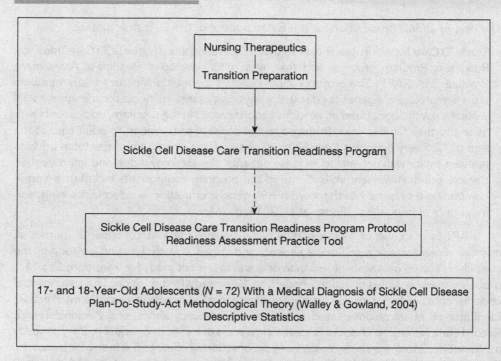

FIGURE 10.4 Conceptual–theoretical–empirical (CTE) structure for a Transitions Framework quality improvement (QI) project—theory of sickle cell disease care transition readiness.

The *non-relational propositions* for the *C component* of the conceptual–theoretical–empirical (CTE) structure are:

- *Nursing Therapeutics* is defined as "all nursing activities and actions deliberately designed to care for nursing clients" (Barnard, as cited in Meleis, 2012, p. 105); especially "those interventions or actions that can modify or influence the outcomes of a transition" (Baird, 2012, p. 259).
- The relevant dimension of Nursing Therapeutics is transition preparation.
  - o *Transition preparation* is defined as "an intervention made by a nurse in collaboration with or referral to other members of the health care team directed toward the client's being informed about and having access to resources for the transition" (J. B. Foust, personal communication, January 6, 2015) and toward promotion of "well-being and mastery of the changes that result from the transition" (Meleis, 2010a, p. 619).

The *non-relational proposition* for the *T component* of the CTE structure is:

- *The Sickle Cell Disease (SCD) Care Transition Readiness Program* is defined as an educational program designed by a multidisciplinary team to determine the readiness of adolescents to move from services of pediatric health care providers to services of adult health care providers.

(continued)

BOX 10.6 An Example of a Conceptual–Theoretical–Empirical Structure for a Transitions Framework Quality Improvement Project *(continued)*

The *non-relational proposition* for the *E component* of the CTE structure is:

- The SCD Care Transition Readiness Program is operationalized by the SCD Care Transition Readiness Program protocol and the investigator-developed Readiness Assessment Practice Tool (RAPT). The protocol stipulates that the multidisciplinary team members are a hematologist, a genetics educator, a physician's assistant, nurse coordinators, social workers, psychologists, and an academic coordinator. "In the program, adolescents with SCD and their families are introduced to the concept of transition to adult care at the age of 12. Every 6 months from 12 to 18 years of age, members of the team address relevant topics with patients to increase patients' disease knowledge and improve their disease self-management skills. Some of the program components include training in completing a personal health record (PHR), genetic education, academic planning, and independent living skills" (Porter et al., 2014, p. 264).

RAPT is made up of four checklists. The medical checklist contains 12 items that address disease literacy, self-management, and organ and dysfunction screening; the checklist is scored on a scale of less than or equal to 5 = not ready for transition, 6 to 11 = probably ready but plan of action needed, to 12 = ready for transition. The psychosocial checklist contains five items that address understanding of necessary resource information, identification of transitions-related concerns, self-advocacy ability, and Personal Health Record completion; the checklist is scored on a scale of less than or equal to 2 = not ready for transition, 3 to 4 = probably ready but plan of action needed, to 5 = ready for transition. The emotional/cognitive checklist contains two items addressing history of emotional/behavioral and cognitive concerns; the checklist is scored on a scale of 0 = not ready for transition, 1 = probably ready but plan of action needed, to 2 = ready for transition. The academic checklist contains five items addressing targeted graduation requirements, plan for education or job training, completion of steps for future planning, knowledge of educational services in the community, and self-advocacy ability for educational or vocational matters; the checklist is scored on a scale of less than or equal to 2 = not ready for transition, 3 to 4 = probably ready but plan of action needed, to 5 = ready for transition.

The Plan-Do-Study-Act (PDSA) methodological theory is used for the QI project. "PDSA is a [quality improvement] method that utilizes small-scale changes to a process…PDSA is executed in cycles and as changes are made, the process acted upon is improved" (Porter et al., 2014, p. 265). Three PDSA cycles are used for the QI project; each cycle includes the four PSDA components—"P = plan/develop; D = do/perform; S = study/learn, A = act/revise" (Porter et al., 2014, p. 266). "The objective of the first cycle [Individualized Tool Implementation] was to assess feasibility and acceptability of the assessment tool….The second cycle [Tool Revision] addressed some of the problems identified during Cycle 1….Following a few months using the assessment process [during the third cycle, Adaptation], each member of the team provided feedback about their observations from the second cycle" (Porter et al., 2014, pp. 265–266). The fourth cycle, Dissemination, which had not been completed at the time of submission of Porter et al.'s (2014) journal article, includes monthly assessments of 17-year-old adolescents with SCD with the RAPT. "Future adjustments and modifications are planned for [the RAPT] as we continue to evaluate its impact and value" (Porter et al., 2014, p. 267).

Source: Porter et al. (2014).

BOX 10.7 Guidelines for Transitions Framework Nursing Research

The purposes of Transitions Framework–based nursing research are to understand, explain, and predict how people experience transitions.

The phenomena to be studied encompass all dimensions and subdimensions of patterns, properties, conditions, and response patterns of developmental, situational, wellness/illness, organizational, and cultural transitions.

The problems to be studied are those emanating from anticipating, experiencing, and completing different types of transitions, patterns of multiple responses rather than single responses, and the effects of "nursing therapeutics designed to prevent negative consequences and enhance health outcomes" (Schumacher & Meleis, 1994, p. 125).

Research participants are people who are anticipating, experiencing, or completing a transition.

Descriptive, correlational, experimental, and mixed-methods research designs are needed to study the phenomena encompassed by the Transitions Framework. A special feature of the Transitions Framework is the contemporary emphasis on the development of situation-specific theories about particular people's experiences of a specific transition (Im, 2014). Data can be gathered in any setting where people are anticipating, experiencing, or completing a transition. Research instruments should reflect the focus and intent of the Transitions Framework and include those instruments that have been directly derived from the Transitions Framework.

Data analysis techniques include qualitative content analysis techniques and nonparametric and parametric statistical procedures.

Transitions Framework–based research facilitates understanding of the processes of transitions and the ways in which Nursing Therapeutics promotes well-being.

Constructed from Coffey (2014); Im (2014); and Schumacher and Meleis (1994).

purpose of their comprehensive literature review was to "explore how the term 'transition' had been used in the health literature" (p. 321).

Kralik et al. (2006) searched the Medline, Comprehensive Index to Nursing and Allied Health Literature Complete (CINAHL), Sociofile, and Psychlit databases using the search term "Transition," which was refined by adding the search terms "Social," "Life Events," "Illness," "Crisis," "Identity," and "Self." Additional searching was done using the search terms "Disruption," "Continuity," and "Self Identity." The database searches were augmented by a review of the reference lists of relevant retrieved articles. Articles in which transition was a central concept and those with a health or social focus were included. Articles addressing molecular or biological transitions were excluded. Inasmuch as Kralik et al.'s (2006) literature review builds on the results of a literature review by Schumacher and Meleis (1994), their review includes journal articles published between 1994 and 2004.

Forty-five full-text articles were retrieved. The final review included 23 of those articles, all of which were deemed relevant because of their focus on "how transition occurred after forced change, for example in chronic illness, where one's reality and one's sense of self were threatened or disrupted" (Kralik et al., 2006, p. 322). All 23 studies were descriptive qualitative research. The content of nonresearch articles among the 22 excluded articles was used for the discussion of transitions theoretical frameworks.

The theory is meaning of transition. The conceptual model concept is Transition. The theory concept that emerged from the literature review is Transition Meaning. The three dimensions of Transition Meaning that were discovered in the literature are movement or passage between two points, transformation or alteration, and process of inner reorientation.

The CTE structure that was constructed from the content of Kralik et al.'s (2006) journal article is illustrated in Figure 10.5. The non-relational propositions for each component of the CTE structure are listed in Box 10.8.

A CTE Structure for Instrument Development

Weiss and Piacentine's (2006) journal article is an example of a report of instrument development that is consistent with the Transitions Framework. The purpose of their study was to estimate the psychometric properties of the Readiness for Hospital Discharge Scale (RHDS) for three patient populations—adult medical–surgical patients, postpartum mothers, and parents of hospitalized children. The RHDS was used in later studies, the reports of which include explicit linkages between concepts of the Transitions Framework and theory concepts (Weiss et al., 2007; Weiss et al., 2008; Weiss & Lokken, 2009).

The theory is readiness for hospital discharge. The conceptual model concept is Nursing Therapeutics, and the relevant dimension is assessment of readiness. The theory concept is Readiness for Hospital Discharge, which represents the assessment of readiness dimension of Nursing Therapeutics. The four dimensions of the theory concept are personal status, knowledge, coping ability, and expected support.

Readiness for Hospital Discharge is measured by the RHDS. Items for the RHDS were generated from discussions with "three clinical teams each consisting of six to 12 nurse clinicians, clinical specialists, and managers in the areas of adult acute, maternal-neonatal, and pediatric care" (Weiss & Piacentine, 2006, p. 167). Weiss and Piacentine reported estimates of adequate psychometric properties for the RHDS, including content validity testing using the Content Validity Index, internal consistency reliability with Cronbach's alpha, construct validity using confirmatory factor analysis and contrasted groups comparison, and criterion-related validity using the predictive validity approach (see Appendix B). The total sample for psychometric testing was 356 participants, 121 of whom were adult medical–surgical patients, 122 of whom were postpartum mothers, and 113 of whom were parents of hospitalized children.

The CTE structure that was constructed from an interpretation of the content of Weiss and Piacentine's (2006) journal article is illustrated in Figure 10.6. The non-relational propositions for each component of the CTE structure are listed in Box 10.9.

BOX 10.8 An Example of a Conceptual–Theoretical–Empirical Structure for a Transitions Framework Literature Review

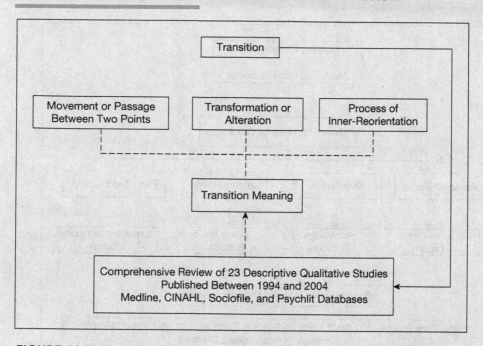

FIGURE 10.5 Conceptual–theoretical–empirical (CTE) structure for a Transitions Framework literature review—theory of meaning of transition.

The *non-relational proposition* for the *C component* of the conceptual–theoretical–empirical (CTE) structure is:

- *Transition* is defined as "a passage of change" (Kralik et al., 2006, p. 323).

The *non-relational propositions* for the *T component* of the CTE structure are:

- *Transition Meaning* is defined as understanding transitions.
- The three dimensions of Transition Meaning are movement or passage between two points, transformation or alteration, and process of inner-reorientation.
  - o *Movement or passage between two points* is defined as "the psychological processes involved in adapting to the change event or disruption" (Kralik et al., 2006, p. 322).
  - o *Transformation or alteration* is defined as involving "incorporation, integration or alteration" (Kralik et al., 2006, p. 324) of the process of transition.
  - o *Process of inner reorientation* is defined as the person's learning "to adapt and incorporate the new circumstances [of the transition] into [his or her] life" (Kralik et al., 2006, p. 324).

The *non-relational proposition* for the *E component* of the CTE structure is:

- Transition Meaning and its dimensions were discovered in a review of 23 journal articles published between 1994 and 2004.

Source: Kralik et al. (2006).

BOX 10.9 An Example of a Conceptual–Theoretical–Empirical Structure for Transitions Framework Instrument Development

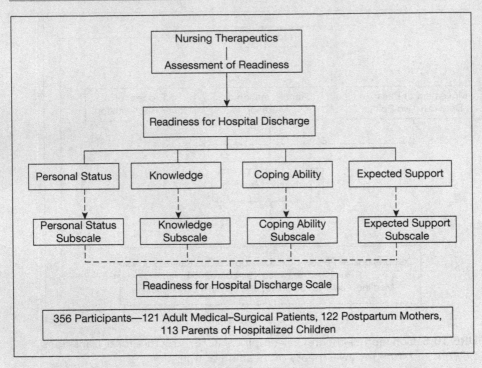

FIGURE 10.6 Conceptual–theoretical–empirical (CTE) structure for Transitions Framework instrument development—theory of readiness for hospital discharge.

The *non-relational propositions* for the *C component* of the conceptual–theoretical–empirical (CTE) structure are:

- *Nursing Therapeutics* is defined as all nursing activities and actions deliberately designed to care for nursing clients" (Barnard, as cited in Meleis, 2012, p. 105), especially "those interventions or actions that can modify or influence the outcomes of a transition" (Baird, 2012, p. 259).
- The relevant dimension of Nursing Therapeutics is assessment of readiness.
  - o *Assessment of readiness* is defined as determination of the person's readiness for the transition experience, which "requires multidisciplinary efforts and should be based on a comprehensive understanding of the client" (Im, 2014, p. 261).

The *non-relational propositions* for the *T component* of the CTE structure are:

- *Readiness for Hospital Discharge* is defined as "a judgment or perception regarding the patient's immediate state and perceived abilities that relate to managing care needs in the home environment" (Weiss & Piacentine, 2006, pp. 166–167).
- The four dimensions of Readiness for Hospital Discharge are personal status, knowledge, coping ability, and expected support.

(continued)

BOX 10.9 An Example of a Conceptual–Theoretical–Empirical Structure for Transitions Framework Instrument Development *(continued)*

- o *Personal status* is defined as "the physical-emotional state of the patient immediately prior to discharge" (Weiss & Piacentine, 2006, p. 167).
- o *Knowledge* is defined as "the perceived adequacy of information needed to respond to common concerns and problems in the posthospitalization period" (Weiss & Piacentine, 2006, p. 167).
- o *Coping ability* is defined as "the perceived ability of the patient to self-manage personal and health care needs after discharge" (Weiss & Piacentine, 2006, p. 167).
- o *Expected support* is defined as "the emotional and instrumental assistance expected to be available following hospital discharge" (Weiss & Piacentine, 2006, p. 167).

The *non-relational proposition* for the *E component* of the CTE structure is:

- Readiness for Hospital Discharge is measured by the Readiness for Hospital Discharge Scale (RHDS; Weiss & Piacentine, 2006). The RHDS is made up of 21 items written as questions and arranged in four subscales—personal status subscale (seven items), knowledge subscale (seven items), coping ability subscale (three items), and expected support subscale (four items). Each item is rated on a scale of 0 to 10. "Anchor words (e.g., *not at all, totally*) were printed at the 0 and 10 poles of the scale to cue the [participant] to the meaning of the numeric scale" (Weiss & Piacentine, 2006, p. 168).

Source: Weiss and Piacentine (2006).

A CTE Structure for Descriptive Qualitative Research

A journal article by Im, Lee, and Chee (2010) is an example of a report of descriptive qualitative research that is consistent with the Transitions Framework. The purpose of their study was "to describe the menopausal symptom experiences of Black midlife women in the United States from their own perspectives in a 6-month online forum" (p. 436).

The theory is meaning of menopause. The conceptual model concept is Transition Type; the relevant dimension of the concept is developmental transition. The theory concept is Inner Power. The four dimensions of Inner Power are raised to be strong, accepting a natural aging process, silent and without knowledge, and our own experience.

The study methodology was guided by a broad feminist perspective (see Appendix A) rather than a specific Black feminist perspective because this study is part of a larger study of menopausal transition experiences of White, Black, Hispanic, and Asian women (see also Im, 2009; Im, Lee, & Chee, 2011; Im, Liu, Dormire, & Chee, 2008). Inner Power and its four dimensions were discovered in Black midlife women's responses to discussion topics about menopausal symptoms posted on an investigator-developed and monitored qualitative online forum. Im et al. (2010) used quota sampling (see Appendix A) to "have an adequate number of early perimenopausal, late perimenopausal, and post-menopausal women from diverse socioeconomic groups" in their sample of 20 Black women (p. 437). Thematic analysis (see Appendix B) was used to identify the concept and its dimensions.

The CTE structure that was constructed from an interpretation of the content of Im et al.'s (2010) journal article is illustrated in Figure 10.7. The non-relational propositions for each component of the CTE structure are listed in Box 10.10.

A CTE Structure for Correlational Research

Weiss et al.'s (2007) journal article is an example of a report of explicit Transitions Framework correlational research. The purpose of their study was to "identify patient characteristics, hospitalization factors, and hospital nursing practices that are predictive of adult medical–surgical patients' perceptions of their readiness to go home at the time of discharge and the relationship of perceptions of discharge readiness to posthospitalization coping and utilization outcomes" (p. 32).

Weiss et al. (2007) used a correlational path model research design (see Appendix A). The 147 research participants were 78 female and 69 male adults who were patients on general medical, surgical, and cardiac units at an urban medical center in the Midwestern region of the United States.

> Patients met study inclusion criteria if they were at least 18 years old, were discharged directly home following hospitalization, had sufficient English-language skills to read and respond to consent forms and study questions, and had telephone access for postdischarge data collection. Patients were excluded if they did not have sufficient cognitive skills to complete the consenting, questionnaire, and interview processes independently or they were discharged home with hospice care. (Weiss et al., 2007, p. 34)

The theory is the relations of hospitalization factors, patient characteristics, and hospital nursing practices to readiness for hospital discharge, coping difficulty, and use of postdischarge support and services. Two conceptual model concepts are Nature of the Transition and Transition Conditions. Two other conceptual model concepts are Nursing Therapeutics and Response Patterns. The relevant dimension of Nursing Therapeutics is transition preparation. The two relevant subdimensions of the Process Indicators dimension of Response Patterns are feeling confident and competent and feeling connected.

The theory concepts are Hospitalization Factors, Patient Characteristics, Hospital Nursing Practices, Readiness for Hospital Discharge, Postdischarge Coping Difficulty, and Utilization of Postdischarge Support and Services. The two dimensions of Hospital Nursing Practices are discharge teaching and care coordination.

Nature of the Transition is represented by Hospitalization Factors, and Transitions Conditions is represented by Patient Characteristics. The transition preparation dimension of Nursing Therapeutics is represented by Hospital

BOX 10.10 An Example of a Conceptual–Theoretical–Empirical Structure for Transitions Framework Descriptive Qualitative Research

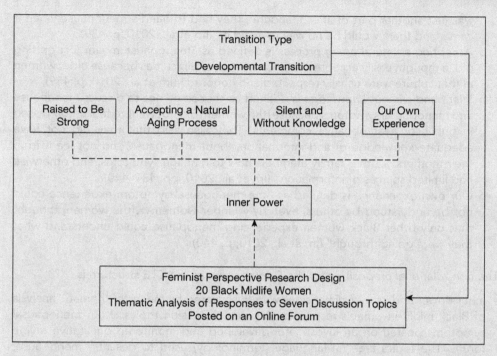

FIGURE 10.7 Conceptual–theoretical–empirical (CTE) structure for Transitions Framework descriptive qualitative research—theory of meaning of menopause.

The *non-relational propositions* for the *C component* of the conceptual–theoretical–empirical (CTE) structure are:

- *Transition Type* is defined as various circumstances that require a process of change.
- The relevant dimension of Transition Type is developmental transition.
  - *Developmental transition* is defined as a normative and dynamic process of biophysical, psychosocial, and spiritual change associated with the stages and phases of maturation throughout the life span (Clayton State University School of Nursing, 2012; Hanna, 2012).

The *non-relational propositions* for the *T component* of the CTE structure are:

- *Inner Power* is defined as a strategy used by Black midlife women "to cope with menopausal symptoms within the contexts of their daily lives as marginalized ethnic minority women" (Im et al., 2010, p. 439).
- The four dimensions of Inner Power are raised to be strong, accepting a natural aging process, silent and without knowledge, and our own experience.
  - *Raised to be strong* is defined as the women's accepting of hardship in their lives. "The women perceived that compared to other difficulties in their lives, menopause

(continued)

BOX 10.10 An Example of a Conceptual–Theoretical–Empirical Structure for Transitions Framework Descriptive Qualitative Research *(continued)*

was just another part of life to 'endure'; they had to handle menopause when it came, and there would be no way to avoid it" (Im et al., 2010, p. 439).

- o *Accepting a natural aging process* is defined as "menopause meant just getting old, a thought easily accepted without emotional difficulties because older women in that culture were usually respected and honored" (Im et al., 2010, p. 439).
- o *Silent and without knowledge* is defined as choosing "not to discuss menopause and menopausal symptoms because [the women] did not want to feel embarrassed in public or hear negative comments. They also said that they did not have adequate knowledge of and information about menopause, did not learn from their mothers or other family members how to manage symptoms, and otherwise had limited sources of information" (Im et al., 2010, pp. 439–440).
- o *Our own experience* is defined as "the menopausal symptom experience could not be understood by others, even by younger women....[the women] thought that only other Black women experiencing menopause could understand what they were going through" (Im et al., 2010, p. 440).

The *non-relational proposition* for the *E component* of the CTE structure is:

- Inner Power and its four dimensions were discovered by means of thematic analysis of Black midlife women's responses to seven discussion topics about menopausal symptoms posted on an investigator-developed and monitored qualitative online forum. The topics are "(a) language (terminology) used to describe menopause, symptoms, and menopausal symptoms and their linguistic meanings; (b) women's daily schedules, and hardships and suffering in their daily lives; (c) culturally universal and specific descriptions of menopausal symptoms; (d) women's ethnic-specific situations and responses to menopausal symptoms; (e) women's perceived ethnic-specific causes of menopausal symptoms and management strategies for menopausal symptoms; (f) factors/life events influencing women's menopausal symptom experience in their daily lives; and (g) women's preferences for symptom management strategies" (Im et al., 2010, p. 437).

Source: Im, Lee, and Chee (2010).

Nursing Practices and its dimensions. Response Patterns is represented by Readiness for Hospital Discharge, Postdischarge Coping Difficulty, and Utilization of Postdischarge Support and Services.

Hospitalization Factors and Patient Characteristics are measured by patient self-report and medical record review. The discharge teaching dimension of Hospital Nursing Practices is measured by the investigator-developed Quality of Discharge Teaching Scale (QDTS), and the core coordination dimension of Hospital Nursing Practices is measured by the investigator-developed Care Coordination Scale (CCS). Readiness for Hospital Discharge is measured by the Readiness for Hospital Discharge Scale-Adult Form (RHDS-Adult; Weiss et al., 2007; Weiss, Ryan, & Lokken, 2006). Postdischarge Coping Difficulty is measured by the investigator-developed Post-Discharge Coping Difficulty Scale (PDCDS), and Utilization of Postdischarge Support and Services is measured by patient self-report. Weiss et al. (2007) tested the path model with multiple regression and logistic regression statistics (see Appendix B).

The CTE structure that was constructed from the content of Weiss et al.'s (2007) journal article is illustrated in Figure 10.8. The non-relational and relational propositions for each component of the CTE structure are listed in Box 10.11.

A CTE Structure for Experimental Research

A journal article by Naylor et al. (2004) is an example of a report of experimental research that is consistent with the Transitions Framework. The purpose of their study was to determine the effect of a transitional care program for older adults with heart failure on hospital readmission date or date of death, reasons for readmission, life quality, level of functioning, study participant satisfaction, and costs of medical care.

Nayor et al. (2004) conducted a randomized controlled trial (Appendix A) comparing outcomes of an APN intervention with outcomes of routine care. Research participants were 65 years of age or older patients with a medical diagnosis of heart failure who were admitted to one of six hospitals in a mid-Atlantic state. Naylor et al. (2004) indicated that the inclusion criteria were that the patient "had to speak English, be alert and oriented, be reachable by telephone after discharge, and reside within a 60-mile radius service area of the admitting hospital" (p. 676). They identified the exclusion criterion as patients "with end-stage renal disease...because of their access to unique Medicare services" (p. 676). Random assignment of the 239 participants to the experimental APN intervention group ($n = 118$) or the control routine care group ($n = 121$) was done "using a computer-generated, institution-specific block 1:1 randomization algorithm" (Naylor et al., 2004, p. 676).

The theory is effects of APN intervention or routine care on rehospitalization, quality of life, functional status, patient satisfaction, and resource use and costs. One conceptual model concept is Nursing Therapeutics; the relevant dimension is creation of a healthy environment. The other conceptual model concept is Response Patterns; the relevant dimension is outcomes indicators, and the four relevant subdimensions are mastery, health outcomes, developmental outcomes, and behavioral outcomes.

One theory concept is Type of Intervention; the two dimensions are APN intervention and routine care. The other theory concepts are Rehospitalization, Quality of Life, Functional Status, Patient Satisfaction, Resource Utilization, and Resource Costs. The Nursing Therapeutics dimension of creation of a healthy environment is represented by Type of Intervention and its two dimensions. The subdimensions of Response Patterns are represented by Rehospitalization,

BOX 10.11 An Example of a Conceptual–Theoretical–Empirical Structure for Transitions Framework Correlational Research

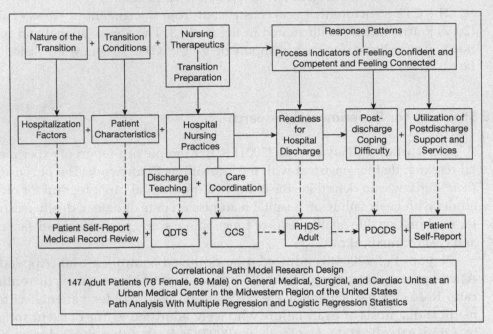

FIGURE 10.8 Conceptual–theoretical–empirical (CTE) structure for Transitions Framework correlational research—theory of relations of hospitalization factors, patient characteristics, and hospital nursing practices to readiness for hospital discharge, coping difficulty, and utilization of postdischarge support and services.

CCS, Care Coordination Scale; PDCDS, Postdischarge Coping Difficulty Scale; QDTS, Quality of Discharge Teaching Scale; RHDS-Adult, Readiness for Hospital Discharge Scale-Adult Form.

The *non-relational propositions* for the *C component* of the conceptual–theoretical–empirical (CTE) structure are:

- *Nature of the Transition* is defined as "Descriptions of the type, pattern, and properties of a transition" (Weiss et al., 2007, p. 33). "A transition is a process of passage from one life phase, condition, or status to another during which changes in health status, role relations, expectations, or abilities create a period of vulnerability" (Weiss et al., 2007, p. 32).
- *Transition Conditions* is defined as "Personal or environmental conditions that facilitate or hinder progress toward achieving a healthy transition" (Weiss et al., 2007, p. 33).
- *Nursing Therapeutics* is defined as focusing on "the prevention of unhealthy transitions, promoting perceived well-being, and dealing with the experience of transitions" (Weiss et al., 2007, p. 33).

(continued)

BOX 10.11 An Example of a Conceptual–Theoretical–Empirical Structure for Transitions Framework Correlational Research *(continued)*

- The relevant dimension of Nursing Therapeutics is transition preparation.
  - o *Transition preparation* is defined as "education targeting assumption of new role responsibilities and implementation of new skills" (Weiss et al., 2007, p. 33).
- *Response Patterns* is defined as "those factors that indicate movement toward enhanced or diminished well-being" (Baird, 2012, p. 259).
- The relevant dimension of Response Patterns is process indicators.
  - o *Process indicators* is defined as responses manifested during and after the process of transition.
  - o The two relevant subdimensions of the process indicators dimension of Response Patterns are feeling confident and competent and feeling connected.
    - *Feeling confident and competent* is defined as "Development of understanding of diagnosis, treatment, recovery, and living with limitations, and strategies for managing" (Weiss et al., 2007, p. 33).
    - *Feeling connected* is defined as "The need to feel and stay connected with, as examples, supportive persons and healthcare professionals" (Weiss et al., 2007, p. 33).

The *non-relational propositions* for the *T* component of the CTE structure are:

- *Hospitalization Factors* is defined as factors associated with hospitalization, including planned admission ("aware of admission date for at least 24 hours prior to admission"), first hospitalization (i.e., no earlier hospitalization or "number of admissions to the hospital"), previous admission for the same health condition, and length of hospital stay (Weiss et al., 2007, p. 34).
- *Patient Characteristics* is defined as patient demographics, including age, gender, race, socioecomonic status, payor, and lives alone (Weiss et al., 2007).
- *Hospital Nursing Practices* is defined as "hospital nursing strategies for preparing patients for discharge" (Weiss et al., 2007, p. 33).
- The two dimensions of Hospital Nursing Practices are discharge teaching and care coordination.
  - o *Discharge teaching* is defined as "the composite of all teaching received by the patient (from the patient's perspective) during the hospitalization in preparation for discharge home and coping with the posthospitalization period" (Weiss et al., 2007, p. 35).
  - o *Care coordination* is defined as "coordination of care through discharge planning activities" (Weiss et al., 2007, p. 33).
- *Readiness for Hospital Discharge* is defined as "a transitional outcome in the continuum of care from hospital to home...Hospital discharge was viewed as a transitional process occurring in 3 sequential phases: (1) the hospitalization phase during which discharge preparation occurs; (2) the discharge when short-term outcomes of the preparatory process can be measured; and (3) the postdischarge period when patients' perceptions of their ability to cope with the demands of care at home and their needs for support and assistance from family and health services provide evidence of positive or adverse outcomes of the patient's transitional process" (Weiss et al., 2007, pp. 32–33).

(continued)

BOX 10.11 An Example of a Conceptual–Theoretical–Empirical Structure for Transitions Framework Correlational Research *(continued)*

- *Postdischarge Coping Difficulty* is defined as "problems and concerns after hospital discharge that reflect lack of readiness for the transition from hospital to home, such as difficulties with activities of daily living, medication and pain management, health maintenance, emotional adjustment, family caregivers, and access to health and social services" (Weiss et al., 2007, p. 33).
- *Utilization of Postdischarge Support and Services* is defined as calls to family, friends, provider, and hospital; visits to provider office, a clinic, and emergency department or urgent care facility; and hospital readmission (Weiss et al., 2007).

The *non-relational propositions* for the *E component* of the CTE structure are:

- Hospitalization Factors of planned admission (0 = no, 1 = yes), first hospitalization (0 = no, 1 = yes), and previous admission for same health condition (0 = no, 1 = yes) are measured by patient self-report at the time of recruitment into the study. Hospitalization Factor of length of hospital stay is measured by medical record review (Weiss et al., 2007).
- Patient Characteristics of chronological age in years, gender (0 = male, 1 = female), race (0 = White, 1 = non-White), socioeconomic status (Hollingshead [1975] 4-Factor Index of Social Status), and lives alone (0 = no, 1 = yes) are measured by patient self-report at the time of recruitment into the study. Patient Characteristic of payor (0 = public, 1 = private) is measured by medical record review (Weiss et al., 2007).
- The discharge teaching dimension of Hospital Nursing Practices is measured by the investigator-developed Quality of Discharge Teaching Scale (QDTS; Weiss et al., 2007). The QDTS is made up of 18 items arranged in two subscales—content and delivery. The six-item content subscale addresses "the amount of 'content received' during teaching in preparation for discharge. The 12-item 'delivery' subscale reflects the skill of the nurses as educators in presenting discharge teaching and includes items about listening to and answering specific questions and concerns, expressing sensitivity to personal beliefs and values, teaching in a way that the patient could understand and at times that were good for patients and family members, providing consistent information, promoting confidence in ability to care for themselves and knowing what to do in an emergency, and decreasing anxiety about going home" (Weiss et al., 2007, p. 35). Each item on each subscale is rated on an 11-point scale of 0 to 10 with anchor words such as "not at all" and "totally."
- The core coordination dimension of Hospital Nursing Practices is measured by the investigator-developed Care Coordination Scale (CCS; Weiss et al., 2007). The CCS contains five items addressing coordination of care during preparation for hospital discharge. Each item is rated on an 11-point scale of 0 to 10 with anchor words, such as "not at all" and "totally."
- Readiness for Hospital Discharge is measured by the Readiness for Hospital Discharge Scale-Adult (RHDS-Adult) Form (Weiss et al., 2007). The RHDS-Adult, which is a modification of the Perceived Readiness for Discharge after Birth Scale (Weiss et al., 2006), contains 22 items. Twenty-one items are from the original RHDS (Weiss & Piacentine, 2006; see Box 10.9); an additional item is "specific to adult medical-surgical patients (knowledge about caring for personal needs). The items form

(continued)

BOX 10.11 An Example of a Conceptual–Theoretical–Empirical Structure for Transitions Framework Correlational Research *(continued)*

four subscales: Personal Status, Knowledge, Coping Ability, and Expected Support" (Weiss et al., 2007, p. 35). Each item is rated on an 11-point scale of 0 to 10 with anchor words such as "not at all" and "totally."

- Postdischarge Coping Difficulty is measured by the investigator-developed Post-Discharge Coping Difficulty Scale (PDCDS; Weiss et al., 2007). The PDCDS includes 10 items about difficulties including "stress, recovery, self-care, self-medical management, family difficulty, help and emotional support needed, confidence in self-care and medical management abilities, and adjustment" (Weiss et al., 2007, p. 35). Each item is rated on an 11-point scale of 0 to 10 with anchor words, such as "not at all" and "totally."
- Utilization of Postdischarge Support and Services is measured by patient self-report given during a telephone interview 3 weeks after hospital discharge. The questions asked are "calls to friends and family for advice and/or support, calls to providers, office or clinic visits, calls to the hospital, urgent care/emergency room visits, and hospital readmission" (Weiss et al., 2007, p. 35). Each question is answered as "yes" or "no."

The *relational propositions* for the C and T components of the CTE structure are:

- Nature of Transition, Transition Conditions, and Nursing Therapeutics are related to Response Patterns (Weiss et al., 2007).
- Therefore, Hospitalization Factors, Patient Characteristics, and Hospital Nursing Practices are related to Readiness for Hospital Discharge.
- Response Patterns are interrelated (Meleis et al., 2000).
- Therefore, Readiness for Hospital Discharge is related to Postdischarge Coping Difficulty and to Utilization of Postdischarge Support and Services.

The *relational propositions* for the E component of the CTE structure are:

- Scores for patient self-report of planned admission, first hospitalization, previous admission for the same health condition, and for medical record review of length of hospital stay are related to scores for the Readiness for Hospital Discharge-Adult Form.
- Scores for patient self-report of age, gender, race, socioecomonic status, and lives alone and for medical record review of payor are related to scores for the Readiness for Hospital Discharge-Adult Form.
- Scores for the QDTS are related to scores for the Readiness for Hospital Discharge-Adult Form.
- Scores for the CCS are related to scores for the Readiness for Hospital Discharge-Adult Form.
- Scores for the Readiness for Hospital Discharge-Adult Form are related to scores for the PDCDS.
- Scores for the Readiness for Hospital Discharge-Adult Form are related to scores for patient self-report of calls to friends and family for advice and/or support, calls to providers, office or clinic visits, calls to the hospital, urgent care/emergency room visits, and hospital readmission.

Source: Weiss et al. (2007).

Quality of Life, Functional Status, Patient Satisfaction, Resource Utilization, and Resource Costs.

The APN intervention dimension of Type of Intervention is operationalized by the APN intervention protocol. The routine care dimension of Type of Intervention is operationalized by the routine care protocol. Rehospitalization is measured by patient records for time of first reshospitalization or death following initial hospital discharge. Quality of Life is measured by the Minnesota Living with Heart Failure Questionnaire (LHFQ; Rector, Kubo, & Cohn, 1987). Functional Status is measured by the Enforced Social Dependency Scale (ESDS; Moinpour, McCorkle, & Saunders, 1992). Patient Satisfaction is measured by an investigator-developed Patient Satisfaction Instrument (PSI). Resource Utilization is measured by data extracted from patient records and bills from physicians, hospitals, and home care agencies. Resource Costs are measured by standardized Medicare reimbursement.

Patient Satisfaction data were collected at 2 and 6 weeks after initial hospital discharge. Data for Rehospitalization, Quality of Life, Functional Status, Resource Utilization, and Resource Costs were collected at 2, 6, 12, 26, and 52 weeks after initial hospital discharge via standardized telephone interviews.

The differential efficacy of the APN intervention and routine care was examined using "Group-specific Kaplan-Meier survival curves...[and] proportional hazards regression" (Naylor et al., 2004, p. 678; see Appendix B). Experimental APN intervention and control routine care group comparisons for Quality of Life, Functional Status, Patient Satisfaction, and Resource Utilization were done using Wilcoxon rank sum tests (see Appendix B). Adjustments in the data were made to account for missing values due to research participants who died during the period of study. Estimates of average Resource Costs were computed separately for the APN intervention group and the routine care group and then calculating the difference in the means for total costs.

The CTE structure that was constructed from an interpretation of the content of Naylor et al.'s (2004) journal article is illustrated in Figure 10.9. The nonrelational and relational propositions for each component of the CTE structure are listed in Box 10.12.

A CTE Structure for Mixed-Methods Research

Ramsay's (2010) doctoral dissertation is an example of a report of mixed-methods research that is consistent with the Transitions Framework. A report of a secondary analysis of the dissertation data placed the study explicitly within the context of the Transitions Framework (Ramsay, Huby, Thompson, & Walsh, 2014). The purpose of Ramsay's (2010) study was to explore experiences and perceptions of prolonged critical illness survivors about their limitations in activities and life quality after hospital discharge.

BOX 10.12 An Example of a Conceptual–Theoretical–Empirical Structure for Transitions Framework Experimental Research

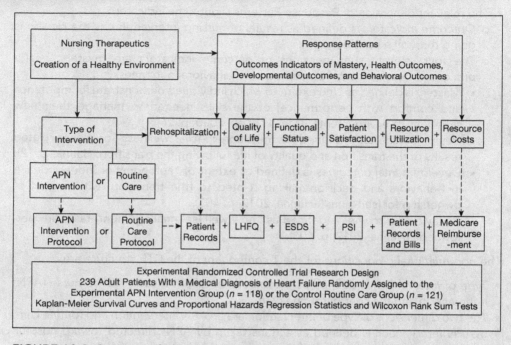

FIGURE 10.9 Conceptual–theoretical–empirical (CTE) structure for Transitions Framework experimental research—theory of effects of APN intervention or routine care on rehospitalization, quality of life, functional status, patient satisfaction, and resource utilization and costs.

APN, advanced practice nurse; ESDS, Enforced Social Dependency Scale; LHFQ, Minnesota Living with Heart Failure Questionnaire; PSI, Patient Satisfaction Instrument.

The *non-relational propositions* for the C component of the conceptual–theoretical–empirical (CTE) structure are:

- *Nursing Therapeutics* is defined as "all nursing activities and actions deliberately designed to care for nursing clients" (Barnard, as cited in Meleis, 2012, p. 105); especially "those interventions or actions that can modify or influence the outcomes of a transition" (Baird, 2012, p. 259).
- The relevant dimension of Nursing Therapeutics is the creation of a healthy environment.
  - *Creation of a healthy environment* is defined as a nursing intervention that involves the nurse working in collaboration with other members of the health care team and with "patient and family to create...healthy...physical, social, political and cultural surroundings...to meet their needs and to promote dignity and personal integrity...[by means of] mobilization of...personal, family, and community...resources" (Coffey, 2014, p. 55).
- *Response Patterns* is defined as "those factors that indicate movement toward enhanced or diminished well-being" (Baird, 2012, p. 259).

(continued)

BOX 10.12 An Example of a Conceptual–Theoretical–Empirical Structure for Transitions Framework Experimental Research *(continued)*

- The relevant dimension of Response Patterns is outcome indicators.
  o *Outcome indicators* is defined as results of nursing intervention as the person is going through a transition.
  o The four relevant subdimensions of outcome indicators are mastery, health outcomes, developmental outcomes, and behavioral outcomes.
    - *Mastery* is defined as "the extent to which individuals demonstrate [competence and comfort with performance] of the skills needed to manage their new situations or environments" (Meleis et al., 2000, p. 26).
    - *Health outcomes* is defined as transition-specific wellness- or illness-related results of the transition and quality of life following the transition (Hanna, 2012).
    - *Developmental outcomes* is defined as extent of "autonomy or independence in behaviors and decision-making related to [the transition] with a goal of ownership for [self-]care" (Hanna, 2012, p. 403).
    - *Behavioral outcomes* is defined as "how well [self-management] tasks are performed" (Hanna, 2012, p. 403).

The *non-relational propositions* for the *T* component of the CTE structure are:

- *Type of Intervention* is defined as the experimental advanced practice nurse (APN) intervention and the control routine care.
- The two dimensions of Type of Intervention are an APN intervention and routine care.
  o *APN intervention* is defined as actions taken by APNs directed toward hospital discharge planning and home follow-up care (Naylor et al., 2004).
  o *Routine care* is defined as heart failure management and discharge planning with home care agency referral if necessary (Naylor et al., 2004).
- *Rehospitalization* is defined as time to first rehospitalization or death after initial hospital discharge (Naylor et al., 2004).
- *Quality of Life* is defined as patient self-assessment of the extent to which heart failure imposes physical, socioeconomic, and psychological impairments (Rector et al. 1987).
- *Functional Status* is defined as the extent to which people need help or assistance from someone else to perform activities that they usually can perform by themselves (Moinpour et al., 1992).
- *Patient Satisfaction* is defined as research participants' expressions of satisfaction with the care they received during the initial hospitalization.
- *Resource Utilization* is defined as number, time, and reasons for readmissions to hospital, unplanned visits for acute care, and visiting nurse or APN care after first discharge from hospital (Naylor et al., 2004).
- *Resource Costs* is defined as estimated costs of care used following initial hospital discharge.

The *non-relational propositions* for the *E* component of the CTE structure are:

- The APN intervention dimension of Type of Intervention is operationalized by the APN intervention protocol. Three master's-prepared APNs, who collaborated

(continued)

BOX 10.12 An Example of a Conceptual–Theoretical–Empirical Structure for Transitions Framework Experimental Research *(continued)*

with physicians, provided an intervention that extended from initial admission to the hospital to 3 months following discharge from the hospital. The APN intervention encompassed a multidisciplinary team-guided program for orientation and training for the APNs, as well as implementation of strategies for management of individualized care and evidence-based heart failure guidelines. The APN visited the patient within the first day following admission to the hospital, at least once a day during hospitalization, at least eight times at home, including once each week for the first month, twice a month for months 2 and 3, and other visits as necessary. The APN was available every weekday from 8 a.m. to 8 p.m., and every weekend from 8 a.m. to 12 p.m. The APN continued daily visits if the patient was readmitted to the hospital during the 3 months after the first hospital admission. The protocol specified the minimum number of APN visits during hospitalization and at home, although flexibility in the protocol promoted individualized care (Naylor et al., 2004).

- The routine care dimension of Type of Intervention is operationalized by the routine care protocol. The patients in the routine care control group received care that is routine for the hospital to which they were admitted, such as management of heart failure, discharge teaching, and referrals to daily home care. The usual care at hospitals in the study included similar policies about and processes for discharge planning, and home care policies and procedures for daily care across agencies were similar (Naylor et al., 2004).
- Rehospitalization is measured by patient records for time of first rehospitalization or death following initial hospital discharge (Naylor et al., 2004).
- Quality of Life is measured by the Minnesota Living with Heart Failure Questionnaire (LHFQ; Rector et al., 1987). The LHFQ is made up of 21 items that address physical, socioeconomic, and psychological impairments related to heart failure. Each item is ranked on a 6-point scale of 0 = no, not related to my heart failure, 1 = very little, to 5 = very much to determine the extent to which it prevents the person from living as he or she wants. Note that lower scores reflect greater quality of life.
- Functional Status is measured by the Enforced Social Dependency Scale (ESDS; Molnpour et al., 1992). The ESDS, which is administered as a semi-structured interview, contains 10 activities arranged in two subscales. The personal competence subscale includes six activities (dressing, eating, walking, traveling, bathing, toileting) that are coded on a 6-point scale of 1 to 6 indicating the extent of help required to perform each activity. The social competence subscale includes four activities; three of the activities (home, work, and social and recreation) are rated on a 4 point scale of 1 = usual activity, 2 = modified activity, 3 = restricted activity, to 4 = no activity (activity no longer performed); the remaining item (communication) is coded on a 3-point scale indicating the extent of help required to communicate. Note that higher scores reflect greater dependency, that is, lower functional status.

(continued)

BOX 10.12 An Example of a Conceptual–Theoretical–Empirical Structure for Transitions Framework Experimental Research *(continued)*

- Patient Satisfaction is measured by an investigator-developed Patient Satisfaction Instrument (PSI). The instrument contains 25 items that are rated on a scale of 0 to 4. Naylor et al. (2004) gave no other information about this instrument.
- Resource Utilization is measured by data about resources used following initial hospital discharge that are extracted from patient records and bills from physicians, hospitals, and home care agencies (Naylor et al., 2004).
- Resource Costs are measured as estimates of the costs of resources used following initial hospital discharge; estimates are based on usual Medicare reimbursement rates (Naylor et al., 2004).

The *relational propositions* for the *C* and *T components* of the CTE structure are:

- Nursing Therapeutics affects Resource Patterns.
- Therefore, Type of Intervention affects Rehospitalization, Quality of Life, Functional Status, Patient Satisfaction, Resource Utilization, and Resource Costs.

The *relational proposition* for the *E component* of the CTE structure is:

- The effects of implementation of the APN intervention protocol are more positive than the effects of implementation of the routine care protocol on scores for patient records for rehospitalization, the LHFS, the ESDS, the PSI, patient records and bills for resource utilization, and Medicare reimbursement for resource costs

Source: Naylor et al. (2004).

Ramsay (2010) used a simple descriptive design for her QUAL + quan mixed-methods study (see Appendix A). Twenty survivors of prolonged critical illness participated in the study at any time up to 6 months following their discharge from intensive care units (ICUs) in hospitals in eastern Scotland. The inclusion criteria were mechanical ventilation for at least 14 days while in an ICU and survival until at least the time of hospital discharge. Exclusion criteria were patients who had an initial diagnosis of a neurological problem or psychiatric illness, patients who were transferred to another facility, and patients who lived too far away from the investigator's home (Ramsay, 2010). The quantitative data were obtained from a mailed fixed-choice questionnaire, and the qualitative data were obtained from responses to an in-person semi-structured interview.

The theory is experiences of prolonged critical illness. The conceptual model concept is Transition Type. Ramsay et al. (2014) identified the three relevant dimensions as situational transition, wellness/illness transition, and organizational transition. One theory concept is Perceived Health-Related Quality of Life. The eight dimensions of this concept are physical functioning, social functioning, role limitations because of physical problems, role limitations because of emotional problems, mental health, energy/vitality, bodily pain, and general health perceptions; general health status is an additional dimension. Ramsay (2010) reconceptualized the eight dimensions of Perceived Health-Related Quality of Life as four dimensions—physical, mental health, social function, and general health perception.

The other theory concepts are Getting By, Moving On, Making Sense of the ICU Experience, Putting Things in Perspective, Leaning on Family and Friends, and I Was Fine, Really. The three dimensions of Getting By are organizing material resources, organizing informal support, and finding new ways of doing things. The three dimensions of Moving On are pacing, resistance, and marking progress and setting goals. The two dimensions of Making Sense of the ICU Experience are filling in the memory gap and making sense of bizarre dreams. The two dimensions of Putting Things in Perspective are it is better than being 6 feet under and there is always someone else worse off. The two dimensions of Leaning on Family and Friends are getting back to normal and being treated differently. The two dimensions of I Was Fine, Really are since I've been ill and I'm probably healthier now.

For the quantitative portion of the study, the three dimensions of Transition Type are represented by Perceived Health-Related Quality of Life, which is measured by the Short Form-36 (SF-36; Ware & Sherbourne, 1992). Ramsay (2010) reported SF-36 subscale raw scores (Appendix B) with comparisons to population norms for each participant.

For the qualitative portion of the study, the theory concepts—Getting By, Moving On, Making Sense of the ICU Experience, Putting Things in Perspective, Leaning on Family and Friends, and I Was Fine, Really—and their dimensions were discovered in the participants' responses to 15 investigator-developed semi-structured interview questions.

Ramsay (2010) used thematic analysis to identify the theory concepts (themes) and their dimensions (subthemes) found in the qualitative data (Appendix B). She then integrated the themes and subthemes with the four reconceptualized dimensions of Perceived Health-Related Quality of Life. For the integration, Ramsay (2010) linked Getting By and Moving On and their dimensions with the physical dimension of Perceived Health Related Quality of Life; Making Sense of the ICU Experience and Putting Things in Perspective and their dimensions with the mental health dimension; Leaning on Family and Friends and its dimensions with the social function dimension; and I Was Fine, Really and its dimensions with the general health dimension.

The CTE structure that was constructed from the content of Ramsay's (2010) dissertation is illustrated in Figure 10.10. The non-relational propositions for each component of the CTE structure are listed in Box 10.13.

BOX 10.13 An Example of a Conceptual–Theoretical–Empirical Structure for Transitions Framework Mixed-Methods Research

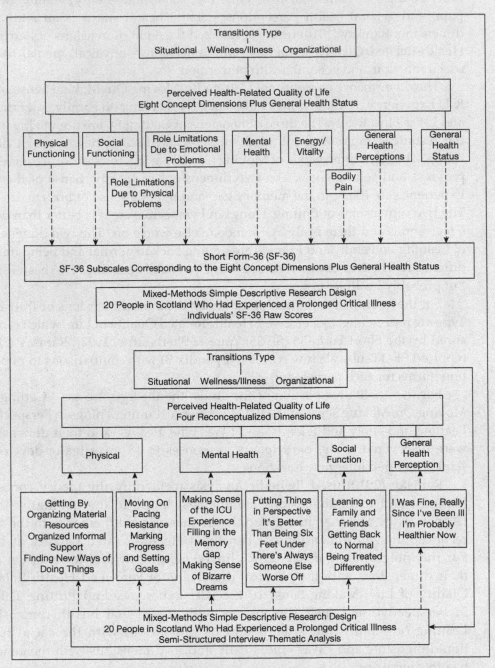

FIGURE 10.10 Conceptual–theoretical–empirical (CTE) structure for Transitions Framework mixed-methods research—theory of experiences of prolonged critical illness—quantitative and qualitative portions.

(continued)

BOX 10.13 An Example of a Conceptual–Theoretical–Empirical Structure for Transitions Framework Mixed-Methods Research *(continued)*

The *non-relational propositions* for the *C component* of the conceptual–theoretical–empirical (CTE) structure are:

- *Transition Type* is defined as various circumstances that require a process of change.
- The three relevant dimensions of Transition Type are situational transition, wellness/illness transition, and organizational transition (Ramsay et al., 2014).
  - o *Situational transition* is defined as a process of change associated with circumstances that represent losses and gains occuring throughout the life span (Im, 2014).
  - o *Wellness/illness transition* is defined as a process of biopsychosocial and spiritual change associated with development, diagnosis, and treatment of disease and full recovery from disease or development of chronic illness.
  - o *Organizational transition* is defined as a process of change within an organization, specifically, "changing environmental conditions that affect the lives of clients and workers" (Im, 2014, p. 257).

The *non-relational propositions* for the *T component* of the CTE structure are:

- *Perceived Health-Related Quality of Life* is defined as the person's evaluation of positive and negative aspects of life that affect physical and/or mental health (Centers for Disease Control and Prevention [CDC], 2011).
- The eight dimensions of Perceived Health-Related Quality of Life are physical functioning, social functioning, role limitations because of physical problems, role limitations because of emotional problems, mental health, energy/vitality, bodily pain, and general health perceptions, plus general health status.
  - o *Physical functioning* is defined as the performance of well persons' normal activities (Ramsay, 2010).
  - o *Social functioning* is defined as the extent to which health problems interfered with normal activities that reflect participation (Ramsay, 2010).
  - o *Role limitations because of physical problems* is defined as the extent to which physical health problems interfered with typical daily activities associated with the person's age-related roles (Ramsay, 2010).
  - o *Role limitations because of emotional problems* is defined as the extent to which depression or anxiety interfered with typical daily activities (Ramsay, 2010).
  - o *Mental health* is defined as the extent to which participants felt nervous, or calm, or peaceful (Ramsay, 2010).
  - o *Energy/vitality* is defined as the extent to which participants felt filled with energy or tired (Ramsay, 2010).
  - o *Bodily pain* is defined as the extent to which pain interfered with usual activities (Ramsay, 2010).
  - o *General health perceptions* is defined as beliefs about one's own health (Ramsay, 2010).
  - o *General health status* is defined as the rating of health over a period of 1 year (Ware & Sherbourne, 1992).

(continued)

BOX 10.13 An Example of a Conceptual–Theoretical–Empirical Structure for Transitions Framework Mixed-Methods Research *(continued)*

- The four reconceptualized dimensions of Perceived Health-Related Quality of Life are physical, mental health, social function, and general health perception.
  - *Physical* is defined as the extent to which survivors' concerns about physical health interfered with their usual activities (Ramsay, 2010). This reconceptualized dimension encompasses the original physical function, role limitations because of physical problems, and energy/vitality dimensions.
  - *Mental health* is defined as survivors' thoughts about experiences of critical care as well as the processes they used to manage continuing symptoms and functional difficulties (Ramsay, 2010). This reconceptualized dimension encompasses the original mental health and role limitations because of emotional problems dimensions.
  - *Social function* is defined as the amount of support and interaction survivors received from family and friends (Ramsay, 2010). This reconceptualized dimension is essentially the same as the original social functioning dimension.
  - *General health perception* is defined as survivors' thoughts and judgments about their overall health (Ramsay, 2010). This reconceptualized dimension is essentially the same as the original general health perceptions dimension.
- *Getting By* is defined as survivors' use of practical methods of managing daily living at home (Ramsay, 2010).
- The dimensions of Getting By are organizing material resources, organizing informal support, and finding new ways of doing things.
  - *Organizing material resources* is defined as the survivors' requirements for mobility aids and organization of the household physical environment (Ramsay, 2010).
  - *Organizing informal support* is defined as survivors' requirements for assistance from spouses, family members, and friends or their surveillance of previously taken-for-granted activities (Ramsay, 2010).
  - *Finding new ways of doing things* is defined as survivors' efforts to identify physical and functional limitations (Ramsay, 2010).
- *Moving On* is defined as methods used by survivors to manage physical and functional limitations as they moved toward a newly normal life (Ramsay, 2010).
- The dimensions of Moving On are pacing, resistance, and marking progress and setting goals.
  - *Pacing* is defined as a complicated method of managing and balancing activity and rest in the context of physical and functional limitations (Ramsay, 2010).
  - *Resistance* is defined as the survivors' awareness of the values and benefits of fighting to overcome symptoms and limitations as they recovered (Ramsay, 2010).
  - *Marking progress and setting goals* is defined as survivors' increasing understanding of their capacities and limitations as they recovered (Ramsay, 2010).
- *Making Sense of the ICU Experience* is defined as survivors' understanding of and rationalizing their experiences, including memories of delusions and gaps in memory (Ramsay, 2010).

(continued)

BOX 10.13 An Example of a Conceptual–Theoretical–Empirical Structure for Transitions Framework Mixed-Methods Research *(continued)*

- The dimensions of Making Sense of the ICU Experience are filling in the memory gap and making sense of bizarre dreams.
  - o *Filling in the memory gap* is defined as survivors' overcoming loss of memory that frequently occurred in the days prior to their critical illness (Ramsay, 2010).
  - o *Making sense of bizarre dreams* is defined as survivors' struggles to understand the strange dreams they had of the acute phase of their critical illness (Ramsay, 2010).
- *Putting Things in Perspective* is defined as survivors' placement of their continuing illness into their everyday living (Ramsay, 2010).
- The dimensions of Putting Things in Perspective are it is better than being 6 feet under and there is always someone else worse off.
  - o *It is better than being 6 feet under* is defined as survivors' perceptions of extreme limitations and illness as a fortunate escape from death (Ramsay, 2010).
  - o *There is always someone else worse off* is defined as situations that survivors regarded favorably compared to others who had more problems (Ramsay, 2010).
- *Leaning on Family and Friends* is defined as methods used by family members and friends to provide support (Ramsay, 2010).
- The dimensions of Leaning on Family and Friends are getting back to normal and being treated differently.
  - o *Getting back to normal* is defined as survivors' resumption of the usual activities that were meaningful to them before the illness (Ramsay, 2010).
  - o *Being treated differently* is defined as survivors' experiences of stigma related to any changes they experienced in their appearance following the critical illness (Ramsay, 2010).
- *I Was Fine, Really* is defined as feeling free from illness and needs for medication and/or hospitalization, and work time off, as well as having no restrictions on usual activities (Ramsay, 2010).
- The dimensions of I Was Fine, Really are since I've been ill and I'm probably healthier now.
  - o *Since I've been ill* is defined as physical and functional limitations and their gratitude for having survived the critical illness (Ramsay, 2010).
  - o *I'm probably healthier now* is defined as survivors' descriptions of self as in better health following the critical illness due to changes in lifestyle (Ramsay, 2010).

The *non-relational propositions* for the *E component* of the CTE structure are:

- Perceived Health-Related Quality of Life is measured by the Short Form 36 (SF-36; Ware & Sherbourne, 1992). The SF-36 contains 35 items arranged in eight subscales—physical functioning (10 items), social functioning (2 items), role limitations due to physical problems (4 items), role limitations due to emotional problems (3 items), mental health (5 items), energy/vitality (4 items), bodily pain (2 items), and general health perception (5 items), plus one item addressing amount of change in general health status during a period of 1 year.

(continued)

> ## BOX 10.13 An Example of a Conceptual–Theoretical–Empirical Structure for Transitions Framework Mixed-Methods Research *(continued)*
>
> The items for the physical functioning subscale are rated as "yes, limited a lot," "yes, limited a little," or "no, not limited at all."
>
> One item for the social functioning subscale and all items for the mental health and the energy/vitality subscales are rated as "all of the time," "most of the time," "a good bit of the time," "some of the time," "a little of the time," or "none of the time."
>
> The other item for the social functioning subscale and one item for the bodily pain subscale are rated as "not at all," "a little bit," "moderately," "quite a bit," or "extremely." The other item for the bodily pain subscale is rated as "none," "very mild," "mild," "moderate," "severe," or "very severe."
>
> Items for the role limitations due to physical problems and role limitations due to emotional problems subscales are rated as "yes," or "no."
>
> Four items for the general health perceptions subscale are rated as "definitely true," "mostly true," "don't know," "mostly false," or "definitely false;" the other item is rated as "excellent," "very good," "good," "fair," or "poor."
>
> The item for general health status is rated as "much better now than one year ago," "somewhat better now than one year ago," "about the same as one year ago," "somewhat worse now than one year ago," or "much worse than one year ago." This item is not included in the total SF-36 score and is "analyzed as a categorical variable or as an ordinal level scale" (Ware & Sherbourne, 1992, p. 477).
>
> • Getting By, Moving On, Making Sense of the ICU Experience, Putting Things in Perspective, Leaning on Family and Friends, and I Was Fine, Really, and their dimensions were extracted by means of a thematic analysis from participant's responses to the investigator-developed semi-structured interview, which includes 15 questions along with prompts and probes to elicit additional information from the research participants (Ramsay, 2010).
>
> *Source:* Ramsay (2010).

CONCLUSION

The examples of the use of the Transitions Framework as a guide for practice, a quality improvement project, and research presented in this chapter underscore the utility of this conceptual model of nursing. The Transitions Framework was introduced to the world of nursing in the early 1990s (Schumacher & Meleis, 1994), a more recent time than all other conceptual models included in this book, with the exception of the Synergy Model, which is an even more recent addition to the discipline of nursing (see Chapter 9).

NOTES

1. The Transitions Framework presented in this chapter is a conceptual model of nursing because of the relatively abstract and general level of concepts and propositions. The Transitions Framework is based on Schumacher and Meleis's (1994) discussion of transitions as a conceptual framework and Meleis's transitions theory (Meleis, 2010b; 2012; Meleis, Sawyer, Im, Messias, & Schumacher, 2000), which others (Coffey, 2014; Im, 2010, 2014) consider a middle-range theory.
2. The Transitions Framework encompasses various perspectives of transitions. Some publications selected for inclusion in this chapter as examples are not directly derived from Meleis's transitions theory, although those publications are reprints of journal articles in Meleis's (2010d) edited book, *Transitions Theory: Middle-Range and Situation-Specific Theories in Nursing Research and Practice*.
3. Baird (2012) pointed out that in an early publication about transitions theory (Chick & Meleis, 1986), "3 phases were identified as entry, passage, and exit, but as the theory progressed, these phases were eliminated" (p. 260).

REFERENCES

Baird, M. B. (2012). Well-being in refugee women experiencing cultural transition. *Advances in nursing science, 35*, 249–263.

Centers for Disease Control and Prevention (CDC). (2011). *Health-related quality of life (HRQOL)*. Retrieved from http://www.cdc.gov/hrqol/concept.htm

Chick, N., & Meleis, A. I. (1986). Transitions: A nursing concern. In P. L. Chinn (Ed.), *Nursing research methodology: Issues and implementation* (pp. 237–257). Rockville, MD: Aspen.

Clayton State University School of Nursing. (2012). *Philosophy*. Retrieved from http://www.clayton.edu/nursing/Philosophy

Coffey, A. (2014). Transitions theory. In J. J. Fitzpatrick & G. McCarthy (Eds.), *Theories guiding nursing research and practice: Making nursing knowledge explicit* (pp. 51–68). New York, NY: Springer.

Foust, J. B. (1994). Creating a future for nursing through interactive planning at the bedside. *Image–The Journal of Nursing Scholarship, 26*, 129–132.

Hanna, K. M. (2012). A framework for the youth with type 1 diabetes during the emerging adulthood transition. *Nursing Outlook, 60*, 401–410.

Hollingshead, A. (1975). *Four factor index of social status*. New Haven, CT: Author. [Working paper.]

Im, E. O. (2009). Ethnic differences in symptoms experienced during the menopausal transition. *Health Care for Women International, 30*, 339–355.

Im, E. O. (2010). Afaf Ibrahim Meleis: Transition theory. In M. R. Alligood & A. M. Tomey (Eds.), *Nursing theorists and their work* (7th ed., pp. 416–433). Maryland Heights, MO: Mosby.

Im, E. O. (2014). Theory of transitions. In M. J. Smith & P. R. Liehr (Eds.), *Middle-range theory for nursing* (3rd ed., pp. 253–276). New York, NY: Springer.

Im, E. O., Lee, S. H., & Chee, W. (2010). Black women in menopausal transition. *Journal of Obstetric, Gynecologic, and Neonatal Nursing, 39*, 435–443.

Im, E. O., Lee, S. H., & Chee, W. (2011). "Being conditioned, yet becoming strong": Asian American women in menopausal transition. *Journal of Transcultural Nursing, 22*, 290–299.

Im, E. O., Liu, Y., Dormire, S., & Chee, W. (2008). Menopausal symptom experience: An online forum study. *Journal of Advanced Nursing, 62*, 541–550.

Kelley, L. S., & Lakin, J. A. (2010). Role supplementation as a nursing intervention for Alzheimer's disease: A case study. In A. I. Meleis (Ed.), *Transitions theory: Middle-range and situation-specific theories in nursing research and practice* (pp. 571–579). New York, NY: Springer. [Reprinted from Kelley, L. S., & Lakin, J. A. (2010). Role supplementation as a nursing intervention for Alzheimer's disease: A case study. *Public Health Nursing, 5,* 146–152.]

Kralik, D., Visentin, K., & van Loon, A. (2006). Transition: A literature review. *Journal of Advanced Nursing, 55,* 320–329.

Meleis, A. I. (2010a). Epilogue. In A. I. Meleis (Ed.), *Transitions theory: Middle-range and situation-specific theories in nursing research and practice* (pp. 619–624). New York, NY: Springer.

Meleis, A. I. (2010b). Transitions as a nursing theory. In A. I. Meleis (Ed.), *Transitions theory: Middle-range and situation-specific theories in nursing research and practice* (p. 11). New York, NY: Springer Publishing.

Meleis, A. I. (2010c). Transitions from practice to evidence-based models of care. In A. I. Meleis (Ed.), *Transitions theory: Middle-range and situation-specific theories in nursing research and practice* (pp. 1–9). New York, NY: Springer Publishing.

Meleis, A. I. (Ed.). (2010d). *Transitions theory: Middle-range and situation-specific theories in nursing research and practice.* New York, NY: Springer Publishing.

Meleis, A. I. (2012). *Theoretical nursing: Development and progress* (5th ed.). Philadelphia, PA: Wolters Kluwer/Lippincott Williams and Wilkins.

Meleis, A. I., Sawyer, L. M., Im, E. O., Hilfinger Messias, D. K., & Schumacher, K. (2000). Experiencing transitions: An emerging middle-range theory. *Advances in Nursing Science, 23,* 12–28.

Moinpour, C. M., McCorkle, R., & Saunders, J. (1992). Measuring functional status. In M. Frank-Stromborg (Ed.), *Instruments for clinical nursing research* (pp. 385–401). Burlington, MA: Jones & Bartlett.

Naylor, M. D., Brooten, D. A., Campbell, R. L., Maislin, G., McCauley, K. M., & Schwartz, J. S. (2004). Transitional care of older adults hospitalized with heart failure: A randomized, controlled trial. *Journal of the American Geriatrics Society, 52,* 675–684.

Naylor, M. D., Feldman, P. H., Keating, S., Koren, M. J., Kurtzman, E. T., Maccoy, M. C., & Krakauer, R. (2009). Translating research into practice. Transitional care for older adults. *Journal of Evaluation in Clinical Practice, 15,* 1164–1170. See also http://www.transitionalcare.info

Porter, J. S., Carroll, Y. M., Anderson, S., Lavoie, P. T., Jr., Hamilton, L., Johnson, M., & Hankins, J. S. (2014). Transition readiness assessment for sickle cell patients: A quality improvement project. *Journal of Clinical Outcomes, 21,* 263–269.

Ramsay, P. (2010). *Quality of life following prolonged critical illness: A mixed methods study* (Unpublished doctoral dissertation). University of Edinburgh, Edinburgh, Scotland.

Ramsay, P., Huby, G., Thompson, A., & Walsh, T. (2014). Intensive care survivors' experiences of ward-based care: Meleis' theory of nursing transitions and role development among critical care outreach services. *Journal of Clinical Nursing, 23,* 605–615.

Rector, T. S., Kubo, S. H., & Cohn, J. N. (1987). Patients' self-assessment of their congestive heart failure. Part 2: Content, reliability and validity of a new measure, the Minnesota Loving with Health Failure Questionnaire. *Heart Failure, 3,* 198–209.

Rossen, E. K. (2010). Assessing older persons' readiness to move to independent congregate living. In A. I. Meleis (Ed.), *Transitions theory: Middle-range and situation-specific theories in nursing research and practice* (pp. 182–187). New York, NY: Springer. [Reprinted from Rossen, E. (2007). Assessing older persons' readiness to move to independent congregate living. *Clinical Nurse Specialist: The Journal for Advanced Nursing Practice, 21,* 292–296.]

Rossen, E. K., & Gruber, K. J. (2007). Development and psychometric testing of the relocation self-efficacy scale. *Nursing Research, 56,* 244–251.

Schumacher, K. L., & Meleis, A. I. (1994). Transitions: A central concept in nursing. *Image–The Journal of Nursing Scholarship, 26*(2), 119–127.

Walley, P., & Gowland, B. (2004). Completing the circle: From PD to PDSA. *International Journal of Health Care Quality Assurance Incorporating Leadership in Health Services, 17,* 349–358.

Ware, J. E., & Sherbourne, C. D. (1992). The MOS 36-item short-form health survey (SF-36). *Medical Care, 30,* 473–483.

Weiss, M., Johnson, N., Malin, S., Jerofke, T., Lang, C., & Sherburne, E. (2008). Readiness for discharge in parents of hospitalized children. *Journal of Pediatric Nursing, 23,* 282–295.

Weiss, M. E., & Lokken, L. (2009). Predictors and outcomes of postpartum mothers' perceptions of readiness for discharge after birth. *Journal of Obstetric, Gynecologic, and Neonatal Nursing, 38,* 406–417.

Weiss, M. E., & Piacentine, L. B. (2006). Psychometric properties of the Readiness for Hospital Discharge Scale. *Journal of Nursing Measurement, 14,* 163–180.

Weiss, M. E., Piacentine, L. B., Lokken, L., Ancona, J., Archer, J., Gresser, S.,...Vega-Stromberg, T. (2007). Perceived readiness for hospital discharge in adult medical-surgical patients. *Clinical Nurse Specialist, 21,* 31–42.

Weiss, M. E., Ryan, P., & Lokken, L. (2006). Validity and reliability of the perceived readiness for discharge after birth scale. *Journal of Obstetric, Gynecologic, and Neonatal Nursing, 35,* 34–45.

METHODS FOR QUALITY IMPROVEMENT PROJECTS AND RESEARCH

This appendix includes descriptions of methodological theories for quality improvement (QI) projects, approaches to literature reviews, the various research designs, and the sampling strategies used by the authors of the examples found in Chapters 2 through 10 of this book.

METHODOLOGICAL THEORIES FOR QI PROJECTS

The methodological theories included in this section of Appendix A are limited to those that were used by the authors of examples of QI projects presented in Chapters 2 through 10 of this book. Additional information about methodological theories for QI projects is available in a journal article by Taylor et al. (2014) and in book chapters by Anderson (2015) and Glanz, Burke, and Rimer (2015).

QUALITY IMPROVEMENT (QI) METHODOLOGICAL THEORIES	DESCRIPTION
Advancing Research and Clinical Practice Through Close Collaboration (ARCC) Model for Quality Improvement (Melnyk & Fineout-Overholt, 2005)	The ARCC model is used to implement and sustain a QI project focused on evidence-based practice (EBP). The ARCC model requires selection of a nurse who is an EBP expert and is willing to assume the role of EBP mentor. As the EBP mentor, the nurse uses findings from an assessment of the readiness of staff nurses and others in an organization to implement and sustain a QI project, develops a strategic plan to increase the staff nurses' knowledge of and skills with EBP, and encourages organization-wide adoption of a culture of best practice.

(continued)

QUALITY IMPROVEMENT (QI) METHODOLOGICAL THEORIES	DESCRIPTION
EBP approach using the PICOT clinical question (Melnyk & Fineout-Overholt, 2005)	PICOT (P = Patient Population, I = Intervention, C = Comparison, O = Outcome, T = Time) is used to clearly identify a clinical question for a QI project. The approach requires identification of a patient population of interest (P); identification of an intervention or an assessment tool (I), determination of a comparison, such as before and after implementation of the intervention or assessment tool or between groups that did and did not receive the intervention or were not assessed using the assessment tool (C); identification of the desired outcome (O); and specification of the time frame for the project (T).
Johns Hopkins Nursing Evidence-Based Practice Model and Guidelines (Newhouse, Dearholt, Poe, Pugh, & White, 2007), and the Practice Question, Evidence, and Translation (PET) Process (Newhouse, Dearholt, Poe, Pugh, & White, 2005, 2007)	The Johns Hopkins Nursing Evidence-Based Practice (EBP) Model and Guidelines are used to evaluate evidence for implementing a QI project. The guidelines encompass six steps: (1) Identify EBP experts within the clinical agency; (2) develop EBP educational programs for nursing staff including history and definitions of EBP, strategies for searching the literature, criteria for evaluating the literature, and strategies for implementing practice changes; (3) develop web-based resources for nursing staff; (4) identify EBP behavioral outcomes and use as criteria for staff job descriptions; (5) identify potential questions for EBP projects; and (6) develop EBP skills and expertise among nursing staff.

The PET process, which is used as a guide for successful implementation of an EBP project, includes formulating the practice question (P); finding, evaluating, summarizing, and rating the strength of the evidence to answer the question (E); and translating the evidence into practice activities if feasible and appropriate (T). |
| Outcomes-focused knowledge translational intervention framework (OFKTIF; Doran & Sidani, (2007) | The OFKTIF includes four components: (1) measurement of patient outcomes and feedback about achievement of outcomes; (2) guidelines for best practices that are reflected in tools for delivery of messages identified from patient assessment; (3) identification of patients' care preferences; and (4) facilitation of the quality improvement project by practice leaders and advanced practice nurses. |

(continued)

QUALITY IMPROVEMENT (QI) METHODOLOGICAL THEORIES	DESCRIPTION
Lewin's (1951) theory of change	Lewin's theory includes three stages: (1) *unfreezing* by identifying a need and desire by nurses for a change in the usual way of practicing; (2) *moving* by involving nurses in selecting and implementing a new way of practicing; and (3) *refreezing* by institutionalizing the new way of practicing.
Plan-Do-Study-Act (PDSA; Gillam & Siriwardena, 2013; Walley & Gowland, 2004)	PDSA is a structured cyclical approach to QI that encompasses four phases for a series of small-scale sequential or parallel cycles: (1) Plan (P)—identify the appropriateness of the change that needs to be made, define the objective for the QI project, and plan how to implement the change; (2) Do (D)—implement the change and collect data about its feasibility and effectiveness; (3) Study (S)—summarize the data to determine what was learned from the implementation of the change; and (4) Act (A)—determine any revisions in the change that need to be made and plan the next cycle. Each cycle repeats the entire PDSA sequence.
Rogers's (2003) theory of planned change	Rogers's theory includes five phases required for successful change: (1) fostering *awareness* of the problem; (2) catalyzing *interest* in a change that will solve the problem; (3) *evaluating* effectiveness of problem solutions found in the literature; (4) conducting a *trial* of the problem solution; and (5) *adopting* the solution as the new way to practice.
Ryan's (2009) integrated theory of health behavior change (ITHBC)	The ITHBC encompasses three phases: (1) enhancing changes in health-related behavior by increasing relevant knowledge of and beliefs about the behavior; (2) increasing skills and motivation required for sustained performance of the behavior; and (3) enhancing social support for and the influence of others on sustained performance of the behavior.

APPROACHES TO LITERATURE REVIEWS

The approaches to literature reviews listed subsequently were used by authors of three examples included in this book. It is noteworthy that most authors did not identify a specific approach, although it is likely that Cooper's (1989) approach was relevant for at least some of those examples.

LITERATURE REVIEW APPROACH	DESCRIPTION
Cooper's (1989) approach	A five-stage approach that guides *systematic reviews* of all types of research. The stages are (1) problem formulation; (2) data collection; (3) data evaluation; (4) analysis and interpretation; and (5) public presentation. Data typically are research results but may include research participant characteristics, sample size, and rigor of the methodology.
Ganong's (1987) approach	A 10-stage approach that guides *integrative reviews* of all types of research. The stages are (1) formulate the purpose of the review as hypotheses to be tested or questions to be answered; (2) identify the criteria for studies to be included in the review; (3) search the literature and select the sample of studies to be reviewed; (4) develop a coding sheet for all relevant information from the studies, such as purpose, conceptual and/or theoretical framework, theory concepts studied, sampling method, sample inclusion criteria, sample size, method of assigning research participants to groups (if applicable), sample characteristics, instruments used to measure theory concepts, data analysis techniques, research results, and methodological issues; (5) identify rules or guidelines for analysis and interpretation of the studies; (6) revise the coding sheet as necessary; (7) read the studies and enter the data on the coding sheet; (8) systematically analyze the findings of the literature reviewed; (9) interpret the results; and (10) prepare a report of the review.
Whittemore and Knafl's (2005) approach	A five-stage approach that guides *integrative reviews* of both qualitative studies (data are words) and quantitative studies (data are numbers), as well as theoretical literature. The stages are (1) problem identification; (2) literature review; (3) data evaluation; (4) data analysis, including data reduction, data display, data comparison, conclusion drawing, and verification; and (5) presentation. Data typically are research results but may include research participant characteristics, sample size, and rigor of the methodology.

RESEARCH DESIGNS

The research designs included in this section of Appendix A are limited to those used by the authors of the examples included in Chapters 2 through 10 of this book. Additional information about research designs is available in Fawcett and Garity's (2009) book, *Evaluating Research for Evidence-Based Nursing Practice*, or another research textbook. Throughout this section of Appendix A, the letters X and Y are used as symbols for theory concepts.

RESEARCH DESIGNS	DESCRIPTIONS
Cross-sectional design	Data are collected once; used with any type of research design—descriptive, correlational, experimental, or mixed methods.
Longitudinal design	Data are collected more than once; used with any type of research design—descriptive, correlational, experimental, or mixed methods.
Secondary analysis of data design	Data that were collected for a primary or larger study are used for another study to investigate a related research question; used with any type of research design—descriptive, correlational, experimental, or mixed methods.
Descriptive qualitative designs	Research that is designed to answer the question, *What is X?* The data collected typically are in the form of *words* found in documents, such as journal articles and book chapters, or expressed by research participants in response to open-ended interview questions.
Concept analysis	Used to enhance understanding of the meaning of a theory concept primarily by means of review of theoretical and research literature but may include collection of data from human beings. The literature constitutes the population or sample of documents for the concept analysis, and the contents of the documents are the data.
Walker and Avant's approach	A frequently used eight-step approach to concept analysis. The steps are (1) select a concept to analyze; (2) identify the purpose of the analysis; (3) review theoretical and research literature, as well as one or more dictionaries, to identify all possible uses of the concept; (4) identify the attributes (dimensions) of the concept; (5) describe a typical (model) instance or case of the concept that includes all of the concept attributes; (6) describe other cases that are similar to or different from the concept (borderline, related, contrary, invented, and illegitimate cases); (7) continue to review theoretical and research literature, as well as one or more dictionaries, to identify the antecedents to and consequences of the concept; and (8) identify ways to measure the concept (i.e., empirical referents, empirical indicators, or research instruments).
Simple descriptive design (Sandelowski, 2000, 2010)	A relatively uncomplicated design used for descriptive qualitative studies that involves a straightforward description of data collected from people or documents to determine the who, what, and/or where of something.
Feminist perspective	Used to understand gender-related discrimination based on issues of control, power, and social class.
Phenomenology	Used to study the meaning of a particular lived experience as perceived and reported by research participants.

(continued)

RESEARCH DESIGNS	DESCRIPTIONS
Hermeneutic phenomenology	Used to study and interpret the meaning of a particular lived experience as perceived and reported by research participants or as found in written documents.
Unitary Field Pattern Portrait Method (UFPP) Research Design (Butcher, 2005)	A type of hermeneutic phenomenology used to identify and understand manifestations of energy field patterns. The researcher selects a human–environmental energy field phenomenon related to well-being and carries out eight phases: (1) initial engagement with the phenomenon; (2) review of existing relevant nursing science literature; (3) immersion in the phenomenon; (4) coming to know and appreciate the pattern manifestations; (5) description of an initial unitary field pattern profile; (6) conferring with research participants to mutually shape and refine the unitary field pattern profile; (7) articulation of a unitary field pattern portrait; and (8) connecting the unitary field pattern portrait with Rogers's Science of Unitary Human Beings.
Descriptive quantitative designs	Research that is designed to answer the question, *What is X?* The data collected typically are in the form of *numbers* from research participants' responses to numeric research instrument items.
Simple descriptive design	A relatively uncomplicated design used for descriptive quantitative studies that involves a straightforward description of research participants' responses to research instruments to determine the how much of something.
Descriptive comparative design	A relatively uncomplicated design used for descriptive quantitative studies that involves a straightforward description of the comparison of two groups of research participants' responses to research instruments to determine the how much of something.
Correlational designs	Research that is designed to answer the question, *What is the relation between X and Y?* The data collected typically are in the form of *numbers* from research participants' responses to research instrument items.
Correlational design or bivariate correlational design	Used to examine the relation between two theory concepts.
Correlational regression model design	Used to examine the relations of two or more concepts to another concept.
Correlational path model research design	Used to test direct and indirect relations of some concepts with other concepts. Direct relations are those that link one or more concepts with another concept. Indirect relations are those that link one or more concepts with another concept and that concept with still another concept.

(continued)

RESEARCH DESIGNS	DESCRIPTIONS
Experimental designs	Research that is designed to answer the question, *What is the effect of X on Y?* The data collected typically are in the form of *numbers* from research participants' responses to research instrument items.
Quasi-experimental research design	Used for studies with no randomization.
Experimental research design	Used for studies involving randomization.
Quasi-experimental one group pretest–posttest research design	Used for study of one group of research participants— the experimental treatment group; research participants respond to the same research instrument items prior to and after implementation of the experimental treatment protocol.
Experimental pretest–posttest research design	Used for study of research participants who are randomly assigned; random assignment may be to experimental treatment and control treatment groups or may be to groups that are then randomly designated as the experimental and control groups; the research participants in each group respond to the same research instrument items prior to and after implementation of the experimental treatment and control treatment protocols.
Randomized controlled trial (RCT) or randomized controlled clinical trial (RCCT)	Similar to the experimental pretest–posttest research design although the design may not include pretest data collection; used to test the effects of an intervention in ideal settings.
Mixed-methods designs (Creswell, 2015)	Research that is typically designed to answer the following questions: *What is X?* and *What is the relation between X and Y?* or *What is the effect of X on Y?* Encompass both descriptive designs (the qualitative portion of a study) and correlational or experimental designs (the quantitative portion of a study). Ideally, the data for the two portions of the study are fully integrated.
QUAL + QUAN	Qualitative and quantitative portions of a study are equally emphasized
QUAL + quan	Qualitative portion of the study is emphasized.
QUAN + qual	Quantitative portion of the study is emphasized.
Concurrent mixed-methods design	Qualitative and quantitative portions of the study are conducted at the same time.
Sequential mixed-methods design	One portion of the study is conducted after data for the other portion of the study has been collected.

SAMPLING

A population is all of the people or documents that are of interest to a researcher. A sample is a portion of a population. There are many strategies for selecting a sample from a population of people or documents. The sampling strategies listed here are those used by the authors of the examples in Chapters 2 through 10 of this book. More detailed information is available in Fawcett and Garity's (2009) book, *Evaluating Research for Evidence-Based Nursing Practice*, or another research textbook.

SAMPLING STRATEGY	DESCRIPTION
Convenience sample	Selection of research participants who are easily available sources of data or easily available documents. Convenience samples typically are not representative of the entire population.
Quota sampling	Designation of certain portions (strata) of interest in a population followed by selection of a certain number of research participants or documents from each portion of the population (quotas). Quota samples may not be representative of the entire population.
Random assignment	Assignment of research participants to groups in a random manner, such that each participant has an equal chance of being assigned to a particular group. Random assignment typically is used to assign research participants to experimental and control groups for experimental research designs.
Opaque envelope technique	An approach to random assignment that involves placing a symbol for experimental and control treatments in the number of opaque envelopes of all people who will be in the sample and randomly selecting an envelope to assign each research participant to the experimental or control group.

REFERENCES

Anderson, P. (2015). Theoretical approaches to quality improvement. In J. B. Butts & K. L. Rich (Eds.), *Philosophies and theories for advanced nursing practice* (2nd ed., pp. 355–373). Burlington, MA: Jones & Bartlett.

Butcher, H. K. (2005). The unitary field pattern portrait research method: Facets, processes, and findings. *Nursing Science Quarterly, 18,* 293–297.

Cooper H. M. (1989). *Integrating research: A guide for literature reviews* (2nd ed.). Newbury Park, CA: Sage.

Creswell, J. W. (2015). *A concise introduction to mixed methods research.* Los Angeles, CA: Sage.

Doran, D., & Sidani, S. (2007). Outcomes-focused knowledge translation: A framework for knowledge translation and patient outcomes improvement. *Worldviews on Evidence-Based Nursing, 4,* 3–13.

Fawcett, J., & Garity, J. (2009). *Evaluating research for evidence-based nursing practice.* Philadelphia, PA: F. A. Davis.

Ganong, L. H. (1987). Integrative reviews of nursing research. *Research in Nursing and Health, 10,* 1–11.

Gillam, S., & Siriwardena, A. N. (2013). Frameworks for improvement: Clinical audit, the plan–do–study–act cycle and significant event audit. *Quality in Primary Care, 21,* 123–130.

Glanz, K., Burke, L. E., & Rimer, B. K. (2015). Health behavior theories. In J. B. Butts & K. L. Rich (Eds.), *Philosophies and theories for advanced nursing practice* (2nd ed., pp. 235–256). Burlington, MA: Jones & Bartlett.

Lewin, K. (1951). *Field theory in social science.* London: Tavistock Publications.

Melnyk, B. M., & Fineout-Overholt, E. (2005). *Evidence-based practice in nursing and healthcare: A guide to best practice.* Philadelphia, PA: Lippincott Williams and Wilkins.

Newhouse, R. P., Dearholt, S. L., Poe, S., Pugh, L. C., & White, K. M. (2005). Evidence-based practice: A practical approach to implementation. *Journal of Nursing Administration, 35,* 35–40.

Newhouse, R. P., Dearholt, S. L., Poe, S., Pugh, L. C., & White, K. M. (2007). *Johns Hopkins nursing evidence-based practice model and guidelines.* Indianapolis, IN: Sigma Theta Tau International.

Rogers, E. M. (2003). *Diffusion of innovations* (5th ed.) New York, NY: Free Press.

Ryan, P. (2009). Integrated theory of health behavior change: Background and intervention development. *Clinical Nurse Specialist: The Journal of Advanced Nursing Practice, 23,* 161–170.

Sandelowski, M. (2000). Focus on research methods. Whatever happened to qualitative description? *Research in Nursing and Health, 23,* 334–340.

Sandelowski, M. (2010) What's in a name? Qualitative description revisited. *Research in Nursing and Health, 33,* 77–84.

Taylor, M. J., McNicholas, C., Nicolay, C., Darzi, A., Bell, D., & Reed, J. E. (2014). Systematic review of the application of the plan–do–study–act method to improve quality in healthcare. *BMJ Quality & Safety, 23,* 290–298.

Walley, P., & Gowland, B. (2004). Completing the cycle: From PD to PDSA. *International Journal of Health Care Quality Assurance, 17,* 349–358.

Whittemore, R., & Knafl, K. (2005). The integrative review: Updated methodology. *Journal of Advanced Nursing 52,* 546–553.

DATA ANALYSIS TECHNIQUES

This appendix includes descriptions of the various data analysis techniques used by the authors of the examples of quality improvement projects and nursing research found in Chapters 2 through 10 of this book. More detailed information about all content in this appendix can be found in Fawcett and Garity's (2009) book, *Evaluating Research for Evidence-Based Nursing Practice,* or another research textbook. More detailed information about statistics can be found in any statistics textbook.

Analysis of Qualitative (Word) Data

NAME OF DATA ANALYSIS TECHNIQUE	DESCRIPTION
Content analysis	A general technique used to extract or discover similarities and differences in word data that may be classified into themes or categories that reflect the meaning of the word data. All techniques used to analyze word data are types of content analysis.
Constant comparative analysis	Used to identify categories of word data in a sequential manner, such that new categories of word data are constantly compared with already identified categories to determine if one or more new categories are evident.
Thematic analysis	Used to identify common themes found in word data.
Miles and Huberman's method	Used to extract and code common themes found in word data.
van Manen's method	Used to interpret word data collected by means of a phenomenological research design.

(continued)

Analysis of Qualitative (Word) Data   *(continued)*

NAME OF DATA ANALYSIS TECHNIQUE	DESCRIPTION
Hermeneutic method of data analysis/hermeneutic phenomenology/ interpretative phenomenological analysis (IPA)	Used to deeply understand and interpret the meaning of transcripts of words spoken by research participants about their experiences of something, or of written documents.
Unitary Field Pattern Portrait Research Method for data analysis	Used to develop a unitary understanding of human energy field pattern manifestations; a unitary field pattern profile is created from word data. The method is similar to the hermeneutic method of data analysis.

Analysis of Quantitative (Number) Data

PSYCHOMETRIC PROPERTIES
Psychometric properties are applied to research instruments that yield number data. Psychometric properties are estimated for each research instrument. Adequate estimates are values equal to or greater than 0.70 or 70%.

NAME OF PSYCHOMETRIC PROPERTY AND SYMBOL	DESCRIPTION
Reliability	An estimate of the extent to which the items making up a research instrument are a *consistent* measure of a theory concept.
Split-half reliability r	A type of *internal consistency reliability* that is an estimate of the extent to which research instrument items are related to each other; the instrument items are divided into two groups, such as the even numbered items and the odd numbered items or the items in the first and last halves of the instrument, and the scores for the two groups of items are then compared by means of a correlation coefficient.
Cronbach's alpha α	A type of *internal consistency reliability*, that is, an estimate of the extent to which research instrument items are related to each other; a statistical procedure that provides an estimate of the split-half reliability for all possible ways of dividing the instrument items into two halves, used when instrument items can be rated on more than two points, such as a 5-point or 10-point rating scale.
Test–retest reliability r	A type of *stability reliability* that requires administering a research instrument to the same research participants two different times. The scores obtained from the two administrations then are compared, typically by means of calculating a correlation coefficient.
Validity	An estimate of the extent to which the items making up a research instrument are an *appropriate* measure of a theory concept, that is, the items measure what they are supposed to measure.

(continued)

Analysis of Quantitative (Number) Data   (*continued*)

NAME OF PSYCHOMETRIC PROPERTY AND SYMBOL	DESCRIPTION
Content validity	An estimate of the adequacy of coverage of the research instrument items generated to measure a specific definition of a theory concept.
Face validity	A weak approach to estimating the content validity of a research instrument, determined by looking at the items and deciding whether the items appear to be measuring the theory concept.
Judgment of experts	A more rigorous approach to estimating content validity is asking people who are considered experts about the theory concept to rate the relevance of each research instrument item to the specific definition of the concept or by comparing research instrument items to relevant literature.
Content Validity Index (CVI)	The CVI is a statistic, expressed as a decimal, indicating the extent of agreement of two or more experts about the relevance of research instrument items.
Popham's average congruency technique	Popham's average congruency technique is a statistic, expressed as a percentage, indicating the extent of agreement of two or more experts about the relevance of research instrument items.
Construct validity	An estimate of what theory concept is measured by the research instrument.
Factor analysis	A statistical technique used to identify clusters of related items (factors) on a research instrument. If the theory concept measured by the instrument is thought to have just one dimension, the factor analysis is expected to yield just one factor. If, however, the concept is thought to have two or more dimensions, the factor analysis is expected to yield the same number of factors as the concept has dimensions.
Exploratory factor analysis (EFA)	Used to determine whether the items on a research instrument cluster together into one or more factors, which form instrument subscales.
Confirmatory factor analysis (CFA)	Used to confirm the clusters of the research instrument items.
Principal component analysis (PCA)	A type of factor analysis used when the factors are thought to be unrelated to each other.
Known groups technique/ contrasted groups technique	An estimate of whether the scores for the research instrument items differ between two or more groups that theoretically should have different scores.
Convergent validity	An estimate of whether there is a high correlation between the scores for the research instrument of interest and the scores for another research instrument thought to measure the same concept.

(continued)

Analysis of Quantitative (Number) Data   (continued)

NAME OF PSYCHOMETRIC PROPERTY AND SYMBOL	DESCRIPTION
Criterion-related validity	An estimate of the results of comparing the scores for a research instrument of interest with the scores for another research instrument regarded as the *best* measure (the "gold standard") of the theory concept.
Predictive validity	A type of criterion-related validity that is an estimate of the ability of the scores for a research instrument to distinguish between people on something specific that will occur in the future.
Rasch analysis	An estimate of the extent to which the total score for a research instrument completely indicates each person's standing on the theory concept, independent of his or her specific score for each item.
Item analysis	Method used to determine the quality of each item on a research instrument.
Item difficulty	The percentage of people who answered a research instrument item correctly.
Item discrimination	The extent to which a research instrument item discriminates or differentiates between people with different levels of knowledge or different characteristics.
Cluster analysis	Used to divide research instrument items into meaningful groups, or clusters

Descriptive Statistics

Descriptive statistics are used to summarize the scores for the research instruments that yield number data.	
NAME OF STATISTIC AND SYMBOL	**DESCRIPTION**
Raw score	The total score for all items on a research instrument or all items on a subscale of the instrument.
Number	A *frequency* statistic that indicates the number of research participants or documents in a sample or population.
N	The total number of research participants or documents.
n	The number of some portion of a sample of research participants or documents with a particular characteristic; or the number of participants who gave a particular response, had a particular score on an instrument, or made up a group of participants.

(continued)

Descriptive Statistics (*continued*)

NAME OF STATISTIC AND SYMBOL	DESCRIPTION
Percent %	A *frequency* statistic. The percentage of participants or documents with a particular characteristic or the percentage of participants who gave a particular response or had a particular score on an instrument.
Absolute risk	A *frequency* statistic. The ratio or percent that an event occurred compared to the event not occurring at a particular time.
Mean *M*	The average score, calculated by adding all scores for a research instrument divided by the total number of scores that were added.
Median	The score at the exact center of all scores from a research instrument, identified by rank ordering all participants' scores and identifying the exact middle score. If the number of participants is uneven, exactly one-half of their scores are above the median score and exactly one-half of their scores are below the median score. If the number of participants is even, the median is the average of the two middle scores.
Standard deviation *SD*	The square root of the extent of the spread of scores from an instrument; the extent to which each score differs from the others and from the average (mean) score.
Range	The highest and lowest scores or the difference between the highest and lowest scores.

Inferential Statistics

Inferential statistics are used to calculate the associations between scores for research instruments that yield number data, including relations between the scores for two or more research instruments or the effect of implementation of a protocol on scores for research instruments that measure outcomes.

Inferential statistics, which are applied to samples of research participants or documents, permit inferences about the research instrument scores for the total population from which the sample was drawn.

NAME OF STATISTIC AND SYMBOL	DESCRIPTION
NONPARAMETRIC STATISTICS	Used to infer the association between the scores for two or more research instruments when the distribution of scores is not normal or the scores are at the nominal or ordinal level of measurement.
	Non-normal distribution: The plot of the distribution—or spread—of scores for a research instrument is not a symmetrical bell-shaped curve.

(continued)

Inferential Statistics   (*continued*)

NAME OF STATISTIC AND SYMBOL	DESCRIPTION
	Nominal level of measurement: Numbers are assigned by the researcher to represent categories, which are artificially created for research participants' responses to the research instrument. The categories must be exhaustive and mutually exclusive. Categories also may be created from word data. The scores are considered *categorical*.
	Ordinal level of measurement: Numbers represent rank order, which is based on the standing of each research participant's score for the research instrument relative to the other research participants' scores. The scores are considered *categorical*.
	Different nonparametric statistics are used for nominal and ordinal levels of measurement.
Correlational statistics Kendall's Tau τ	Used to infer the relation between scores for two research instruments, when the scores are at the ordinal level of measurement.
Differences statistics Chi-square χ^2	Used to infer the difference in the research instrument scores between two or more groups when the scores are at the nominal level of measurement.
McNemar's test	Used to infer the direction of change in the scores for a research instrument that is administered twice to one group of research participants, when the scores are at the nominal level of measurement.
Mann–Whitney U	Used to infer the difference between research instrument scores for two groups when the scores are at the ordinal level of measurement.
Wilcoxon rank sum test	Used to infer the difference in the direction (positive, negative) and magnitude of scores between two matched groups or the same group at two different times, when the scores are at the ordinal level of measurement.
Survival analysis	Used to calculate the risk of surviving an event, such as a health condition.
Kaplan–Meier survival curve	The Kaplan–Meier survival curve is a nonparametric estimation of the risk of surviving the occurrence of an event.
Proportional hazards regression	Proportional hazards regression is used to calculate the extent of the influence of scores for two or more research instruments on the risk of the occurrence of an event or the efficacy of an intervention.

(continued)

Inferential Statistics   (*continued*)

NAME OF STATISTIC AND SYMBOL	DESCRIPTION
PARAMETRIC STATISTICS	Used to infer the association between scores for two or more research instruments when the distribution of scores is normal and the scores are at the interval or ratio level of measurement.
	Normal distribution: The plot of the distribution—or spread—of scores for a research instrument is a symmetrical bell-shaped curve.
	Interval level of measurement: Numbers are separated by a meaningful interval, and each interval between any two numbers is equal to every other interval between two numbers. The scores are considered *continuous*.
	Ratio level of measurement: Numbers represent an absolute value or score, and are relative to a possible and *meaningful* zero value. The scores are considered *continuous*.
	All parametric statistics may be used for either the interval or ratio level of measurement.
Correlational statistics	
Pearson Product Moment Coefficient of Correlation *r*	Used to infer the relation between scores for two research instruments.
Multiple regression R, R^2	Used to infer the relations of scores for two or more research instruments (that measure the independent variables) to the score for another research instrument (that measures the dependent variable), when the scores for all research instruments are at the interval or ratio level of measurement.
Hierarchical regression R, R^2	A special case of multiple regression used to enter scores for two or more research instruments (that measure the independent variables) into the analysis in a certain order singly or in sets, based on a theoretical rationale.
Logistic regression R, R^2	A special case of multiple regression used when the score for the other research instrument (that measures the dependent variable) has two or more categories.
Path analysis R, R^2	A type of regression analysis used when the scores for some research instruments (that measure the independent variables) form a path to the scores for another research instrument (that measures the intervening variable) and then to the scores for another research instrument (that measures the dependent variable). Path analysis typically is done with multiple regression.
Path coefficient	The correlation coefficient for the relation between the scores for two research instruments in the path.
Structural equation modeling (SEM)	A complex type of path analysis that is used when the scores for two research instruments are theoretically interrelated. SEM also may be used in place of path analysis with multiple regression statistics.

(*continued*)

Inferential Statistics (*continued*)

NAME OF STATISTIC AND SYMBOL	DESCRIPTION
Test of mediation	A mediator is a concept that comes between two or more other concepts and influences the direct relation between those concepts; the direct relation is regarded as contingent on the concept that comes between the other concepts. The existence of a concept as a mediator may be tested using a regression data analysis method developed by Baron and Kenny (1986; Kenny, 2016). The four steps of the mediation method are:
	Step 1. Determine the relation between the research instrument scores for the independent variable (X) and the research instrument scores for the dependent variable (Y). $X \rightarrow Y$
	Step 2. Determine the relation between the research instrument scores for the hypothesized mediator variable (Z) as the dependent variable and the research instrument scores for the independent variable. $X \rightarrow Z$
	Step 3. Determine the relation between the research instrument scores for the hypothesized mediator variable as the independent variable and the research instrument scores for the dependent variable. $Z \rightarrow Y$
	Step 4. Repeat Step 1 but hold constant the research instrument scores for the hypothesized mediator variable.
	$X \rightarrow Y$ (Z held constant)
	If the relation between the research instrument scores for the independent and dependent variables is not significant, the hypothesized mediator variable is, indeed, the mediator variable.
Differences statistics	
t-test	Used to infer the difference in research instrument scores between two groups.
Paired t-tests	Used to infer the difference in scores for a research instrument administered twice to one group or between research instrument scores for two matched groups.
Analysis of variance (ANOVA) F ratio	Used to infer the difference in the scores for one research instrument between two or more groups.
Repeated measures ANOVA F ratio	Used to infer the difference in scores for repeated administrations of a research instrument between one or more groups. The *linear mixed-model* approach to repeated measures ANOVA is used when the scores for the repeated administrations of the instrument may be correlated or when participants who have some missing data are to be included in the analysis.
Analysis of covariance (ANCOVA) F ratio	Used to infer the difference in research instrument scores between two or more groups, controlling for the influence of one or more other research instrument scores (the covariates).
Repeated measures ANCOVA F ratio	Used to infer the difference in scores for repeated administrations of a research instrument between two or more groups, controlling for the influence of one or more other research instrument scores (the covariates).

REFERENCES

Baron, R. M., & Kenny, D. A. (1986). The moderator-mediator variable distinction in social psychological research: conceptual, strategic, and statistical considerations. *Journal of Personality and Social Psychology, 51,* 1173–1182.

Fawcett, J., & Garity, J. (2009). *Evaluating research for evidence-based nursing practice.* Philadelphia, PA: F. A. Davis.

Kenny, D. A. (2016). *Mediation.* Retrieved from http://davidakenny.net/cm/mediate.htm

INDEX

Printed in the United States
By Bookmasters